ELEMENTS
of
MOLECULAR
NEUROBIOLOGY

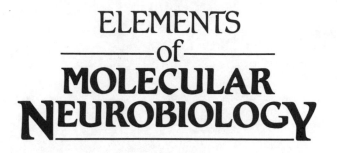

ELEMENTS
of
MOLECULAR
NEUROBIOLOGY

C. U. M. Smith

Department of Vision Sciences
Aston University, UK

A Wiley Medical Publication

JOHN WILEY & SONS

Chichester · New York · Brisbane · Toronto · Singapore

Library of Congress Cataloging in Publication Data:
Smith, C.U.M. (Christopher Upham Murray)
  Elements of molecular neurobiology.
  (A Wiley medical publication)
  Bibliography: p.
  Includes index.
  1. Molecular biology, I. Title. II. Series.
QH506.S615 1989   599'.0188   89-5763
ISBN 0 471 92124 6

British Library Cataloguing in Publication Data:
Smith, C.U.M.
  Elements of molecular neurobiology.
  1. Neurobiology. Molecular biology
  I. Title
  591.1'88

  ISBN 0 471 92124 6

Printed and bound in Great Britain by
Courier International Ltd, Tiptree, Essex

Contents

Preface

This book is intentionally entitled 'elements'. It is intended as an introductory account of what is now a vast and rapidly expanding subject. Indeed so rapid is the advance that any writer finds difficulty in steering between the Scylla of up-to-dateness (with its danger of rebuttal) and the Charybdis of received understanding (with its danger of obsolescence). I hardly expect to have safely navigated between these twin sirens at first attempt. But I hope to have avoided shipwreck to the extent that further attempts can be made in subsequent editions. To this end I would welcome critical (I hope constructively critical) comments so that the text can be updated and improved in the years ahead.

The elements upon which I have based my account have been relevant parts of molecular biology, biophysics and neurobiology. Several themes have wound their way through the book as if they were leitmotivs. Any biologist must see his subject from an evolutionary perspective and this theme is never far from the surface. Any biophysicist must recognise that the operation of nervous systems depends on the flows of ions across membranes; this theme, also, recurs throughout the text. Any molecular biologist must approach the subject in terms of the structure and function of great and complex molecules. From the beginning to the end of the book the operation of these intricately beautiful structures is a central concern. They are shown to underly not only action potentials and synaptic transmission but also, multiplied up through the architecture of the brain, to determine such holistic phenomena as memory and psychopathology.

Because of the interdisciplinary nature of the subject I have tried to make the book accessible to as broad a readership as possible. It is for this reason that I have started with an introductory account of animal brains, in particular mammalian brains, and it is for this reason that I have included an extensive glossary and a list of the acronyms with which the subject abounds. After the introductory chapter I have attempted to start at the beginning, at the molecular level, and work upwards through considerations of membrane, ion fluxes, sensory transduction, nerve impulses and synaptic biochemistry to end with such higher level phenomena as neuroembryology, memory and neuropathology. I have hoped to show that the molecular approach is beginning to provide a coherent theory of the brain's structure and functioning. At the same time I have hoped to emphasise that the complexity of the 'two handfuls of porridge' within our skulls precludes any crass and over-hasty reductionism. Molecular approaches to the brain are, nevertheless, beginning to give us considerable power: in order to use it well our decisions must be informed with an understanding of the underlying science.

Leonardo da Vinci annotated one of his anatomical drawings thus: 'O Writer, with what words will you describe with like perfection the entire configuration as the design here makes. . . and the longer you write, minutely, the more you will confuse the mind of the auditor. . .' (trans. Keele). Accordingly I make no apology for supplementing my text with numerous illustrations. This, moreover, is the place to repay a debt of gratitude to the illustrator at my publishers who was able to transform my pencil sketches into finished and stylistically consistent figures. I hope that these, as Leonardo insisted, go some way to clarifying the written descriptions. Equally I owe an immense debt of gratitude to the many scientists who kindly allowed me to reprint their half-tones and line drawings. These latter debts are acknowledged in the figure legends.

Last, but far from least, I would like to acknowledge the anonymous reviewers who read the first drafts of many of my chapters. I have benefited greatly from their comments though hardly dare to hope that all my errors have thereby been eliminated. This is also the place to thank the editorial staff at John Wiley who provided indispensable help in integrating a complicated typescript. I cannot finish, however, without acknowledging the generations of students who have listened to my lectures (without too much complaint) and who by their conscious and unconscious reactions have taught me what little I know of developing a subject in a consistent and coherent fashion. Nor can I finish without acknowledging the help of my wife who, as with previous books, has put up with absences of mind and company and remained the most loyal of critics.

C.U.M.S. February, 1989

Chapter 1
Introductory orientation

The nervous system and, in particular, the brain is commonly regarded as the most complex and highly organised form of matter known to man. Indeed it has sometimes been said that if the brain were simple enough for us to understand, we ourselves would be too simple to understand it! This, of course, is a play on the word 'simple' and, moreover, seems in the long perspective of scientific history unnecessarily pessimistic.

Our task in this text is, anyway, far less ambitious. We do not hope to achieve any total 'understanding' of the brain in the following pages. All we shall attempt is an exposition of the elements of one very powerful approach to its structure and functioning—**the molecular approach**. It is always important to bear in mind that this is but one of several approaches. A full understanding (if and when that comes) will emerge from a synthesis of insights gained from many different disciplines. In this respect the brain is very like a ravelled knot. Indeed Schopenhauer, in the nineteenth century, famously alluded to the mind/brain problem as '**the world knot**'.

Molecular neurobiology is a young subject. But, like all science, its roots can be traced far back into the past. It has emerged from the confluence of a number of more classical specialisms: **neurophysiology**, **neurochemistry**, **neuroanatomy**. Whilst neurophysiology and neuroanatomy may be traced back into the mists of antiquity, neurochemistry originated comparatively recently. Thudichum is generally regarded as having founded the subject in 1884 with the publication of his book *The Chemical Constitution of the Brain*. This comparatively recent origin has, of course, to do with the great difficulty of studying the chemistry of living processes, especially those occurring in the brain. Biochemistry itself, although originating in the nineteenth century, only began to gather momentum in the middle decades of the twentieth.

Perhaps the decisive moment came almost exactly midway through the twentieth century when, in 1953, James Watson and

Francis Crick published their celebrated solution to the structure of **DNA**. From this date may be traced a vast and still explosively developing science—molecular biology—which has informed the work of all biologists, not least those who have been concerned with the biology of the nervous system.

Molecular biology itself originated by the coming together of two very different strands of scientific endeavour. It combined the work of **biophysicists** interested in the molecular structure of biological materials, especially the structure of proteins and nucleic acids, with the work of **geneticists**, especially microbial geneticists, concerned with understanding the nature of heredity and the genetic process. Although molecular biology has undergone a huge development and diversification in the decades since 1953 these concerns still remain at its core. The conjunction of these two apparently dissimilar interests has led in the 1980s to a new high-tech industry—**biotechnology**. Biology is no longer a descriptive subject: the understandings flowing from molecular biology are beginning to allow us to manipulate living material in powerful and fascinating ways. The first company to be founded explicitly to exploit this manipulative ability (Genentech) was valued at over $200 million by the New York stock exchange in 1981; in 1987 the world-wide sales of genetically engineered chemicals were upwards of $700 million; a multibillion dollar industry is confidently predicted for the 1990s.

This new-found ability to manipulate has very recently begun to be applied to the nervous system. It is this development which lies at the root of the subject to be outlined in this book—**molecular neurobiology**. It is beginning to be possible to manipulate basic features of the nervous system both to aid understanding and, as knowledge is often power, to bring about desirable change. The brain is man's most precious possession and to a large extent makes him what he is and can become. The birth of molecular neurobiology thus brings prospects of enormous practical importance—for good or ill. We have every reason to study it carefully.

1.1 OUTLINE OF NERVOUS SYSTEMS

There are many excellent accounts of the nervous system. Some recommended texts are indicated in the bibliography. This introductory section is merely designed to present some of the salient points in a convenient form.

It is possible to argue that the nervous system developed to serve the senses. Heterotrophic forms such as animals necessarily have to seek out their nutriment. The information gathered by the sensory cells has to be collated and appropriate responses

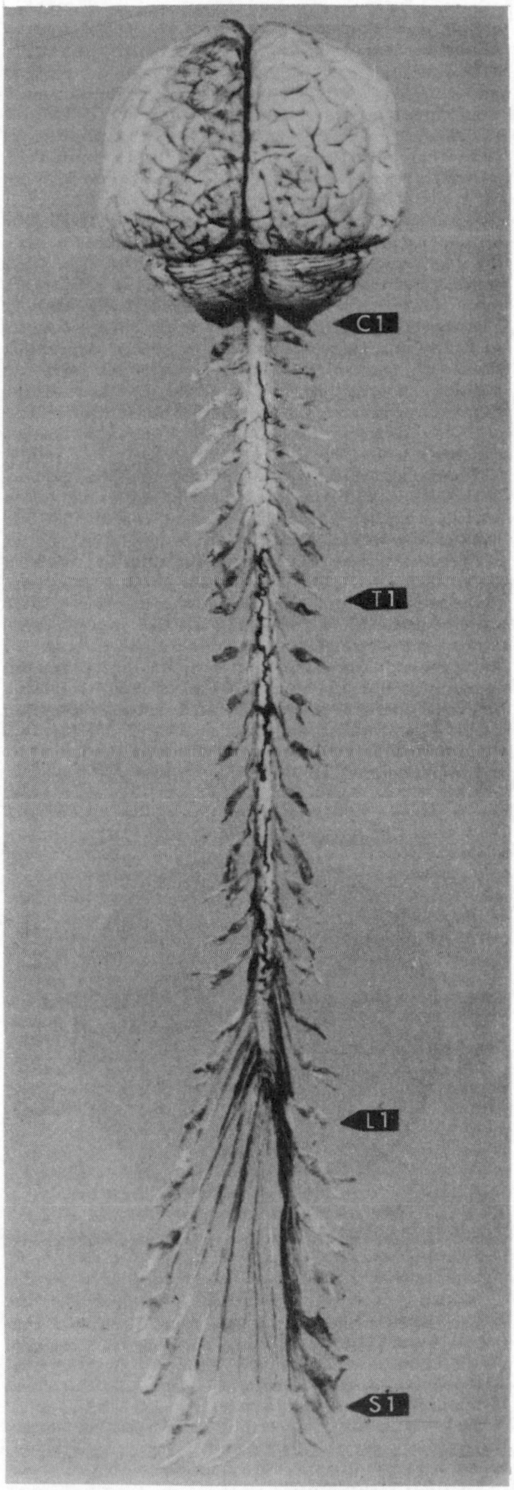

Figure 1.1   Human brain and spinal cord showing roots of the spinal nerves. The central nervous system is viewed from behind. The posterior view of the brain shows the two large cerebral hemispheres resting on top of the two cerebellar hemispheres. Spinal nerves emerge between the vertebrae of each segment of the cord (8 cervical, 12 thoracic, 5 lumbar and 5 sacral). The spinal cord ends between the twelfth thoracic and the second lumbar segment and continues as the cauda equina. In the figure the latter has been fanned out on the left and left undisturbed on the right. C1 = first cervical vertebra; T1 = first thoracic vertebra; L1 = first lumbar vertebra; S1 = first sacral vertebra. (From Warwick and Williams, eds., 1973, *Gray's Anatomy*: reproduced by permission of Churchill Livingstone, Edinburgh.)

computed. Hence the nervous system. It also follows that, to an extent, the nature of the nervous system which an animal possesses reflects its life-style. Active animals develop large and elaborate nervous systems; quiescent forms make do with minimal nervous tissue. In general animals cannot afford to carry more nervous system than they actually need.

A glance at any zoology text is enough to remind us of the huge variety of animals with which we share the globe. It follows that there is a huge number of different nervous system designs. Many of these designs provide opportunities to investigate neurobiological problems which are difficult to solve in mammalian systems. An awareness of the wealth of different systems presented by the animal kingdom is a valuable asset for any neurobiologist and, in particular, as we shall see, for any molecular neurobiologist.

One general design feature is found in all nervous systems above the level represented by the Porifera (sponges) and Cnidaria (jelly fish, sea anemones, hydroids). This is the separation of the nervous system into a **central** 'computing' region and a **peripheral** set of nerve fibres carrying information to and from the centre. In the chordates the 'central region', or **central nervous system (CNS)**, consists of the brain and spinal cord, and the **peripheral nervous system (PNS)** consists of the cranial and spinal nerves.

Other animals show other designs. Often we can dimly discern evolutionary reasons for these differences. One major difference which is worth mentioning at this stage is that which obtains between the chordates and the great assemblage of heterogeneous forms grouped for convenience under the title 'invertebrates' or 'animals without backbones'. The CNS of chordates (this phylum includes all the vertebrates) always develops in the dorsal position whilst that of the invertebrates develops in the ventral position. It is believed that this striking difference is due to the fact that chordates originated in the warm upper layers of palaeozoic seas whilst invertebrates originated as forms crawling over the bottoms of equally or yet more ancient seas and lagoons. The major sensory input for the chordates would have thus come from above, that for the invertebrates from below. Hence the different positioning of their central nervous systems. We shall see, in later chapters, that evolutionary considerations also play a significant role in molecular neurobiology. Here, as elsewhere, they help us answer the question of *why* things are as they are.

Whilst the nervous systems of all animal phyla are of great interest, neurobiologists have tended to concentrate their attention on a few phyla in particular. The phylum **Nematoda** (roundworms) provides forms with extremely simple nervous systems and quick generation times. The worm *Caenorhabditis elegans* has provided a nervous system simple enough (just 302

A

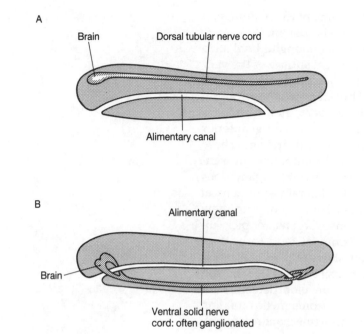

Brain   Dorsal tubular nerve cord

Alimentary canal

B

Alimentary canal

Brain

Ventral solid nerve
cord: often ganglionated

Figure 1.2 (A) Schematic sagittal section through idealised chordate to show position of CNS. (B) Schematic diagram to show the position of the CNS in a typical non-chordate. It should be borne in mind that whereas chordates form a homogeneous group, sharing a common design principle, non-chordates are many and various. The schematic diagram in (B) fits the worms and the Arthropoda but is quite inappropriate for radially symmetrical groups such as the Cnidaria and Echinodermata and can only with difficulty accommodate the Mollusca

cells) to have its genetics, development and anatomy mapped in its entirety. The phylum **Annelida** (segmented worms) contains forms such as the leech *Hirudo* whose ganglionated CNS has also provided a simple system for intensive investigation. The phylum **Mollusca** has also been much studied. The squid has provided excellent experimental preparations. More recently, the sea-hare *Aplysia* has been the focus of a great deal of interest at the molecular level. The phylum **Arthropoda** provides many insect and crustacean preparations and in recent years the fruitfly *Drosophila*, long a favourite with geneticists, has become central to those interested in the genetics and embryology of the nervous system. Finally, of course, we come to the phylum **Chordata**— the phylum to which we, along with all the other vertebrates, belong. Although disinterested curiosity has always motivated scientists and animal nervous systems are worth investigating in their own right 'because they're there', the major thrust of neurobiological endeavour (and its funding agencies) has always been to illuminate the workings of the human brain. Invertebrates, as indicated above, frequently provide particularly convenient preparations for investigating problems which are difficult to tackle in mammalian and *a fortiori* human brains, but at the end of the day it is an understanding of the human nervous system which is sought.

Further information about invertebrate nervous systems can be obtained from the books listed in the bibliography. Here we shall confine ourselves to a very brief resumé of the mammalian and, especially, the human central nervous system.

The CNS of all vertebrates begins life as a longitudinal strip of **neurectoderm** which appears on the dorsal surface of the very early embryo. Does embryology recapitulate phylogeny here as Ernst Haeckel long ago suspected? This strip of neurectoderm soon sinks beneath the surface of the embryo, first forming a gutter and then rolling up to form a neural tube. At the anterior end of this tube three swellings (or vesicles) appear. These constitute the embryonic fore-, mid-, and hindbrains (**prosencephalon, mesencephalon and rhombencephalon**). Again, does embryology recapitulate phylogeny? All bilaterally symmetrical animals move with one end of their bodies entering new environments first. It follows that sense organs to pick up information from and about the environment tend to be concentrated on that anterior end. It also follows that specialisation of these sense organs to pick up the principal types of information is likely to occur. Thus animals tend to develop detectors for chemical substances (**chemoreceptors**), electromagnetic radiation (**photoreceptors**) and mechanical disturbance (**mechanoreceptors**). It turns out that the three primary vesicles mentioned above are initially concerned with the analysis of these three primary senses—olfaction, vision, vibration—respectively.

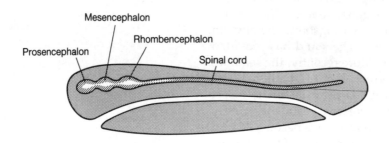

Figure 1.3   Embryology of the vertebrate brain: idealised sagittal section of three-vesicle stage

As embryological development continues the early three-vesicle brain subdivides to form a five-vesicle structure. This happens by the hindbrain (the rhombencephalon) subdividing into a posterior **myelencephalon** and a more anterior **metencephalon** and the forebrain (the prosencephalon) also subdividing into an anterior **telencephalon** and a more posterior **thalamencephalon** (or **diencephalon**). The midbrain remains undivided. The cavity within the metencephalon now expands somewhat to form the **fourth ventricle** joined by a narrow canal, the iter or cerebral aqueduct, to the **third ventricle** within the thalamencephalon. This in turn communicates with the **lateral ventricles** within the **cerebral hemispheres**, which develop from the telencephalon.

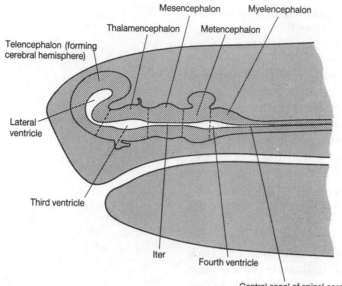

Thalamencephalon

Telencephalon (forming cerebral hemisphere)

Mesencephalon

Metencephalon

Myelencephalon

Lateral ventricle

Third ventricle

Iter

Fourth ventricle

Central canal of spinal cord

Figure 1.4 Embryology of the vertebrate brain: idealised sagittal section of five-vesicle stage. The figure shows the telencephalon growing backwards over the surface of the thalamencephalon. This only occurs in animals which develop large cerebral hemispheres, such as mammals. From the roof of the thalamencephalon grows the pineal gland whilst from its floor develops the neural part of the pituitary. The cerebellum grows from the roof of the metencephalon whilst the floor of this region expands to form the pons. The whole structure contains a cavity continuous with the central canal of the spinal cord and filled with cerebral spinal fluid (CSF)

Further development of the brain does not involve any further major subdivision. The fundamental architecture of the brain remains essentially as shown in Figure 1.4. Great developments, however, occur principally from the roof of this five-vesicle structure. From the roof of the metencephalon grows the **cerebellum**. This structure, as it is involved in the orchestration of the muscles to produce smooth behavioural movements, is always large in active animals. In primates, such as ourselves, it is thus extremely well developed. Survival of 30 million years or so of arboreal life demanded an extreme of neuromuscular co-ordination. In ourselves it is the second largest part of the brain. Associated with the cerebellum, in the floor of the metencephalon, is another large structure, the **pons**. The pons acts as a sort of junction box where fibres to and from the cerebellum can interact with fibres running to and from other parts of the central nervous system.

The roof of the midbrain forms the **tectum** in the lower vertebrates. It is to this region, as indicated above, that the visual information is directed. This information is so important that, in the fish and amphibia, it also attracts fibres carrying information from the other senses, so that the tectum becomes the major brain area for association and cross-correlation of sensory information. The tectum in these animals is perhaps the most important part of the brain. In the mammals, however, this importance is lost. Visual information, as we shall see, is mostly directed to the cerebral cortex. The roof of the midbrain in mammals is thus quite poorly developed. Four smallish swellings can be detected there—two inferior and two superior **colliculi**. The inferior colliculi are part of the auditory pathway from the cochlea whilst the superior colliculi still play a small, though important, role in the analysis of visual information.

It is the forebrain, however, which has undergone the most dramatic development in the mammals and especially in the primates. A number of important nerve centres are located in the thalamencephalon (the **lateral geniculate, medial geniculate** and **thalamic nuclei**) which act as 'way stations' for fibres running from the senses towards the cerebrum. From the roof of this region grows the **pineal** organ (in the mammals an important endocrine gland of which we shall have more to say later), and from the floor (the hypothalamus) grows the neural part of the **pituitary**.

But by far the greatest development occurs in the telencephalon. This grows enormously and becomes reflected back over the thalamencephalon which it ultimately covers and encloses (Greek *thalamos* = inner room). It divides into two great 'hemispheres', the **cerebral hemispheres**, each of which contains a ventricle—the lateral ventricle. In the mammals information from all the senses is brought to the cerebrum and it is here that it is collated and analysed.

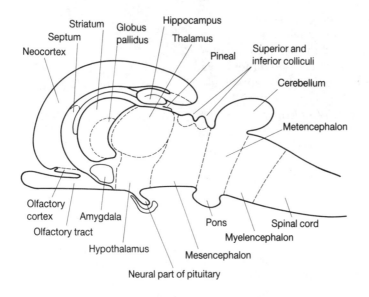

Figure 1.5 Ground plan of the mammalian brain. The schematic figure shows the basic architecture of the mammalian brain. Notice how the neocortex has grown back over the thalamencephalon. In humans this enlargement reaches a climax so that the neocortex grows back as far as the cerebellum and hides the more ancient parts of the brain. (After Nauta and Feirtag, 1986, *Fundamentals of Neuroanatomy*, New York: Freeman.)

In *Homo sapiens* the cerebrum has become gigantic and overgrows and obscures the other (more ancient) regions of the brain. The anatomy is also made more difficult to understand by man's assumption of an upright stance. This causes the brain to bend through nearly a right angle—a characteristic called **cerebral flexure**.

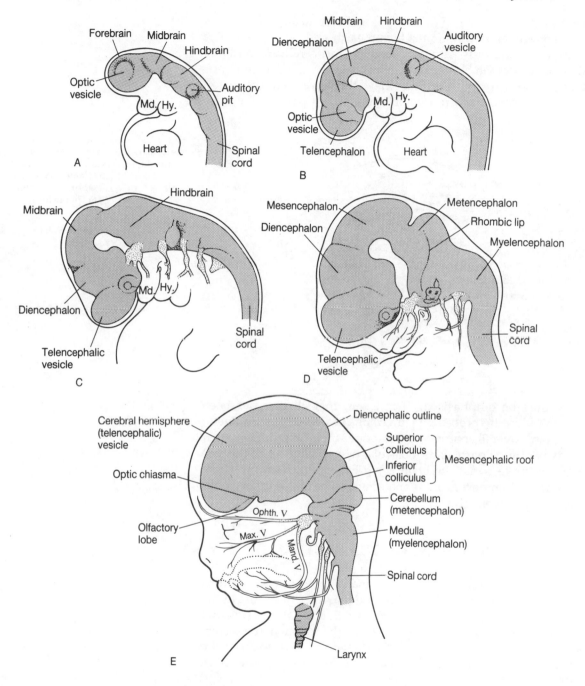

One other feature of the general anatomy of the human brain should be mentioned. This is the existence of a series of structures which lie between the cerebrum and the thalamencephalon. These structures constitute the **limbic system**—so called from the Latin

Figure 1.6 Development of the human brain showing flexure. (From Patten and Carlson, 1974, *Foundations of Embryology*, New York: McGraw Hill; with permission)

limbus meaning 'edge' or 'border', as in the Dantean limbo, which was conceived as a region between earth and hell. The limbic system is not only situated between the cerebrum and the thalamencephalon but is also believed to be involved in emotions and emotional responses. Some have therefore seen this region as a relic from our infra-human evolutionary past.

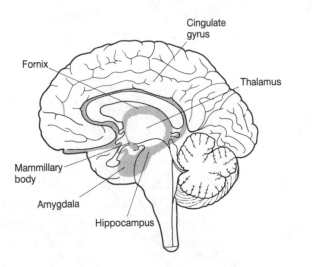

Figure 1.7 Parasagittal section through the human brain to show some elements of the limbic system. (From *Biological Psychology*, 2/E, by James W. Kalat © 1984, 1981 by Wadsworth, Inc. Reprinted by permission of the publisher.)

It must be emphasised, once again, that all that has been attempted in the preceding paragraphs is a very brief outline of the brain's overall anatomy. It is important, however, that in their study of minute particulars molecular neurobiologists do not lose sight of the fact that the brain is a great, complex and intricate system. Further details of the anatomy may be found in the books listed in the bibliography.

1.2 CELLS OF THE NERVOUS SYSTEM

The nervous system is built of two major types of cell: **neurons** and **neuroglia (= glia)**. Both play essential roles in the life of the system. It is only the neurons, however, that are able to transmit messages from one part of the CNS to another or out of the system altogether to the muscles and glands, and vice versa from the sense organs into the CNS. Let us consider each type of cell in turn.

1.2.1 Neurons

Histologists have described many different types of neuron: pyramidal cells, stellate cells, Purkinje cells, Martinotti cells, mitral cells, granule cells, etc. Szentágothai recognises over 50 major types and there are many subtypes. All, however, share a common basic design. All possess a metabolic centre (**cell body/cyton/perikaryon**) from which one or more processes spring. The number of processes provides a useful classification. Thus we can distinguish between **monopolar, bipolar** and **multipolar** neurons.

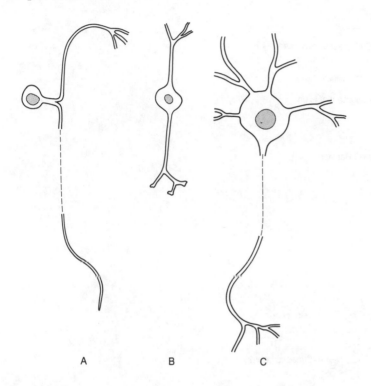

A   B   C

Figure 1.8 Classification of neurons. A simple way of classifying neurons is by noting the number of processes springing from the perikaryon. The figure shows (A) unipolar neuron (e.g. mammalian somaesthetic sensory neuron); (B) bipolar neuron (e.g. retinal bipolar neuron); (C) multipolar neuron (e.g. mammalian motor neuron)

Another useful classification of neurons is into **principal** or **projection** neurons and **local circuit** or **inter-** neurons. Principal neurons transmit messages out of the local region where their cell bodies are located, whilst local circuit neurons interact closely with their near neighbours.

As much of the remainder of this book is concerned with the molecular biology of neurons it is important to give an introductory outline of the major features of a typical neuron. The **multipolar neuron** is by far the commonest type of neuron in animal nervous systems. Let us therefore look at it in a little detail.

Figure 1.9 shows that two types of process emerge from the perikaryon: the short, branching **dendrites** and the long unbranched (except at its terminal) **axon**. Both the foregoing statements (as most statements in biology) have many exceptions. Monopolar neurons have unbranched dendrites, and in many cases the axons of multipolar neurons branch.

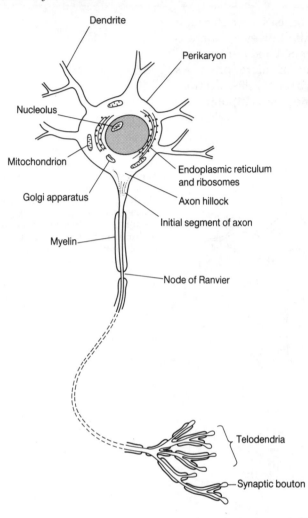

Figure 1.9 Multipolar neuron

Dendrite

Perikaryon

Nucleolus

Mitochondrion

Endoplasmic reticulum
and ribosomes

Golgi apparatus

Axon hillock

Initial segment of axon

Myelin

Node of Ranvier

Telodendria

Synaptic bouton

Neurons are **physiologically 'polarised'**. Messages flow down the dendrites to the perikaryon and away from the perikaryon along the axon. Furthermore in the multipolar neuron only the axon transmits the message by means of action potentials (impulses). The dendrites, as we shall see, do not *in general* develop action potentials.

The perikaryon itself shows all the ultrastructural features of intense biochemical activity. There is a large nucleus, well-developed nucleolus (sometimes more than one), rich rough endoplasmic reticulum, prominent Golgi apparatus (again sometimes more than one), abundant mitochondria, whilst lysosomes, peroxisomes and multivesicular bodies are frequently visible. In addition to this wealth of organelles, neurons exhibit a well-developed cytoskeleton. Neurotubules, neurofilaments and intermediate filaments are all present and, as we shall see, play vital roles in the life of the neuron. The neuron should never be mistaken for the simple on/off relay of which computers are made. Indeed it has been pointed out that neurons are much more like multi-functional silicon chips than simple yes/no gates.

In many neurons, especially large multipolar neurons, the axon (= nerve fibre) emerges from a conical part of the perikaryon termed the **axon hillock**. It then generally runs without varying in diameter to its final destination. In many cases, as shown in Figure 1.9, it is encased in a **myelin sheath**. The myelin, as we shall see, is formed by neuroglial cells and plays a vital role in determining the rate of impulse conduction. The junctions between the neuroglial cells constitute the **nodes of Ranvier**. It is only at these junctions that the axonal membrane is exposed to the intercellular medium. At its termination the axon branches into a more or less large number of **telodendria**. The endings of these telodendria make synaptic 'contact' with other neurons or, if the axon is a motor fibre leading out of the CNS, with muscle fibres.

The axon again must not be mistaken for a passive conducting 'wire'. It is true, as we shall see in detail later, that an impulse once initiated at the **initial segment** (see Figure 1.9) runs without decrement to the telodendrial terminations, yet the axon itself has an intricate ultrastructure. It has been shown to possess a complex and dynamic cytoskeleton in which are embedded mitochondria, vesicles of transmitter substances en route to the synaptic termini, and numerous other biochemical entities. All these elements are moving more or less slowly (**axoplasmic flow**) in both directions, either towards the telodendria or, vice versa, from the telodendria back to the perikaryon. Again we shall have much more to say about the ultrastructure of axons and axoplasmic flow later in the book (Chapter 14).

Following the axon out to its termination we ultimately arrive at the **synaptic 'bouton'**, **'knob'** or **'end foot'**. In some cases this termination is far more elaborate than a simple swelling and may form a complicated claw or other intricate structure. Within the termination the electron microscopist can usually detect **mitochondria** and **synaptic vesicles**; other organelles are, however, scarce. We shall return to the structure of synapses later in this chapter.

Finally, in this introductory section on neurons, let us turn our attention to those other processes which emerge from the perikaryon—the dendrites. In many multipolar neurons these have a much greater diameter than the axon. We shall see the reason for this in Chapter 11, where we discuss electrotonic conduction. Again, as Figure 1.9 shows, dendrites unlike axons are extensively branched. Indeed the dendrites of the large Purkinje cells of the cerebellum resemble nothing so much as the

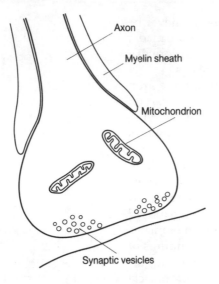

Axon

Myelin sheath

Mitochondrion

Synaptic vesicles

Figure 1.10   Synaptic bouton

branches of an espaliered fruit tree. In addition to arboraceous branching, dendrites often develop tiny protuberances commonly known as **spines**. These, as again we shall see, are the sites of synaptic 'contact'. Lastly, it is worth emphasising once again that dendrites are in no way passive or inert. Like axons they possess a complex ultrastructure formed, in this case, principally of neurotubules.

1.2.2 Glia

Glial cells outnumber neurons ten to one in the CNS. Unlike neurons they have not finished multiplication at birth. Although they do not conduct impulses they play many other important roles in the nervous system. Not least, they are able to invade damaged regions and clear away necrotic material, producing a glial scar.

On the other hand they resemble neurons in showing a large number of different structural forms. It is usual to recognise three major types: **astroglia**, **oligodendroglia** and **microglia**. Each type has an important role in the life of the nervous system. Let us review each in turn.

Astroglial cells (= astrocytes), as the name implies, possess a number of radiating (star-like) processes from a large central cell body (c. 20 μm in diameter) which contains the nucleus. It is frequently found to be the case that some of these radiating processes end on the endothelial walls of cerebral blood vessels whilst others are closely adposed to neurons. In other cases (or sometimes the same case) the feet of astroglial cells abut the ependymal cells lining a cerebral ventricle or, alternatively, the cells of the innermost of the brain's meningeal membranes—the pia mater. It has been suggested, in consequence, that astroglial cells are involved in the movement of materials between **cerebro-spinal fluid (CSF)**, **blood** and **neuron**—perhaps with some metabolic elaboration en route. This, however, has yet to be firmly established and we shall return to it later.

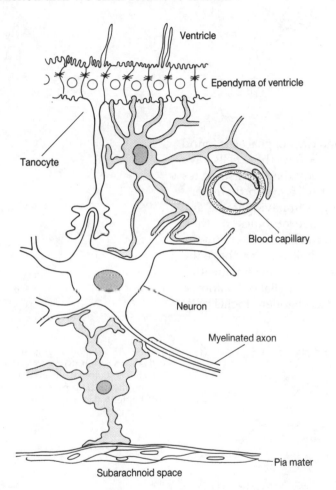

Figure 1.11 Astroglial cells. The schematic diagram shows two astrocytes (stippled). The upper astrocyte stretches from the ependymal epithelium lining the cavity of the ventricle to the perikaryon and dendrites of a neuron. It also invests a blood capillary. The lower astrocyte reaches from the flattened epithelium of the pia mater (which abuts the subarachnoid space) to the neuron. Note that this is a schematic diagram: it is unlikely that a neuron will have astrocytic connections with both the ventricle and the subarachnoid space. (After Warwick and Williams, eds, 1973, *Gray's Anatomy*, Edinburgh: Churchill Livingstone.)

Another important feature of astrocytes is the strong development of fibres (= **neurofilaments**) in the cytoplasm. Generally speaking these fibres are more strongly developed in the astrocytes located in the white matter than in those located in grey matter. These two types of astrocyte are consequently called **fibrous** and **protoplasmic** astrocytes respectively. The neurofilaments are believed to confer a certain tensile strength and as astrocytes are often firmly bound to each other and to neurons by way of **tight junctions** (see Chapter 6) they may be regarded as giving structural support to nervous tissue.

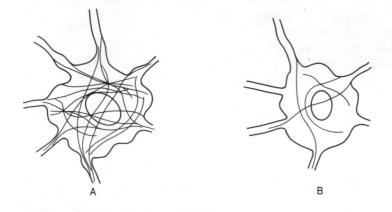

A   B

Figure 1.12   Fibrous and protoplasmic astrocytes

Oligodendroglial cells constitute a second class of glial cells found in the CNS. As the name indicates (*oligos* = few) these cells have fewer processes radiating from the cell body than do astrocytes and the cell body is itself much smaller (c. 5 μm in diameter). Oligodendroglia also differ from astrocytes in having few if any neurofilaments but large numbers of neurotubules in their cytoplasm. These cells are found in both the grey matter and the white matter. In the white matter, as we shall see, they have the very important role of investing axons in their myelin sheaths.

It is appropriate at this point to indicate that glial cells, known as **Schwann cells**, although not classified as oligodendroglial cells,

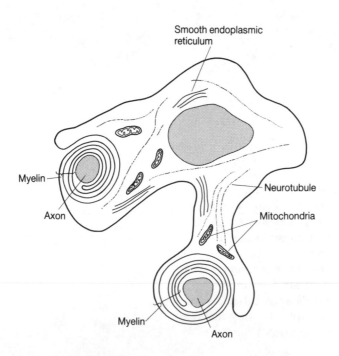

Smooth endoplasmic reticulum

Myelin

Axon

Neurotubule

Mitochondria

Myelin

Axon

Figure 1.13   Oligodendroglial cells. The cell is shown with two processes, each of which has wrapped a central axon in its myelin sheath. This process is described in Chapter 6 (see Fig. 6.15)

carry out the business of enveloping **peripheral** axons in their myelin. Peripheral and central myelin is not laid down in precisely the same way, as we shall see, but the end result is much the same.

Microglial cells constitute the last major class of glia to be found in the adult nervous system. Their cell bodies are smaller than the other types of glia, seldom exceeding 3 μm in diameter. They make up for their lack of size by their large numbers. They probably have numerous functions. It has been suggested that they are of importance in maintaining the **ionic environment** surrounding neurons—of the greatest importance to the biophysics of the action potential. It is probable, also, that they are involved in the **uptake and disposal** of unwanted end-products of synaptic activity. Last, but far from least, it is the microglia which proliferate and move to any site of injury to **phagocytose** necrotic tissue.

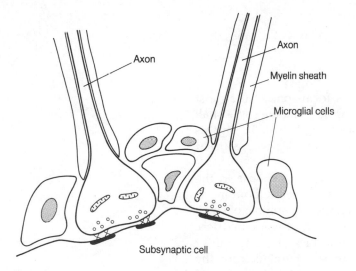

Axon

Axon

Myelin sheath

Microglial cells

Subsynaptic cell

Figure 1.14   Microglial cells. A group of microglial cells is shown surrounding a synaptic junction. They are positioned to remove excess transmitter or the breakdown products of transmitters which would otherwise accumulate in the synaptic cleft. Microglial cells may also be involved in resynthesising fresh transmitter from these breakdown products and passing it back into the synaptic terminal (see Chapter 15)

Before completing this introductory section on glia it is worth noting that in the embryonic nervous system another class of glia is present: **radial glia**. These cells develop long processes, sometimes extending across the whole width of the brain, from the cerebral ventricle to the pial surface, and guide the migration of neurons during embryonic development (see Chapter 17). Radial glia, for the most part, disappear or are transformed into astroglia in adult brains. However, they remain virtually unchanged in two regions—the retina, where they are known as **Müller cells**, and the cerebellum, where they are called **Bergmann glia**.

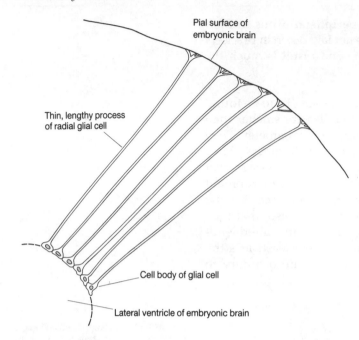

Pial surface of
embryonic brain

Thin, lengthy process
of radial glial cell

Cell body of glial cell

Lateral ventricle of embryonic brain

Figure 1.15 Radial glia in the early development of the telencephalon. The figure shows that these glial cells develop extraordinarily lengthy processes which extend from the cell body (next to the ventricle) right across the width of the developing brain to the pial surface

1.2.3 Organisation of Synapses

The structure and function of synapses forms one of the most important areas of research in molecular neurobiology. We shall discuss the molecular detail in Chapters 14, 15 and 16. In this section we shall merely look in an introductory way at their organisation in the brain.

Figure 1.16 shows the structure of a **typical synapse** in the CNS. The termination of the axon swells to form a 'bouton' as we noted in Section 1.2.1. The bouton contains a number of small (20–40 nm) vesicles which are believed by most workers (there are some exceptions) to contain the molecules of a transmitter substance. The **presynaptic membrane** is separated from the **postsynaptic** (= **subsynaptic**) **membrane** by a gap of some 30–40 nm. Characteristically the postsynaptic membrane appears denser and thicker in the electron microscope than the presynaptic membrane. The presence of synaptic vesicles and this **post-synaptic thickening** enables the physiological polarity of the synapse to be determined: i.e. transmission always occurs across the synaptic gap in one direction—**from** pre- **to** postsynaptic membrane.

Just as there are many different types of neuron and many different types of glia, so there are many different types of synapse. Indeed it would be somewhat strange if there were not for, at a conservative estimate, there are some 10^{14} synapses in

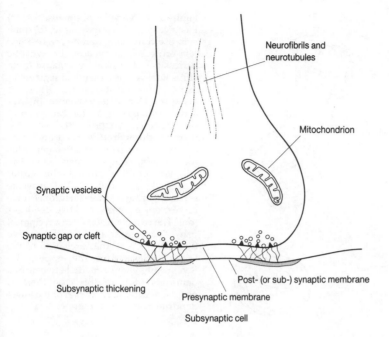

Neurofibrils and neurotubules

Mitochondrion

Synaptic vesicles

Synaptic gap or cleft

Subsynaptic thickening

Post- (or sub-) synaptic membrane

Presynaptic membrane

Subsynaptic cell

Figure 1.16 'Classical' synapse. (Description in text). The figure shows that there is often evidence of some material filling the synaptic cleft. The figure also shows ridges projecting upwards from the presynaptic membrane. These ridges form part of the presynaptic grid (see Chapter 14)

the human brain. The structural and biochemical diversity is gigantic. Some of the different structures and arrangements are shown in Figure 1.17. The structures range from simple **electrical** synapses (= 'gap junctions', see Chapter 6), through classical synapses, to synapses made **en passant** (sometimes called '**varicosities**'), to **reciprocal** synapses and complicated groups of synapses.

One simplifying feature of synaptic appositions was first proposed by the pharmacologist Henry Dale in the 1930s. **Dale's principle** states that any given neuron synthesises only one type of transmitter molecule—hence all the terminations of that neuron contain only that one type of transmitter. Although many exceptions to Dale's principle are nowadays known (see Chapter 15) it remains a good first approximation. It is also to some extent possible to relate the transmitter molecules present in a synaptic terminal to the form of the presynaptic vesicles. Thus small spherical translucent vesicles are believed to contain excitatory transmitters such as acetylcholine or aspartate, whilst small translucent ellipsoidal vesicles contain inhibitory transmitters such as glycine or GABA. Larger, dense-cored, vesicles are believed to contain catecholamine transmitters, whilst large translucent vesicles probably contain peptide transmitters.

Classical neurophysiologists understood the connectivity of the nervous system to be one-way only—from axon to dendrite or perikaryon. It remains true that most synapses are **axo-dendritic**

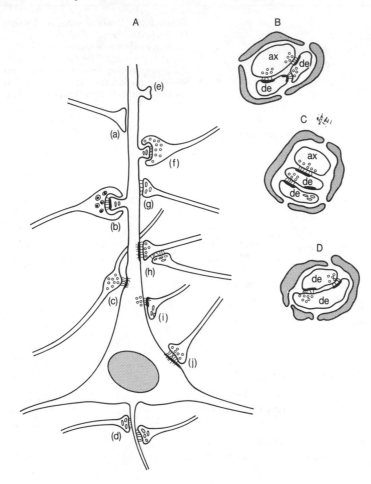

Figure 1.17   Varieties of synapse. (A) (a) Electrically conducting synapse, (b) spine synapse containing dense-core vesicles, (c) 'en passant' synapse or synaptic varicosity, (d) inhibitory synapse (note ellipsoidal vesicles) on initial segment of axon, (e) dendritic spine, (f) spine synapse, (g) inhibitory synapse, (h) axo-axonic synapse, (i) reciprocal synapse, (j) excitatory synapse. (B) Transverse sections through three neuronal processes: one axon (ax) and two dendrites (de) showing complex organisation. The stippled profiles around the group represent glial cells. (C) Transverse section through three neuronal processes: one axon (ax) and two dendrites (de). The two dendrites form a reciprocal pair. They are arranged in a negative feedback loop so that excitation of the lower switches off the upper, (D) Reciprocal synapse made between two dendrites (de). In this case there is positive feedback. Excitation of the lower dendrite re-excites the upper

or **axo-perikaryal** (= **axo-somatic**), but in recent years other arrangements have been discovered. **Axo-axonic** synapses are quite common. This arrangement allows one neuron to control the synaptic activity of another. More recently it has been shown that dendrites also make synapses. **Dendro-dendritic** synapses have been demonstrated in the olfactory bulb, in the retina, in the superior colliculi and elsewhere. Finally it appears that synapses are sometimes made between perikarya. It seems, therefore, that all the possible permutations between neuronal processes are made somewhere or other in the brain. Some of these 'non-classical' arrangements are shown in Figure 1.18.

It is clear from the foregoing paragraphs that the synaptic organisation of the brain is exceedingly complex and as yet far from completely understood. The dendritic and perikaryal surfaces of many neurons are densely covered with synaptic endings of various sorts. It has been computed that the large

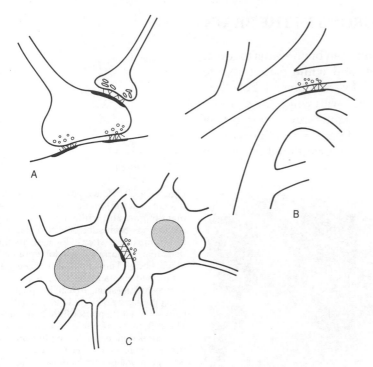

Figure 1.18 'Non-classical' synapses. (A) Axo-axonic synapse. The termination of one axon may control the activity of another terminal. (B) Dendro-dendritic synapse. Synaptic appositions are sometimes found between the dendritic processes of neighbouring neurons. (C) Perikaryo-perikaryal synapse. Very occasionally synaptic junctions are made between adjacent perikarya

Purkinje cells of the cerebellum are exposed to over 100 000 synaptic appositions. The dense investment by synaptic endings of various different sizes of the perikaryon of a spinal motor neuron is shown in Figure 1.19.

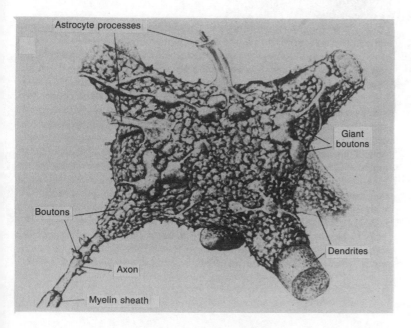

Figure 1.19 Synaptic contacts on the perikaryon of a spinal motor neuron. This reconstruction from serial electron micrographs shows how densely covered the perikaryon of a motor neuron is with large and small synaptic endings. (From Poritsky, 1969, *Journal of Comparative Neurology*, **135**, 423–452; with permission.)

1.3 ORGANISATION OF NEURONS IN THE BRAIN

To the naked eye a section of the mammalian brain seems to reveal two types of substance: **grey matter** and **white matter**. White matter is composed of huge numbers of nerve fibres. In bulk they appear white because the myelin sheaths with which the majority are enveloped reflect and glisten in the light. Grey matter, on the other hand, consists of the dendrites and perikarya of the neurons plus numerous glial cells. These are not surrounded by myelin and hence in bulk appear greyish.

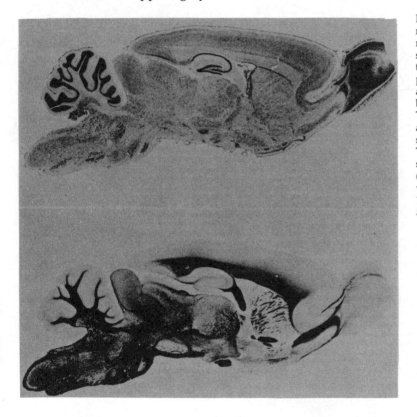

Figure 1.20 Parasagittal section of mammalian (rat) brain to show arrangement of grey and white matter. The top section has been subjected to a staining technique (Nissl stain) which stains the perikarya of neurons. Each dot represents a cell body. The Loyez technique has been used to stain the middle section. This technique stains myelin but does not affect perikarya. The middle section thus shows the white matter fibre pathways. The bottom diagram maps the anatomical structures delineated by the two stains. (Courtesy of Drs. H.F. Hall and D. Major, with permission from Nauta and Feirtag, 1979, 'The organisation of the brain', *Scientific American*, **241**, 78 – 105.

In the early embryo the grey matter is situated in the **centre** of the CNS immediately surrounding the central fluid-filled cavity (central canal in spinal cord, ventricle in brain). It retains this primitive position throughout life in the spinal cord, but in the brain many of the neurons migrate during embryological development along the processes of radial glia to form surface cortices or 'rinds' (see Figure 1.15 and Chapter 17). This occurs especially in the cerebrum and the cerebellum and gives rise to the cerebral and cerebellar cortices. Other groups of perikarya, however, remain deep within the brain, forming islands of grey matter amongst the fibre tracts: these constitute nuclei and ganglia. An outline of this organisation is shown in Figure 1.20.

Grey matter, especially that of the cerebral cortex, has an extremely complex and little-understood organisation. Silver staining by the Golgi-Cox technique shows an elaborate interconnectivity (Figure 1.21). It is known, moreover, that this staining technique impregnates only about one per cent (at random) of the neurons present. The true interconnectivity is thus almost unimaginably intricate. Electron micrographs of the cortex reveal densely packed masses of cells and cell processes with apparently rather little intercellular space. The 'wiring' of the cortex remains one of the most difficult research frontiers in neuroscience. The pattern of synaptic connection and interaction is of almost inconceivable complexity. Indeed the cortex has been compared to a hologram, implying that information is not held in discrete localities but 'smeared' throughout.

Against this idea of a 'randomised' cortex there has always been a strong tradition which envisages the cortex as consisting of a number of functionally and structurally distinct units or **modules**. This tradition gained prominence at the end of the nineteenth and beginning of the twentieth century in the functional topography of Ferrier and in the cortical architectonics of Brodmann and the Vogts. In the mid-twentieth century this tradition has gathered momentum. Neurophysiologists interested in sensory cortices (Mountcastle—somaesthetic cortex; Hubel and Wiesel—visual cortex) have shown that the neocortex consists of functional **columns** or **slabs**.

The most obvious feature of the neocortex when viewed under the optical microscope is its layered stratification. This layering is shown in Figure 1.22. Traditionally **six laminae** have been distinguished. Layer four is conventionally further subdivided into three sublayers: a, b and c. The stratification of the neocortex is more obvious in some regions (e.g. visual cortex) than others (e.g. association cortex). Cortical modules lie, however, **orthogonal** to this stratification. The first histological hints of this vertical organisation were provided by Lorente de No in his classical research during the 1930s. Nowadays cortical modules are believed to consist of columns of cells with an overall diameter of some 300 – 500 μm. The neocortex appears to be a mosaic of such columns which, moreover, vary very little in diameter throughout the mammals, from mouse to monkey.

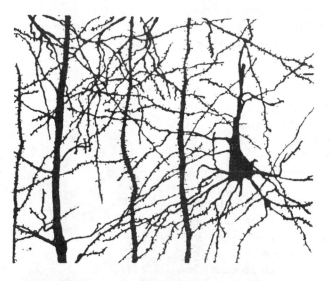

A

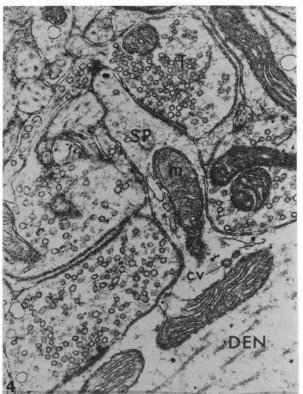

Figure 1.21   Structure of grey matter. (A) Silver-stained section of cerebral cortex ($\times$250). A pyramidal neuron can be seen on the right hand side of the picture and three large, vertically running dendrites to its left. The surfaces of the dendrites are covered in spines. (B) Electron micrograph of the oculomotor nucleus of the cat ($\times$26 000). In the lower right hand corner the pale expanse is a dendrite (DEN) from which springs a spine (SP). Synaptic boutons filled with vesicles surround the spine and the dendrite. The bouton labelled T makes a particularly well-imaged synaptic contact with the spine. m = mitochondrion; cv = cytoplasmic vesicle. (From Pappas and Waxman, 1972, in *Structure and Function of Synapses*, ed. G.D. Pappas and D.P. Purpura, Amsterdam: North Holland; with permission.)

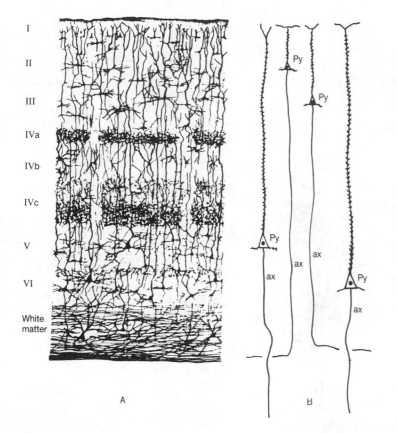

I

II

III

IVa

IVb

IVc

V

VI

White matter

A   B

Figure 1.22   Stratification of the cerebral cortex. (A) Cortical neurons stained by the Golgi–Cox silver technique (×75). The figure shows that incoming axons terminate in complex ramifications in layers IVa and IVc. These ramifications are some 350 to 450 μm in diameter. One complete ramification is shown in the centre of the figure flanked by two half ramifications. (From Rakic, 1979, in *The Neurosciences, Fourth Study Program*, eds F.O. Schmitt and F.G. Worden, Cambridge, Mass.: MIT Press, pp. 109–127; with permission) (B) Output from the cortex. The figure shows that the axons (ax) from the small pyramidal cells (Py) in layers ll and lll mostly pass out of the cortex to run in the subcortical white matter to re-enter the cortex at some other place. The axons from pyramidal cells in layers V and VI, however, run to subcortical nuclei or out of the cerebrum altogether to the brain stem or spinal cord

Figure 1.22(b) shows that the output from the cerebral cortex is carried by axons leaving the bases of the pyramidal cells. These axons may course through the white matter and re-enter the cortex at some more-or-less distant location, or may cross from one hemisphere to the other via the corpus callosum and re-enter the cortex on the opposite side. Other axons run out of the cortex altogether and terminate in some distant part of the brain or spinal cord. It is interesting to note, however, that the latter are in the minority. Of axons leaving or entering the cortex by far the greater number go to or come from other parts of the cortex. Indeed Braitenberg estimates that cortico-cortical fibres outnumber non-cortico-cortical fibres by a factor approaching 10 000 : 1. Each part of the cortex is thus influenced by every other part—each module, it has been argued, contains, like the fragment of a holograph, a fuzzy representation of the whole.

Figure 1.23 shows the neuronal structure of a cortical module as envisaged by Szentágothai. This is not the place to enter into a detailed description of this neuronal meshwork. Interested readers should examine Szentágothai's account. Figure 1.23 is included merely to give some 'feel' for the complexity which undoubtedly exists at the histological level.

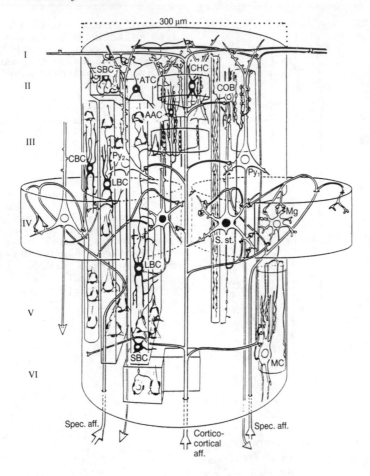

Figure 1.23 Neocortical module. The diagram represents a cortico-cortical column 300μm in diameter. The six horizontal layers of the cortex are numbered to the left of the figure. The two flat cylinders in lamina IV correspond to the termination territory of a specific afferent. (From Szentágothai, 1979, in *The Neurosciences: Fourth Study Program*, eds F.O. Schmitt and F.G. Worden, Cambridge, Mas.: MIT Press, pp. 399–415; with permission.)

Figure 1.23 emphasises that the intricate juxtaposition of neurons and neuroglia in the cortex provides innumerable possibilities for the synaptic contacts discussed in the previous section and for the neurochemistry to be outlined in the subsequent chapters of this book. Neurons cannot be regarded as discrete, 'introspective', units such as the transistors and resistors of a circuit board but as interacting together in rich and diverse ways. The long-axon 'principal' neurons of classical neurophysiology are not typical of the intricate webs of dendrites, short axons and perikarya, neuroglia of various sorts, which are characteristic of grey matter. Here the full complexity of submillivolt cable conduction (Chapter 11), of subtle shifts of baselevel resting potentials and postsynaptic sensitivities (Chapter 16), of heterogeneous membrane patches (Chapter 6), of molecular transfer between cells via gap junctions (Chapter 6), of changes in ambient ion concentration, of complicated sculpturing of electric fields by the three-dimensional geometries of dendritic arbors and spine morphologies and so forth and so on, can occur. The state of matter in the cerebral cortex is of mind-boggling complexity.

Yet in spite of the analyses of the structural biologists—the anatomists, histologists, cytologists, molecular biologists—the cortex can perhaps best be regarded, to quote Szentágothai again, 'as something of a continuous medium'. As in all areas of scientific endeavour so with the cerebral cortex: analysis comes first. The reconstruction of the whole from its constituent fragments follows later—in this case very much later, some time in the yet-unforeseeable future. The observer surveying the cortex naturally wishes to see edges, modules, demarcations, levels—this is the only hope of progress. In reality, however, there is an immensely complex, extended pattern of material activity, a flow of activity comparable, as Freeman puts it, to the 'continuum of a chemical reaction'. Moreover the cortex, as we have already emphasised, is linked together so that each part of the immense sheet is affected by what is happening in every other part. It is this complex interconnectivity which makes the brain unique among living tissues.

Chapter 2
The conformation of informational macromolecules

In Chapter 1 we reminded ourselves of the great structural complexity of the brain, from its 'naked-eye' anatomy to its cellular and subcellular detail. There was no need to labour the point that this intricacy of structure has to do with its central function: information processing—the computing of life-preserving responses to the challenges of the biotic and abiotic environment.

In this chapter we start from the other end of the scale of neurobiological magnitudes, the molecular end. But once again the same feature stands out. Biological molecules often have extremely complicated structures and these structures are basic to their biological function. This, indeed, is the fundamental insight of molecular biology.

Two types of biological macromolecule are central to molecular biology: the **proteins** and the **nucleic acids**. These molecules are sometimes called **informational macromolecules**. Other molecular species also play a crucial role—e.g. the carbohydrates and the lipids—but they are of lesser importance. We shall discuss the role of the latter in the formation of biomembranes in chapter 6. In this chapter and the next we shall concentrate on the proteins and nucleic acids. These are the molecules which bring about the information processing upon which the cell, just as much as the brain, depends.

2.1 PROTEINS

Proteins, like all informational macromolecules, are **polymers** built of a large number of monomeric units. In the case of proteins these monomeric units are **amino acids**. Molecular biologists recognise **20** different types of amino acid. These are shown in

Figure 2.1. Except for **proline** they all share a common structure differing only in their side chains. This structure is shown below:

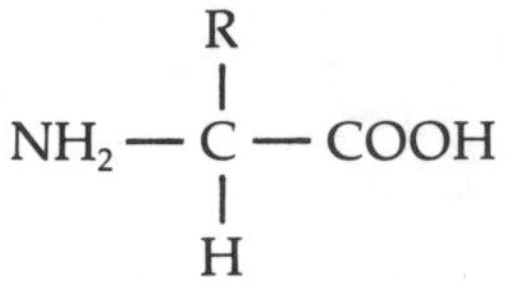

$$NH_2 - \overset{\displaystyle R}{\underset{\displaystyle H}{\overset{\displaystyle |}{\underset{\displaystyle |}{C}}}} - COOH$$

The side chains of the amino acids are, however, of great importance. Table 2.1 shows some of their more important properties. The side chain of proline bends round, as shown, and unites with the amino group by removing one of its hydrogens. This, as we shall see, has significant consequences for some of the conformations into which amino acid chains are twisted. Another even more significant feature so far as the conformation of proteins is concerned is the **hydrophilicity** or **hydrophobicity** of the side chains. We shall see that the solubility or insolubility of different parts of a protein in water is of great importance in molecular neurobiology. The sheer **bulkiness** of the side chains is also significant. Glycine, with just a single hydrogen, has the smallest side chain of all, and alanine with a methyl group is not much bigger; in contrast tyrosine, phenylalanine and in particular tryptophan have bulky aromatic side chains. Finally two amino acids, methionine and cysteine, contain sulphur atoms in their side chains. Both play important roles in molecular biology. The sulphydryl (SH) group of cysteine is particularly important. The three-dimensional form of many proteins is stabilised by the formation of disulphide linkages between the SH groups of neighbouring cysteines. Table 2.1 also shows that each amino acid has been assigned a three-letter abbreviation and a one-letter symbol.

The conformation of protein molecules can be extremely complex. For convenience it is usual to treat it as if it had four different levels: **primary**, **secondary**, **tertiary** and **quaternary**. Only the first of these levels can be determined by conventional biochemical techniques (chromatography, electrophoresis, etc.); in recent years, as we shall see, the techniques of genetic engineering have also been increasingly used to determine this level of structure. Higher levels are investigated principally by the technique of X-ray diffraction but electron microscopy also plays a part. The determination of protein structure is a laborious and time-consuming process. Nevertheless more than 4000 primary structures are now known and more than 200 secondary and higher structures.

Table 2.1 Amino acids

Name and abbreviations	Formula	Comment
1. Polar (hydrophilic) side chains		
Glycine, Gly, G	$$H-\underset{\underset{COOH}{\mid}}{\overset{\overset{NH_2}{\mid}}{C}}-H$$	Simplest and smallest side chain
Aspartic acid, Asp, D	$$H-\underset{\underset{COOH}{\mid}}{\overset{\overset{NH_2}{\mid}}{C}}-CH_2-\underset{\underset{O^-}{\mid}}{\overset{\overset{O}{\parallel}}{C}}$$	Acidic, negatively charged side chain
Asparagine, Asn, N	$$H-\underset{\underset{COOH}{\mid}}{\overset{\overset{NH_2}{\mid}}{C}}-CH_2-\underset{\underset{NH_2}{\mid}}{\overset{\overset{O}{\parallel}}{C}}$$	
Glutamic acid, Glu, E	$$H-\underset{\underset{COOH}{\mid}}{\overset{\overset{NH_2}{\mid}}{C}}-CH_2-CH_2-\underset{\underset{O^-}{\mid}}{\overset{\overset{O}{\parallel}}{C}}$$	Acidic, negatively charged side chain
Glutamine, Gln, Q	$$H-\underset{\underset{COOH}{\mid}}{\overset{\overset{NH_2}{\mid}}{C}}-CH_2-CH_2-\underset{\underset{NH_2}{\mid}}{\overset{\overset{O}{\parallel}}{C}}$$	
Cysteine, Cys, C	$$H-\underset{\underset{COOH}{\mid}}{\overset{\overset{NH_2}{\mid}}{C}}-CH_2-SH$$	SH (sulphydryl) group frequently involved in disulphide (S—S) linkages
Serine, Ser, S	$$H-\underset{\underset{COOH}{\mid}}{\overset{\overset{NH_2}{\mid}}{C}}-CH_2-OH$$	Hydroxyl group often phosphorylated by protein kinases
Threonine, Thr, T	$$H-\underset{\underset{COOH}{\mid}}{\overset{\overset{NH_2}{\mid}}{C}}-\overset{\overset{CH_3}{\mid}}{CH}-OH$$	Hydroxyl group often phophorylated by protein kinases

Table 2.1   Amino acids (*continued*)

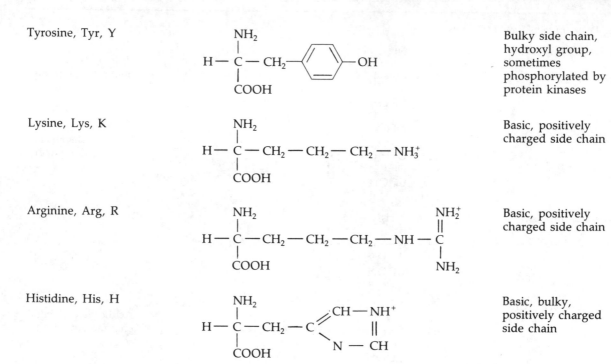

Tyrosine, Tyr, Y		Bulky side chain, hydroxyl group, sometimes phosphorylated by protein kinases
Lysine, Lys, K		Basic, positively charged side chain
Arginine, Arg, R		Basic, positively charged side chain
Histidine, His, H		Basic, bulky, positively charged side chain

2. *Non-polar (hydrophobic) side chains*

Alanine, Ala, A		Small side chain
Valine, Val, V		
Leucine, Leu, L		

Table 2.1   Amino acids (*continued*)

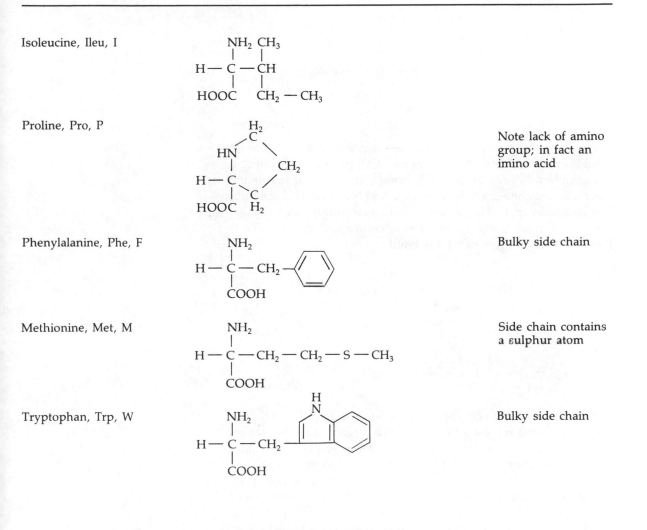

Isoleucine, Ileu, I	(structure)	
Proline, Pro, P	(structure)	Note lack of amino group; in fact an imino acid
Phenylalanine, Phe, F	(structure)	Bulky side chain
Methionine, Met, M	(structure)	Side chain contains a sulphur atom
Tryptophan, Trp, W	(structure)	Bulky side chain

2.1.1 Primary structure

It is well known that amino acids are able to link together by the elimination of the elements of water between the carboxylic acid ($-COOH$) group and the amino ($-NH_2$) group. In this way it is possible to form long chains of amino acids (often called **residues** when incorporated in a chain) linked by **peptide bonds**. Peptide bonds are covalent forces caused by the sharing of valency electrons and are hence very strong. An energy input of about

70 kcal/mol is required to break them. Hence the primary structure of a protein or polypeptide is tough and difficult to disrupt.

$$NH_2\cdots - \overset{\overset{\displaystyle H}{|}}{\underset{\underset{\displaystyle R}{|}}{C}} - \overset{\overset{\displaystyle O}{||}}{C} - \overset{}{\underset{\underset{\displaystyle H}{|}}{N}} - \overset{\overset{\displaystyle R}{|}}{\underset{\underset{\displaystyle H}{|}}{C}} - \cdots COOH$$

It is worth noting at this stage that resonance occurs between the double covalent bond of the **carbonyl (CO) group** and the single covalent bond of the **imino (NH) group**. In other words valency electrons are shared between the O, C and N atoms. This seeming detail ensures that all the atoms in the **amide group** are **co-planar**. This, in turn, restricts the number of conformations into which the amino acid chain can be twisted.

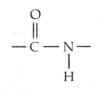

Planar amide group

The sequence in which the amino acids are linked together is called the **primary sequence** or **primary structure**. The amino acids in a primary sequence are numbered from the N-terminal end of the chain. The distinction between **polypeptides** and **proteins** is rather arbitrary. Traditionally sequences of more than about fifty residues were regarded as proteins; sequences of less than that number of residues were termed polypeptides. That tradition has broken down. Nowadays there seems to be little or no distinction between what is termed a polypeptide and what is termed a protein. Many proteins have considerably more than 100 amino acids in their primary structure. As there are 20 different amino acids it follows that primary sequences could, theoretically, be almost infinitely various. The number of different sequences possible for a primary structure of 100 amino acids is 20^{100}, i.e. 1 followed by about 130 zeros! In other words there are more possible primary sequences than there are atoms in the universe. Needless to say only a very small subset of this immense number of sequences is synthesised by living cells. The primary sequences of some neuroactive peptides are shown in Table 2.2.

Table 2.2 Primary structure of some neuroactive peptides

Cholecystokinin 8 (CKK 8)	asp-tyr-met-gly-trp-met-asp-phe
Cholecystokinin 4 (CCK 4)	trp-met-asp-phe
β-Endorphin	*tyr-gly-gly-phe-met*-thr-ser-glu-lys-ser-gln-thr-pro-leu-val-thr-leu-phe-lys-asn-ala-ile-lys-ile-lys-asn-ala-tyr-lys-lys-gly-glu
Leu-enkephalin	tyr-gly-gly-phe-leu
Met-enkephalin	tyr-gly-gly-phe-met
Neurotensin (NT)	glu-leu-tyr-glu-asn-lys-pro-arg-arg-pro-tyr-ile-leu
Angiotensin (AT)	asp-arg-val-tyr-ile-his-pro-phe
Somatostatin 14 (ST)	ala-gly-cys-lys-asn-phe-phe-trp-lys-thr-phe-thr-ser-cys
Substance P (SP)	arg-pro-lys-pro-glu-glu-phe-phe-gly-leu-met
Substance K (SK) (neurokinin A (NKA)	his-lys-thr-asp-ser-phe-val-gly-leu-met
Neuromedin K (NK) (neurokinin B (NKB)	asp-met-his-asp-phe-phe-val-gly-leu-met
Bradykinin (BJ)	arg-pro-pro-gly-phe-ser-pro-phe-arg
Bombesin (BB)	glu-gln-arg-leu-gly-asn-glu-trp-ala-val-gly-his-leu-met
Vasopressin (VP)	cys-tyr-phe-gln-asn-cys-pro-arg-gly
Oxytocin (OT)	cys-tyr- ile - gln-asn-cys-pro-leu-gly

Inspection of this table will show that several of these neuroactive peptides share common amino acid sequences. We shall see in Chapters 3 and 4 that this is no mere coincidence. Families of neuroactive peptides are often derived from a single mother or precursor polypeptide

Glycoproteins. Before completing this section it is important to describe the structure of glycoproteins. We shall see in subsequent chapters that many of the most important neurobiological proteins are **glycosylated**. This means that attached to the polypeptide chain are oligosaccharide side chains. Such proteins are defined as glycoproteins. The most common saccharide units in glycoproteins are **galactose (Gal)**, **mannose (Man)** and **fucose (Fuc)** (= **6-deoxygalactose**). In addition the amino sugars ***n*-acetyl-galctosamine (GalNAc)** and ***n*-acetylglucosamine (GlcNAc)** are very common as is **sialic acid (*n*-acetylneuraminic acid (NANA))**.

Only certain amino acids form points of attachment for oligosaccharide chains. *O*-Glycosidic links are formed with the hydroxyl terminals of side chains of **serine**, **threonine**, **hydroxy-lysine (Hyl)** and **hydroxyproline (Hyp)**, whilst *n*-glycosidic links are made to the terminal amino group of **asparagine's** side chain. These linkages and structures are shown in Figure 2.1. The cell biology of glycosylation will be described in Chapter 14.

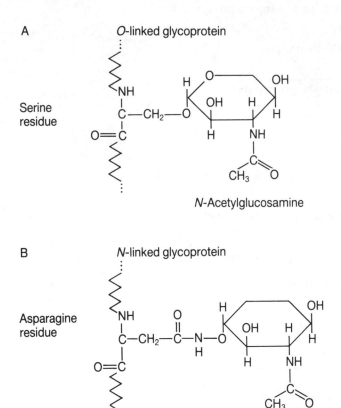

Figure 2.1 Glycoproteins and glycosidic links. In (A) *n*-acetylglucosamine is linked to a serine residue by an *o*-glycosidic bond; in (B) *n*-acetylglucosamine is linked to an asparagine residue by an *n*-glycosidic bond

2.1.2 Secondary structure

Secondary structure is somewhat difficult to define. In effect it consists of the structure conferred by **hydrogen bonding** between contiguous parts of a primary structure. H-bonds can occur between the hydrogen atoms of imino groups and the oxygen atoms of carbonyl groups. This is because electronegative atoms such as N attract hydrogen's lone electron, leading to a fractional negative charge (δ-) on N and a fractional positive charge (δ+) on H. H is thus open to electrostatic attraction from another electronegative atom such as O:

$$C = O \ \text{IIII} \ H - N$$
$$\delta + \quad \delta - \quad \delta + \quad \delta -$$

The electrostatic force between the partial charges is very weak. It is computed to be about **three percent of the covalent-bond force, i.e. 1–5 kcal mol^{-1}**.

Carbonyl and imino groups are, as we saw in Section 2.1.1, repeated features of a protein's primary structure. Consequently it is possible for very large numbers of H-bonds to form if amino acid chains are correctly aligned. It follows that although each H-bond may be easy to break, the force exerted by large numbers may be quite strong. But, as indicated, this does depend on correct alignments of the bonded chains. Here we meet for the first time one of the themes which run throughout molecular biology: **the 'stickiness' of complementary surfaces**.

There are three important secondary structures: β-pleated sheets, 'collagen'-like triple helices and α-helices. Let us briefly consider each in turn.

The β-pleated sheet. Beta-pleated sheets come in two varieties: **parallel** and **antiparallel**. The antiparallel type is the most stable. Here amino acid chains run in opposite directions. In Figure 2.2(A) the chain from N to C runs right to left above and from left to right below. When this alignment occurs the imino hydrogens and the carbonyl oxygens are all optimally positioned for H-bond formation.

Figure 2.2(B) shows that when the amino acid chains run in the same direction the hydrogen bonding potentialities are not quite so easily satisfied. Nonetheless alignment is possible and the result is the 'parallel' β-pleated sheet. Because of the slight strain in the hydrogen bond alignments the sheet tends to twist in a right handed sense. This twist can be seen in the α/β tertiary structure shown in Figure 2.8.

The best-known example of an extensive antiparallel β-pleated sheet is found in **silk fibroin**. Silk is built up from layer upon layer of pleated sheet. It is clear that if the pleated sheets are to fit snugly together the amino acid side chains cannot be too bulky. It is thus no surprise to find that silk fibroin consists almost entirely of gly and ala residues.

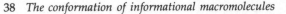

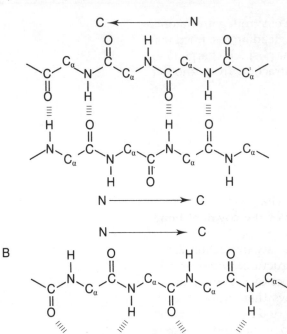

Figure 2.2 Antiparallel and parallel β-pleated sheets. (A) Antiparallel pleated sheet. The figure shows that if the two polypeptide chains run in opposite directions they can be aligned so that their hydrogen-bonding potentialities are easily satisfied. The side chains attached to the α-carbon atoms are not shown: they project in the third dimension, above and below the plane of the paper. (B) Parallel pleated sheet. The figure shows that if two polypeptide chains both run in the same direction they can nevertheless be aligned so that hydrogen bonds are formed between their imino hydrogens and carbonyl oxygens. The alignment between carbonyl oxygen and imino hydrogen is, however, not so precise as it is in the antiparallel sheet. In consequence the parallel sheet tends to develop a right-hand twist

Figure 2.3 Stacking of antiparallel pleated sheets in silk fibroin. The figure gives a three-dimensional view of a small portion of the antiparallel pleated β-sheet structure of silk fibroin. The hydrogen bonding between imino nitrogen and carbonyl oxygen (in contrast to Fig. 2.2) is shown in the third dimension, above and below the plane of the paper. The small side chains of alanine and glycine nestle neatly between the sheets

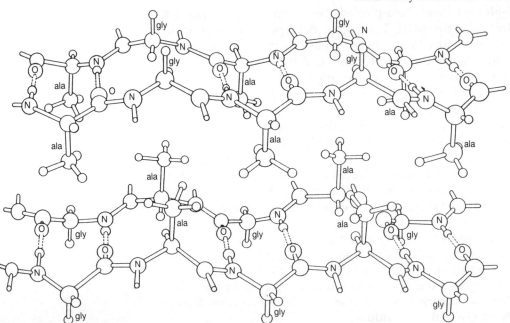

β-Pleated sheets are by no means restricted to fibrous proteins such as silk. We shall see that they often form structural domains within large globular proteins.

Collagen and collagen-like structures. A second well-understood example of secondary structure is provided by **collagen**. Collagens are found throughout the Metazoa and in the mammals they constitute some 25% of all the body's proteins.

There are several different types of collagen. As the molecule plays rather little part in neurobiology we shall consider only its

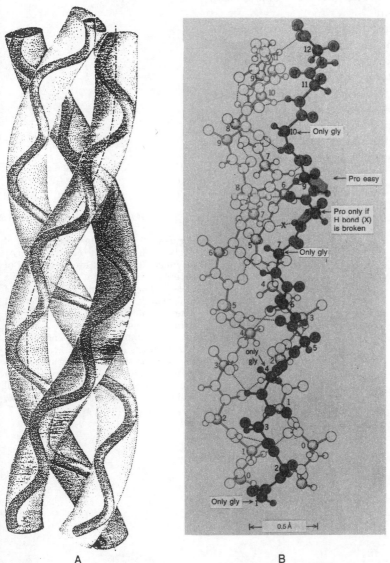

A   B

Figure 2.4 Collagen (A) The three-stranded 'rope' of a portion of a tropo-collagen molecule. Each strand is itself a twisted amino acid chain. (B) The detailed molecular structure of the three-stranded rope shown in (A). The numbers refer to α-carbon atoms; two of every three imino hydrogens and carbonyl oxygens are hydrogen-bonded to another chain (dotted lines). This gives a structure with a high tensile strength. (After Dickerson and Geis, 1969, *The Structure and Action of Proteins*, Menlo Park, California: Benjamin/Cummings.)

general structure. Unlike silk fibroin the amino acid chain is not extended in the β-conformation. Instead each amino acid is rotated through 120° with respect to its predecessor in the chain. This produces a twisted thread. Next three of these twisted threads are wound together and held by intra-chain hydrogen bonds. For this complex structure to be possible only certain amino acids can be incorporated into the chains. Glycine, because it is small, forms every third residue and there are large quantities of hydroxyproline and hydroxylysine. Hydroxyproline is believed to be involved in the formation of the intra-chain H-bonds, whilst the hydroxylysine is frequently glycosylated by the addition of two carbohydrate residues—galactose and glucose. Collagen can thus be classified as a 'glycoprotein'.

Although, as we have already noted, collagens play little part in the structure and functioning of the brain another molecule which shares the collagen structure does: this is the synaptically important enzyme **acetylcholinesterase (AChE)**.

We shall consider the important role of this enzyme in Chapter 15 and again in Chapter 16. Here we shall restrict ourselves to noting that AChE is found in two major configurations. In some cases it consists of globular units, often grouped together to form dimers and tetramers. In other cases it is strongly asymmetrical with a pronounced 'tail'.

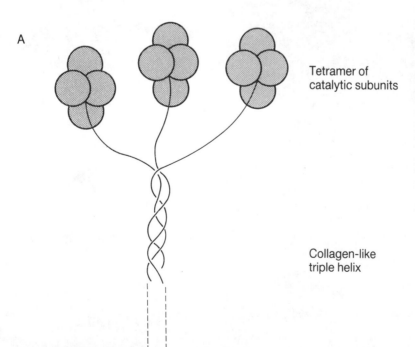

A

Tetramer of catalytic subunits

Collagen-like triple helix

Figure 2.5 Molecular structures of acetylcholinesterase (AChE). (A) Asymmetric AChE. Three tetramers of catalytic subunits are attached to a collagen-like triple helix. This helix is not hydropathic and consequently is not inserted into the lipid phase of a cell membrane but into a protein-based basement membrane. (B) Independent catalytic subunits of AChE. (C) Sometimes the catalytic subunits of AChE possess glycophospholipid 'tails' which anchor the enzyme by inserting into the cell membrane. (After Taylor *et al.*, 1986, *Trends in Pharmacological Science*, **7**, 321–23.)

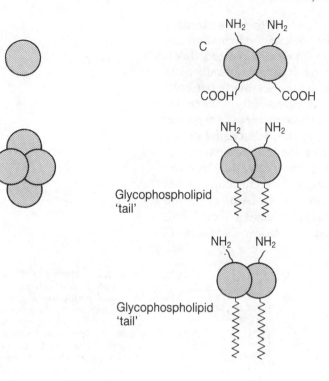

The globular unit is the known as the **catalytic unit**. It is this part of the molecule which possesses the AChE activity. The catalytic unit is found not only in the nervous system but on the membranes of other cells (e.g. erythrocytes) as well. Often, but not always, the catalytic unit may possess a glycophospholipid side chain which confers solubility in the lipid phase of a cell membrane (see Chapter 6).

Of greater interest in this section, however, is the finding that in many cases, especially at neuromuscular junctions, the catalytic units are joined to a lengthy 'collagen-like' tail. This tail consists, like collagen, of three polypeptide chains, each with a 'threefold screw' axis, twisted around each other to form a three-stranded 'rope'. Further confirmation of the collagen-like nature of the tail comes from the finding that, like collagen itself, there is much hydroxyproline and hydroxylysine and that the whole structure is sensitive to enzymic digestion by collagenase. Finally it should be noted that this 'asymmetrical' form of AChE is a huge molecule: the molecular weight being computed at roughly 1000 kDa. It is believed that the collagen-like tail is inserted into the basement membrane which is strongly developed in the folds of the neuromuscular junction (Figure 14.16). In this way the catalytic units are held in place, optimally positioned to carry out their enzymic activity.

The α-helix. Last, but very far from least, of these 'secondary structures' is the **α-helix**. This is an important conformation not only in many fibrous proteins but also (like the β-pleated sheet) in regions of numerous globular proteins. It differs radically from the previous structures in that the H-bonds are made between the imino hydrogens and the carbonyl oxygens of the *same* chain. All possible H-bonds are made so that the structure is energetically very stable and, most importantly, the side chains of the amino acids project outwards away from the longitudinal axis of the helix. Thus, with the sole exception of proline, the structure can incorporate every one of the twenty different amino acids Proline, it will be remembered, does not possess an imino hydrogen and hence is unable to form the requisite H-bond with the carbonyl oxygen in the spiral above or below its position.

A

B

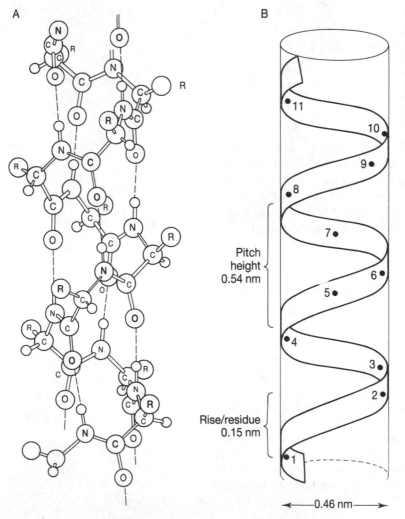

Pitch
height
0.54 nm

Rise/residue
0.15 nm

←——0.46 nm——→

Figure 2.6   α-Helix. (A) Atomic structure of the right-handed α-helix. Note that the hydrogen bonds are aligned with the longitudinal axis of the molecule and that the amino acid side chains project outwards. (B) Schematic diagram of a right-handed α-helix. The diameter is 0.46 nm, the rise per residue is 0.15 nm and the pitch height is 0.54 nm (i.e. 3.6 × 0.15 nm). The α-carbon atoms are numbered

Figure 2.6 shows a right-handed α-helix. This is more stable than the left-handed form. It also shows that the rise per residue is 1.5 Å and that there are about 3.6 residues per turn. It turns out that an isolated α-helix is rather unstable in an aqueous environment. In consequence α-helices are usually stabilised by the interaction of their side chains with neighbouring groups. These neighbours may be other regions of the same molecule or

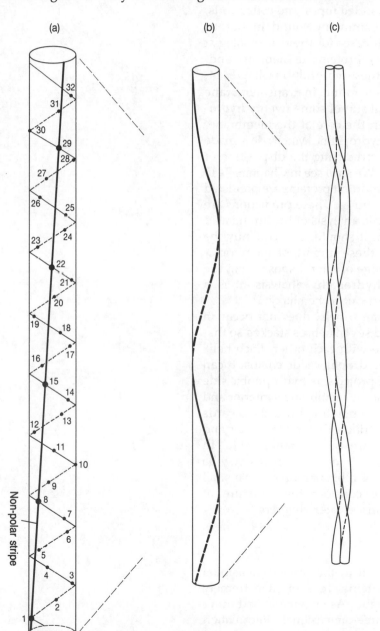

(a)   (b)   (c)

Non-polar stripe

Figure 2.7   Non-polar 'stripes' and two-stranded α-helical 'ropes'. (A) Schematic diagram to show a 32-residue length of α-helix. If every seventh residue possesses a non-polar side chain a non-polar 'stripe' develops along the length of the helix. (B) A lengthy segment of α-helix showing the way in which a non-polar stripe may twist around the molecule. (C) Schematic to show how two α-helices each possessing a non-polar stripe may twist around each other, being held together by hydrophobic forces in the ambient aqueous environment

other molecules altogether. It is sometimes found that every seventh residue in an α-helix is non-polar. Because there are about 3.6 residues per turn this so-called **heptad** repeat results in a non-polar stripe forming at a slight inclination to the long axis of the helix. It follows that if another α-helix with a non-polar heptad repeat is laid alongside the first, twisting gently round it in left-handed sense, then its non-polar residues can fit against the first's non-polar stripe. In this way **two-stranded ropes**, and **coiled coils**, can form. These coils are quite commonly found in fibrous proteins and particularly important cases for the neurobiologist are the **intermediate filament (IF)** proteins of neurons and, especially, axons. We shall consider these more fully in Chapter 14.

α-Helical domains are also often found in transmembrane proteins. In these cases an α-helical run of some twenty **hydrophobic** residues is believed to span the core of the membrane. These domains are usually termed hydropathic. Much use is made of these hydropathic sequences in predicting the disposition of a polypeptide chain in a membrane. We shall see in Chapters 7–10 that numerous neurobiologically important proteins are predicted to span the membrane five or more times. These predictions are made on the strength of hydropathic analysis of the amino acid sequence in the polypeptide chain. It should, consequently, be borne in mind, when examining these important membrane-bound structures, that our knowledge of their disposition in the membrane is based mainly on hydropathy analysis: it is a foundation which could easily turn out to be shaky.

In other cases it is found that an α-helix does not occur in isolation. It is quite common to find seven helices stacked so that their long axes are at a small angle with each other. Each helix may have both hydrophobic and hydrophilic side chains. It can then be arranged that each α-helix projects its hydrophobic side chains into the lipid environment of the membrane's interior and maintains its hydrophilic side chains pointing inwards towards its six neighbours. Helices which distribute their hydrophobic and hydrophilic residues in this way are called **amphipathic**. In consequence it is possible to see how hydrophilic pores may be developed across the lipid bilayer of a biomembrane. We shall return to this concept when we consider the structure of membranes and membrane proteins in later chapters.

2.1.3 Tertiary Structure

Tertiary structure is the name given to the three-dimensional conformation of the globular proteins. It is often extremely intricate and always extremely fragile. As enzymatic and other biological activities depend on this three-dimensional conformation it is also extremely important.

The tertiary structure of a protein is believed to be determined by its primary structure. The most important forces involved are **hydrophobic** and **hydrophilic** forces. We have already emphasised the significance of hydrophobic and hydrophilic amino acid side chains above. In globular proteins situated in an aqueous environment (i.e. most proteins), hydrophobic residues will tend to end up in the interior, whilst hydrophilic residues will cluster on the surface where they can enter the surrounding water structure. Some have therefore likened a globular protein to a tiny oily droplet covered by hydrophilic hairs. In addition non-specific **van der Waals' forces** between complementary '**docking**' surfaces also play an important role in maintaining the three-dimensional structure. Finally **disulphide linkages** between neighbouring cysteine residues and **ionic (salt) linkages** between neighbouring polar side chains may be formed and thus help to stabilise the conformation. Even so the structure is often, as indicated above, on the edge of unravelling into instability. The energy state associated with the conformation of a typical small globular protein such as egg-white lysozyme is only **10 kcal mol^{-1}** below that of a random organisation; in other words only that quantity of energy is required to **denature** the molecule.

Table 2.3   Energies of chemical bonds

Single covalent bonds	$\Delta E = -50$ to -110 kcal/mol
Double covalent bonds	$\Delta E = -120$ to -170 kcal/mol
Triple covalent bonds	$\Delta E = -195$ kcal/mol
Ionic interactions ('salt bridges')	$\Delta E \sim -4$ kcal/mol
Hydrogen bonds	$\Delta E = -1$ to -5 kcal/mol
Van der Waals' interactions	$\Delta E \sim -1$ kcal/mol
Hydrophobic interactions	$\Delta E \sim -1$ kcal/mol

It is largely the last four forces which hold the higher structures of biological macromolecules together

A large protein molecule frequently consists of several different regions: these are known as **domains**. The domains normally consist of structurally well-formed regions, for instance stacks of β-pleated sheets or lengths of α-helix. The domains are held to each other by lengths of nondescript polypeptide chain. Some instances of the most common domain structures are shown in Figure 2.8. It can be seen that it almost appears as if large globular proteins are **modularised**.

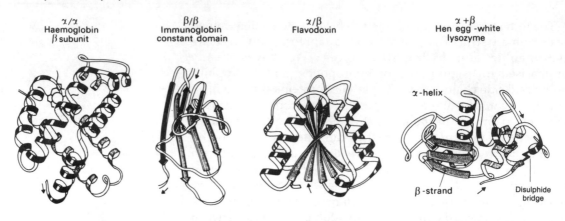

| α/α Haemoglobin β subunit | β/β Immunoglobin constant domain | α/β Flavodoxin | $\alpha + \beta$ Hen egg -white lysozyme |

This notion of modularisation may, in fact, not be so far wide of the mark. It begins to seem probable that some of the large protein structures synthesised by cells have evolved by the union of genes which programme the synthesis of individual domains. We shall return to this concept in Chapter 4, where we discuss molecular evolution.

Before leaving the topic of tertiary structure we must emphasise once more that the integrity of this fragile three-dimensional conformation is essential for the biological activity of the protein. The **active site** of an enzyme is, for instance, normally some specific region of the protein's surface which is rather precisely 'tailored' to fit its substrate. This accurate stereochemical fit depends on the maintenance of tertiary structure. Any denaturation (= degradation) destroys biological activity. But this seeming disadvantage is made use of in living cells for the purposes of control. Because the tertiary structure is so fragile small molecules (**allosteric effectors**) can be used to change it and thus alter the catalytic or other properties of the active site. In a sense, perhaps, one can detect at this level a primordial instance of sensitivity, of response to environment. The enzyme alters the activity of its active site when ambient conditions affect another part of its structure. This very important process is shown in Figure 2.9

Finally it is important, in the context of this book, to note that not only are alterations in three-dimensional conformation significant in the control of enzyme activity but that they are also responsible for a whole raft of neurobiological phenomena. We shall see, as we proceed through the following pages, that phosphorylation alters the conformation of proteins, especially membrane proteins, thus altering their functional state; that transmitter/modulator molecules act by changing the conformation of their proteinaceous membrane receptors; that

Figure 2.8   Domain structure of globular proteins. Globular proteins can be classified into four major classes depending on the organisation of the internal α-helical and β-sheet domains. In the figure α-helices are represented by coiled ribbons, and β-pleated sheets by flat arrows which indicate the direction in which the polypeptide chain runs. In the α/α organisation the protein consists almost entirely of α-helices; the β/β structure, in contrast, consists almost entirely of β-pleated sheets (in the figure, antiparallel) and no α-helix; the α/β structure is built from alternating regions of α-helix and β-sheet (regions of α-helix commonly surround the β-sheet); finally in the $\alpha + \beta$ structure the α-helices and β-sheets tend to develop in different parts of the molecule. (From Rees and Sternberg, 1984, *From Cells to Atoms*, Oxford: Blackwell Scientific Publications; with permission.)

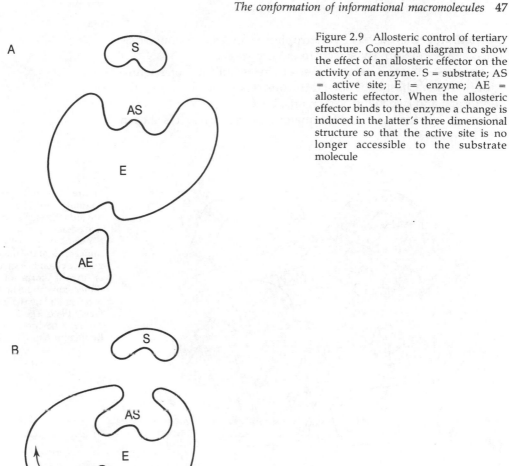

Figure 2.9 Allosteric control of tertiary structure. Conceptual diagram to show the effect of an allosteric effector on the activity of an enzyme. S = substrate; AS = active site; E = enzyme; AE = allosteric effector. When the allosteric effector binds to the enzyme a change is induced in the latter's three dimensional structure so that the active site is no longer accessible to the substrate molecule

photons affect the 3-D conformation of opsins; that cAMP and other 'second messengers' affect membrane channels; and that voltage changes control the opening and shutting of membrane gates. Controlled alterations of the 3-D conformation of proteins is indeed a continuing theme in molecular neurobiology.

2.1.4 Quaternary structure

Many proteins consist of more than one subunit. The organisation of the subunits to form one coherent molecule constitutes the molecule's **quaternary** structure. Unlike the domain structure discussed above the subunits of a quaternary structure are not joined by a continuous polypeptide chain. Such proteins are termed **multimeric**. In most cases the subunits are held (or pushed!) together merely by **hydrophobic forces**. It follows that, once again, quaternary structure is very fragile.

The best-known quaternary structure is still that of **haemoglobin**—the earliest to be solved. It consists of four subunits, two identical α and two identical β chains. Because it is so well known it has come to form a model for quaternary structures. It is shown in Figure 2.10.

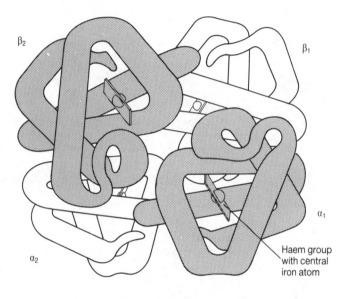

Figure 2.10 Quaternary structure of haemoglobin. The α_1 and β_2 chains face towards the viewer in this representation of oxyhaemoglobin. The identical α_2 and β_1 chains are partially hidden. The figure indicates that the major part of the polypeptide chain in each of the four subunits is in the form of an α-helix. The dimensions of the molecule are $6.4 \times 5.5 \times 5.0$ nm. (After I. Geis in Dickerson and Geis, 1969, *The Structure and Action of Proteins*, Menlo Park, California: Benjamin/ Cummings.)

Haemoglobin's subunits each have a molecular weight of about 16 000 Da and consist of 141 amino acids (α-chains) and 146 amino acids (β-chains). The molecular weight of the entire molecule is about 68 000 Da. Many multimeric globular proteins are far bigger. The nicotinic acetylcholine receptor (nAChR), which we shall discuss in Chapter 9, consists of five large subunits, whilst ferritin is built of 20 identical subunits, each consisting of 200 amino acids, and weighs in at a total molecular weight of 480 000 Da. We shall look in some detail at the tertiary and quaternary structures of some proteins of neurobiological importance in later chapters.

The principle of building larger and larger structures by making use of the complementary surfaces of smaller units can of course be extended from proteins to other molecules. The structures of viruses and such ubiquitous organelles as ribosomes consist of assemblages of globular proteins and nucleic acids. It seems likely that eukaryotic chromosomes are built on similar principles and the structure of cell membranes (as we shall see in Chapter 6) can be understood in much the same way.

2.2 NUCLEIC ACIDS

There are two major classes of nucleic acid: **deoxyribonucleic acid**, **DNA** (largely but not exclusively confined to the nucleus in eukaryotic cells) and **ribonucleic acid**, **RNA** (largely but not exclusively confined to the cytoplasm). Both, like the proteins,

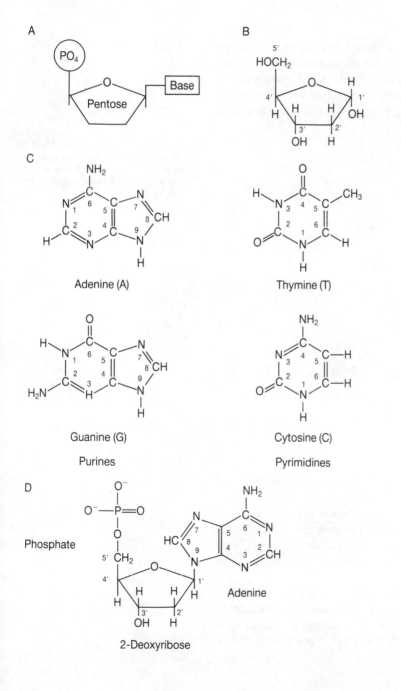

Figure 2.11 Structure of deoxyribo-nucleotides. The figure shows how deoxyribonucleotides are built from a phosphate group, a sugar (deoxyribose) and one of four nitrogenous bases. The latter come in two sizes: the purines and the smaller pyrimidines. The purines are attached to the pentose sugar through nitrogen atom 9 while the pyrimidines are attached through nitrogen atom 1. (A) Schematic diagram of a nucleotide. (B) The pentose sugar, 2-deoxyribose. (C) The four different bases. (D) A typical deoxyribonucleotide: deoxyadenosine monophosphate (dAMP)

are polymers. The monomers of which they are constituted are called nucleotides. Since at least 1944, when Avery, MacLeod and McCarty showed that DNA was responsible for pneumococcal transformation, and certainly from 1953 when Watson and Crick published their solution to the structure of DNA, it has been clear that nucleic acids store and transmit the cell's genetic information.

2.2.1 DNA

The nucleotides of which nucleic acids are built consist of three parts: a **phosphate group**, a **sugar** and a **nitrogenous base**. In the case of DNA the sugar is **deoxyribose** (hence the nucleotide is a **deoxyribonucleotide**) and four different bases are involved— two purines and two pyrimidines. The purine bases are **adenine**

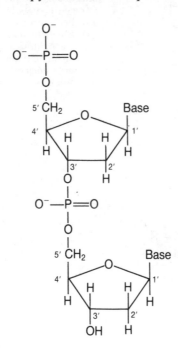

Figure 2.12 Phosphodiester bond between two deoxyribonucleotides. Note how the phosphate group connects the 3′ carbon of one pentose sugar to the 5′ carbon of the next

(A) and **guanine (G)** and the pyrimidines are **cytosine (C)** and **thymine (T)**. The structure of these molecules is shown in Figure 2.11. It should be noted that the purine bases are considerably bigger than the pyrimidines, that both purines and pyrimidines show considerable conjugation (i.e. alternation of single and double covalent bonds) and that they are all planar and hydrophobic.

The deoxyribonucleotides are strung together to form long polynucleotide chains. The connection between one nucleotide and the next is made through the phosphate group of one bonding (by elimination of the elements of water) with the 3′

carbon of the deoxyribose sugar of the other. The phosphate group thus connects the **3' carbon of one deoxyribose with the 5' carbon of the next deoxyribose**. This bonding, a **phosphodiester** bonding, is shown in Figure 2.12.

A

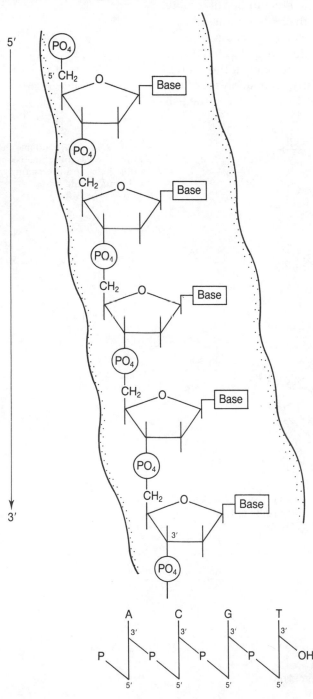

B

Figure 2.13 (A) Portion of a polynucleotide chain. Note the direction of the chain: from 5' to 3'. (B) Short-hand form for writing the formula of a polynucleotide strand. P represents the phosphate group; a vertical line represents the pentose sugar; an appropriate letter represents the base

It is clear that this bonding can be continued (analogously to peptide linkages) to build up long chains of nucleotides. Figure 2.13 shows that the resulting polynucleotide consists of a ...**– phosphate – sugar – phosphate – sugar –** ... 'backbone' to which are attached the nitrogenous bases. It is important to note that the backbone (again analogous to the polypeptides) has a polarity. Conventionally one proceeds along the chain from **5' carbon to 3' carbon.** The initial nucleotide is thus located at the 5' end of the sequence and the terminal nucleotide at the 3' end.

The great contribution of the X-ray diffraction analyses of the early 1950s (Franklin, Wilkins, Watson, Crick) was to establish

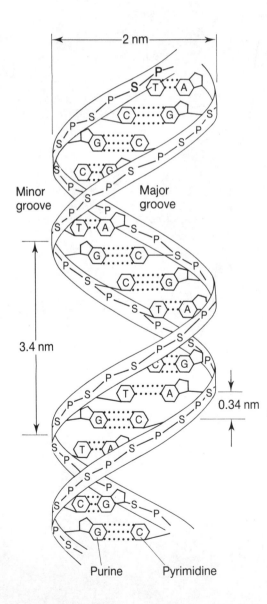

Figure 2.14 DNA double helix. The figure shows the dimensions of the double helix and the pairing properties of the nucleotide bases

the conformation of these polynucleotide strands in nucleic acids, especially DNA.

The Watson–Crick double helix is now almost a cliché. Two polynucleotide strands wind around each other, one proceeding in the 5′ to 3′ direction, the other in the 3′ to 5′ direction. The bases project inwards toward each other, pyrimidines always partnering purines: thus ensuring that the two phosphate–sugar backbones are always at a constant distance (1.085 nm) from each other. The structure is a brilliant solution to the X-ray diffraction data, the requirement of chemical stability (the hydrophobic bases project inwards and the hydrophilic sugar–phosphate backbone outwards toward the aqueous environment), and last, but very far from least, the requirements of a genetic molecule.

Hereditary information is stored in the sequence of bases. Figure 2.15 shows that **adenine (A) always partners thymine (T)** and **guanine (G) always partners cytosine (C)**. These pairings (the so-called Watson–Crick pairings) are established by the selective stickiness of hydrogen bonds—two such bonds, as the figure shows, being formed between A and T and three between G and C.

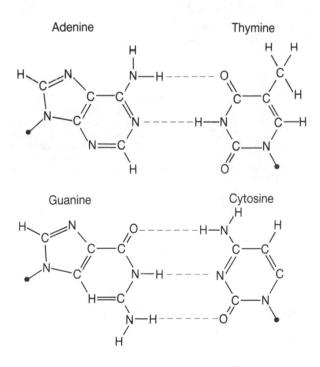

Figure 2.15 Watson–Crick pairings of nucleotide bases. The figure shows that when properly aligned two hydrogen bonds can be formed between A and T and three between C and G. The 'cocktail sticks' attached to the nitrogen atoms of the four bases indicate where the bond uniting them to the doxyribose and thus the rest of the polynucleotide strand is formed

The processes of information transfer in the living cell in which DNA plays so central a role will be discussed in Chapter 3.

2.2.2 RNA

Although the DNA double helix can exist in three different forms (A, B and Z) it mostly exists in the classic Watson–Crick A-form in the living cell. The forms which RNA takes in the cell are far more varied. Let us, however, first look at its 'primary' structure. Like DNA it is composed of nucleotides strung together by phosphodiester linkages. However, the nucleotides differ from those constituting DNA in two respects. **First**, the sugar is not deoxyribose but **ribose**. As Figure 2.16 shows it carries a bulky hydroxyl group at the 2' position instead of deoxyribose's single hydrogen atom. Again this is more than a detail. Because of this bulkiness at the 2' position RNA is unable to stack its bases perpendicular to the long axis of a polynucleotide double helix as can DNA. If a double helix is formed the bases are stacked awkwardly at 20° to the long axis, as they are in the B-configuration of DNA. **Second**, one of the pyrimidine bases differs from those found in DNA. Instead of thymine (T), **uracil (U)** (having the same Watson–Crick pairing properties) is found. This, too, is not an accidental detail. We shall see in the next chapter that T, although it requires more energy to synthesise, is necessary if repair enzymes are to keep DNA's message undegraded. Because of its far more transient existence this is not important in RNA. The latter can thus make do with the less energy-demanding U.

A

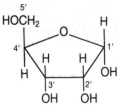

B

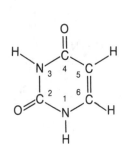

Figure 2.16 Structure of ribonucleotides. The figure shows how ribonucleotides are built from a pentose sugar (ribose), a nitrogenous base and a phosphate group. (A) The pentose sugar, ribose. (B) Uracil (U) replaces thymine. (C) A typical ribonucleotide, adenosine monophosphate (AMP)

C

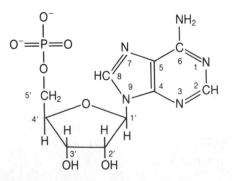

Three major types of RNA are found in the cell: **messenger RNA (mRNA)**, **transfer RNA (tRNA)** and **ribosomal RNA (rRNA)**. A fourth type, **heteronuclear RNA (hnRNA)** is found in the nuclei of eukaryotic cells. This latter type is in fact a precursor of mRNA. We shall see in Chapter 3 that they are all involved in the information transfer process (central to molecular biology) whereby the message held in the structure of DNA is expressed in the structure (and hence activity) of proteins. Here we shall look briefly at their conformations

mRNA hardly has a conformation at all. It is but a single stranded transcript of the appropriate base sequences of DNA. It ranges in length from 75 to over 3000 ribonucleotides.

tRNAs, on the other hand, do have a complex conformation. As we shall see in the next chapter each amino acid has a specific tRNA assigned to it. Thus we refer to $tRNA_{phe}$ $tRNA_{ala}$ etc. It follows that there are at least 20 different types of tRNA molecule. However they all have much in common. To begin with their molecular weights are all about 25 000 Da, which means that they all consist of about 75 nucleotides. Second, they are all believed to have a somewhat similar tertiary structure—rather like a clover leaf. Third, at the end of the clover leaf's 'stem' there is always a group of 'free' (i.e. non-hydrogen bonded) bases. These form the so-called **anticodon** which, as we shall see in the next chapter, recognises the genetic message carried by mRNA from the nuclear DNA. Finally all tRNAs have a group of three ribonucleotides (C, C and A) at the opposite end of the molecule from the anticodon 'stem'. The appropriate amino acid is attached to the final ribonucleotide of this triplet. This attachment is made via the 3' carbon of the adenosine's ribose moiety. This complicated conformation is shown in Figure 2.17.

The complexity of the tertiary structure of tRNAs reflects the difficulty of the job they have to do in the cell. They act as a go-betweens betwixt the proteins and the nucleic acids. Each type of tRNA requires a complex and highly individual conformation so that it can be 'recognised' by the active site of an enzyme—an **aminoacyl synthetase enzyme**. Yet each tRNA has also to recognise an appropriate triplet of nucleotide bases in the mRNA transcript. Proteins and nucleic acids are two very different types of molecule; although both make use of complementary surfaces for recognition the sorts of complementary surface (as must by now be very clear) are radically different. tRNAs must be able to recognise, or be recognised by, both. The means by which this is achieved are considered in the next chapter (Section 3.2.3).

rRNA is transcribed from nuclear DNA as a very large molecule (about 13 000 ribonucleotides in length) known as **45S rRNA**. *S*

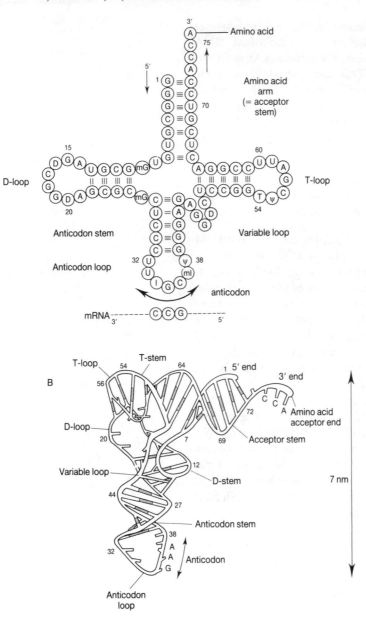

Figure 2.17   The conformation of yeast alanine tRNA (tRNA$_{ala}$). (A) Conventional 'clover-leaf' representation. The majority of the nucleotides are the classical Watson – Crick U, G, C or A but there are a few non-classical types present. These are often found in the loops, where they may play a role in the recognition of the tRNA by the aminoacyl synthetase enzyme. The non-classical bases are ψ = pseudouridine; D = dihydrouridine; I = inosine; T = thymine; m = methyl group. Inosine (I) in the anticodon recognises C (it will also recognise A and U). It will also be noted that in positions 3 and 13 G/U pairs are formed. (After Darnell, Lodish and Baltimore, 1986, *Molecular Cell Biology*, New York: Scientific American Books.) (B) This shows the three-dimensional form of tRNA$_{phe}$ as deduced by X-ray diffraction. The compact and intricate L-shaped structure is stabilised not only by Watson – Crick hydrogen bonding between bases but also by numerous hydrophobic forces. (From Rees and Sternberg, 1984, *From Cells to Atoms*, Oxford: Blackwell Scientific Publications; with permission.)

is an abbreviation for the Svedburg, a sedimentation coefficient. The larger the value of this coefficient the greater the molecular weight. 45*S* rRNA is, however, soon cleaved into three smaller fragments—28*S* (c. 5000 ribonucleotides), 18*S* (c. 2000 ribonucleotides) and 5.8*S* (c. 160 ribonucleotides). In addition to 45*S* rRNA and its cleavage products an entirely separate 5*S* rRNA is also synthesised. All of these various types of rRNA are assembled with a large array of different proteins to form the two subunits of the **ribosome**. This intricate assembly occurs in the nucleolus and the finished products (the two ribosomal subunits) are passed separately out of the nucleus into the cytoplasm. It is notable, as mentioned in Chapter 1, that neurons are distinguished by their large nuclei and prominent nucleoli. It is clear that neurons are very active in the synthesis of ribosomes and thus in the whole business of protein biosynthesis.

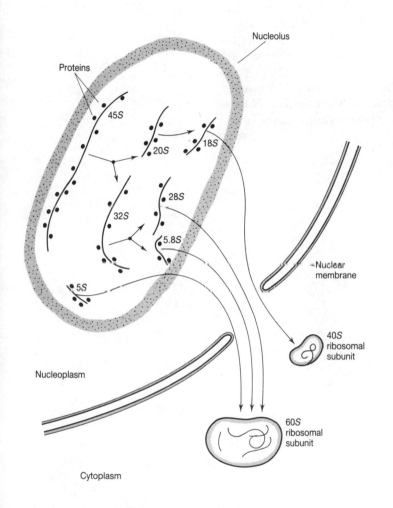

Figure 2.18 Assembly of ribosomes from rRNA and proteins in the nucleolus (explanation in text). The figure shows that the 45S rRNA is progressively split into three fragments: 18S, 28S and 5.8S rRNA. A separate 5S rRNA is transcribed independently from the DNA. The figure shows that all of these rRNA moieties are from the beginning associated with proteins. The two ribosomal subunits are assembled within the nucleolus and passed (probably through a pore in the nuclear membrane) into the cytoplasm. (After Darnell, Lodish and Baltimore, 1986, *Molecular Cell Biology*, New York: Scientific American Books.)

2.3 CONCLUSION

In this chapter we have looked, all too briefly, at the conformation of the most important of the molecules which we shall meet as we proceed with our subject. The biological activity of these molecules emerges from their three-dimensional conformation, just as the biological activity of the brain emerges from its anatomy. It is also worth noting once again the deep significance of complementary surfaces and selective 'stickiness'. The three-dimensional structure responsible for these complementary surfaces and selective stickinesses depends on the presence of multitudinous, in themselves negligible, forces—the H-bonds, hydrophobic forces, van der Waals' attractions, etc. Finally the great difference in the conformation of the two types of macro-molecule we have been considering in this chapter should be borne in mind. The whole complexity of the molecular biology which we shall consider in the next chapter arises from the necessity to translate between one type of informational macromolecule and the other. This is a necessity as each type of molecule depends on the other, they are symbiotically related. On their own they would be comparatively ineffective. Nucleic acids make very poor enzymes (if they possess any catalytic power at all); proteins cannot replicate.

Chapter 3
Information processing in cells

In Chapter 2 we briefly reviewed the nature of the cell's 'informational macromolecules' and also emphasised that cells, like brains, are deeply involved in information processing. In contrast to the brain, however, most (though by no means all) of the information available to the cell is hereditary information. It has been accumulated over two or three billion years of trial-and-error interaction with the environment. By far the greatest amount is stored in the base sequences of DNA.

We also emphasised in Chapter 2 that the two informational macromolecules—the nucleic acids and the proteins—were very different from each other and yet interacted symbiotically in the life of the cell. Each type of molecule is especially good at one of life's necessities—the nucleic acids at preserving and transmitting genetic information (in particular information which determines the structure of proteins), the proteins at catalysing metabolic reactions (including those which lead to the replication of DNA)—but both are required if the cell is to survive.

The central area of molecular biology is thus the study of the interaction of nucleic acids and proteins. Francis Crick summarised the essence of this area in what he memorably called **the central dogma of molecular biology**: 'DNA makes RNA and RNA makes protein'. We now know that the 'dogma' has exceptions. As we shall see, we now know that in some cases information flows from RNA to DNA. A complete reversal of the dogma has, however, never been observed; indeed, as we shall see, there appear to be good molecular reasons for thinking that a flow of information all the way from protein to nucleic acid is impossible. Thus Crick's 'dogma' remains essentially uncontroverted: the major flow of information progresses from nucleic acids to proteins and never vice versa.

It might be added in parenthesis here that Crick's 'dogma' merely states in molecular terms what orthodox biology has been saying since the publication of Charles Darwin's *Origin of Species* in 1859. Information flows from the 'germ plasm' or 'genotype', to the 'somatoplasm' or 'phenotype', and never in the contrary direction. Any reversal of the direction of this information flow would amount to an instance of Lamarckism—the inheritance of acquired characteristics. In spite of much effort and ingenuity Lamarckian inheritance has never yet been observed.

3.1 THE GENETIC CODE

As we saw in Chapter 2, there are up to 20 different amino acids in a protein but only four different nucleotides in DNA. **How can four different nucleotides specify 20 different amino acids?** This is the essence of the 'coding problem' of the late 1950s and early 1960s.

It is clear that four different nucleotides, taken on their own, could only specify four different amino acids; it is also clear that taken in groups of two there would be $4^2 = 16$ different **pairs** of nucleotides, still not sufficient to specify 20 different amino acids; if, however, they were grouped in threes then there would be $4^3 = 64$ different possible **triplets**, more than enough to code for the 20 amino acids. Clever experiments by Crick, Brenner and others in the early 1960s established that the DNA genetic code was indeed a **triplet code**. Each amino acid was specified by one or usually more than one nucleotide triplet. These triplets became known as **codons**. Figure 3.1 shows the genetic code as it is nowadays understood.

First position (5'-end)	Second position of codon				Third position (3'-end)
	U(T)	C	A	G	
U(T)	UUU ⎫ Phe UUC ⎬ UUA ⎫ Leu UUG ⎭	UCU ⎫ UCC ⎬ Ser UCA UCG ⎭	UAU ⎫ Tyr UAC ⎬ UAA ⎫ Term UAG ⎭	UGU ⎫ Cys UGC ⎬ UGA Term UGG Trp	U(T) C A G
C	CUU ⎫ CUC ⎬ Leu CUA CUG ⎭	CCU ⎫ CCC ⎬ Pro CCA CCG ⎭	CAU ⎫ His CAC ⎬ CAA ⎫ Gln CAG ⎭	CGU ⎫ CGC ⎬ Arg CGA CGG ⎭	U(T) C A G
A	AUU ⎫ AUC ⎬ Ile AUA ⎭ * AUG Met	ACU ⎫ ACC ⎬ Thr ACA ACG ⎭	AAU ⎫ Asn AAC ⎬ AAA ⎫ Lys AAG ⎭	AGU ⎫ Ser AGC ⎬ AGA ⎫ Arg AGG ⎭	U(T) C A G
G	GUU ⎫ GUC ⎬ Val GUA * GUG ⎭	GCU ⎫ GCC ⎬ Ala GCA GCG ⎭	GAU ⎫ Asp GAC ⎬ GAA ⎫ Glu GAG ⎭	GGU ⎫ GGC ⎬ Gly GGA GGG ⎭	U(T) C A G

* is initiation

Figure 3.1 The genetic code. Bases are given as ribonucleotides. For deoxyribonucleotides substitute T for U

There are several features of the code which should be noted. First it is read continuously from the 5' to the 3' end of the polynucleotide strand. There are, in other words, no commas, colons or semicolons separating one codon from the next. There are, however, start and stop signals ('capital letters' and 'full stops'). Figure 3.1 shows that **AUG**, in virtue of the fact that it codes for met, often (but not always) acts as a **start signal** (this is sometimes also the case with GUG), whilst **UAA, UAG** and **UGA** act as full stops and terminate the message. Apart from the 'stop' codons all the others specify an amino acid. There is thus considerable redundancy or **degeneracy**—amino acids such as arg, leu and ser being assigned no less than six codons, whilst thr, pro, ala, gly and val are assigned four codons each. In this connection it is worth noting that the first two nucleotides in the triplet are the most important—suggesting, perhaps, that the triplet code has evolved from a primordial duplex code. Finally, the chemical nature of the amino acid is to some extent reflected in its codon. Every codon with a **U** in the second position specifies a **hydrophobic** amino acid and every (meaningful) codon with an **A** in the middle specifies a **hydrophilic** residue.

3.2 'DNA MAKES RNA AND RNA MAKES PROTEIN'

Let us take Francis Crick's 'central dogma' a step at a time. The process whereby 'DNA makes RNA' is called **transcription**; the process by which 'RNA makes protein' is called **translation**. The idea behind these two terms is that whilst DNA and RNA are variants of the same nucleic acid 'language', RNA and protein are two quite different languages.

3.2.1 Transcription

We saw in Section 3.1 that the genetic code is an uninterrupted sequence of nucleotides read continuously from one end to the other. It will probably already have occurred to you that as DNA consists of two polynucleotide chains both cannot carry the message. After all, one is in effect the 'mirror image' of the other. You are right. Only one strand, the ($-$) or '**antisense**' strand is read; the other, the ($+$) or '**sense**' strand is left alone. The ($+$) strand only comes into its own at replication. Then, of course, it is required as a template for the formation of a daughter double helix. It is, however, conventional to refer to this, the ($+$) strand, as the coding or 'sense' strand because, as we shall see below, the message transcribed on to the mRNA is identical to this strand saving only that U substitutes for T.

Much of our understanding of transcription comes from studies in prokaryotic systems, especially *E.coli*. Transcription in eukaryotes is known to be more complicated. Nevertheless the essential features are much the same. The following brief account is thus based principally on findings in *E. coli*, with additions where it is known that the eukaryotes differ.

Initiation of transcription requires an enzyme, **DNA-dependent RNA polymerase**, to gain access to a special region of the (−) DNA strand some ten or so nucleotides 'upstream' of the site at which the genetic message begins. This special region (about 40 bases in length) is called the **promoter** region. In *E.coli* the DNA-dependent RNA polymerase is a huge multimeric enzyme consisting of five subunits—two α, one β, one β′ and a σ, i.e. ($α_2ββ′σ$)—and has a molecular weight of about 500 kDa. The σ subunit is essential for the recognition of the promoter region of the DNA double helix. In eukaryotic cells such as neurons and glia the situation is considerably more complicated. There are four

Figure 3.2 Transcription in a pro-karyocyte. (A) The multimeric DNA-dependent RNA polymerase 'explores' the DNA double helix until it happens upon the promoter region (about 40 base pairs in length) of a gene. (B) The σ subunit recognises this region and the polymerase enzyme binds to the DNA. (C) The σ subunit is released and the two strands of the double helix unwind. The remainder of the polymerase enzyme moves along the (-) strand using it as a template for synthesising a comple-mentary RNA strand from rNTPs. The DNA double helix re-forms behind. (D) The synthesis of mRNA continues until a terminator sequence on the (-) strand is reached. The polymerase enzyme then detaches. In prokaryocytes translation of the mRNA message into protein structure then occurs directly without any further modification of the mRNA strand

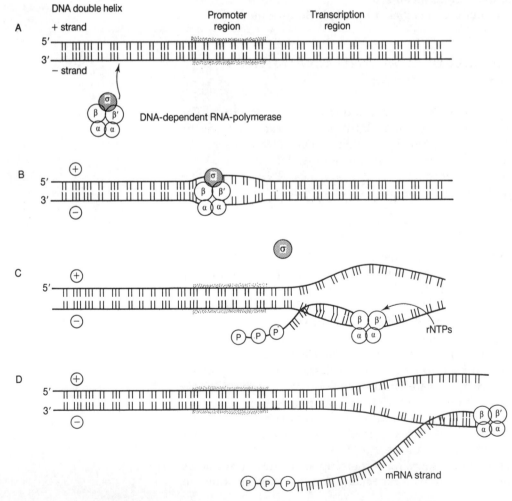

different kinds of DNA-dependent RNA polymerases. Three are located in the nucleus and one in the mitochondria. Of the three located in the nucleus **polymerase 1** is found in the nucleolus and is responsible for transcribing the 45S rRNA of ribosomes (see Chapter 2), **polymerase 2** is located in the nucleoplasm and transcribes hnRNA (i.e. pre-mRNA) and **polymerase 3**, also found in the nucleoplasm, transcribes 5S rRNA and the tRNAs.

Figure 3.2 shows the process of transcription in *E.coli*, where it is well understood. The figure shows that after the σ subunit has done its job of recognising the promoter region it falls away and the remaining polymerase is able to unwind the double helix

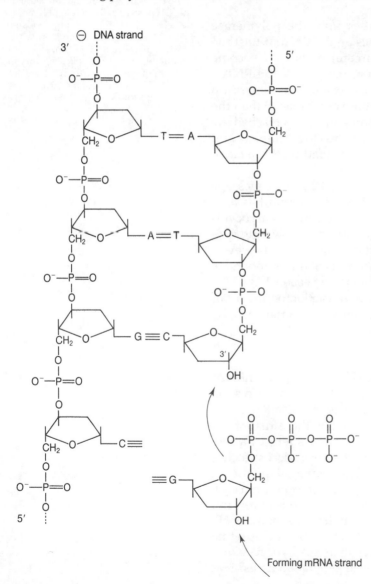

Figure 3.3 Synthesis of an mRNA strand alongside the (-) DNA strand. An rNTP (guanosine triphosphate) is shown approaching at the bottom of the figure. Cytosine on the DNA template ensures that it is acceptable. The RNA polymerase enzyme is then able to connect it by way of a phosphodiester link to the nucleotide immediately above. The energy for this synthesis comes from breaking an energy-rich phosphate bond in the triphosphate. The two terminal phosphate groups of the triphospate and the hydrogen of the the hydroxyl group form pyrophosphate which is released

and to synthesise on the template provided by the (−) strand a complementary strand of RNA. In order to carry out this **elongation** phase of the transcription process the polymerase, of course, requires raw materials and these take the form of **ribonucleoside triphosphates (rNTPs)**. Figure 3.2 also shows that the (−) strand is transcribed from the 3′ to the 5′ end. You will, however, remember that we stated in Section 3.1 above that the code is read from 5′ to 3′. Don't be alarmed. Because base pairing in polynucleotide strands is 'antiparallel' (see section on the DNA double helix in Chapter 2) the RNA strand is laid down in the 5′ to 3′ direction and, as we shall shortly see, is read in this direction at the ribosome.

The process of elongation continues until the polymerase enzyme reaches a termination sequence on the DNA. Whilst the RNA chain is growing, earlier (upstream) parts of it become displaced from the (−) strand. This occurs because the RNA–DNA duplex is thermodynamically less stable (see remark on difference between ribose and deoxyribose in Chapter 2) than the DNA–DNA duplex. When a termination sequence is reached the RNA becomes completely detached from the DNA template and the polymerase enzyme also falls free, able to bind another σ factor and initiate another synthesis.

The process of transcription is now over. The genetic message encoded in the base sequence of the DNA (+) strand has now been transferred to a sequence of RNA bases. In prokaryocytes this message passes directly to the ribosomes, where it is 'translated' into protein structure. In the eukaryocytes, however, the situation is more complicated. The results of transcription are the lengthy hnRNA or pre-mRNA strands (see Section 2.2) which accumulate in the nucleoplasm. Before translation occurs a fair amount of **post-transcriptional processing** is undertaken.

3.2.2 Post-transcriptional processing

Post-transcriptional processing of all three types of RNA—mRNA, tRNA and rRNA—occurs in eukaryotic cells. We shall restrict ourselves to the post-transcriptional processing of mRNA.

The first point to notice is that, unlike the situation in prokaryotic cells, eukaryotic DNA contains large stretches where the base sequences code nonsense. These nonsensical stretches are called **introns** (an abbreviation for 'intervening sequences'). They separate the meaningful sections of DNA or **exons** from each other. Practically all eukaryotic genes have at least one intron and some, for instance the collagen gene, may have as many as 50. What is the significance of this eukaryotic characteristic? Is it that prokarocytes have been around longer than eukaryocytes and, moreover, usually have much more rapid generation times? Has

Figure 3.4   Post-transcriptional processing of eukaryotic mRNA. (A) The DNA double helix is schematised as two parallel lines with the exons drawn lightly and the introns bold. DNA-dependent RNA polymerase 2 is represented as a stippled circle. (B) RNA polymerase attaches to the promoter region and opens the DNA double helix. Transcription commences. The newly synthesised mRNA strand is capped by guanosine triphosphate and methylated. (C) The process of transcription continues. Both exons and introns are transcribed. (D) On reaching a termination signal on the DNA strand the RNA polymerase detaches. A lengthy 'tail' of adenosines (150–200) is attached to the 3′ end of the newly transcribed hnRNA. Enzymes now cut out the introns and splice together the cut ends of the exons to form the finished mRNA. The remains of the introns form small loops known (from their shape) as 'lariats'   ⟶

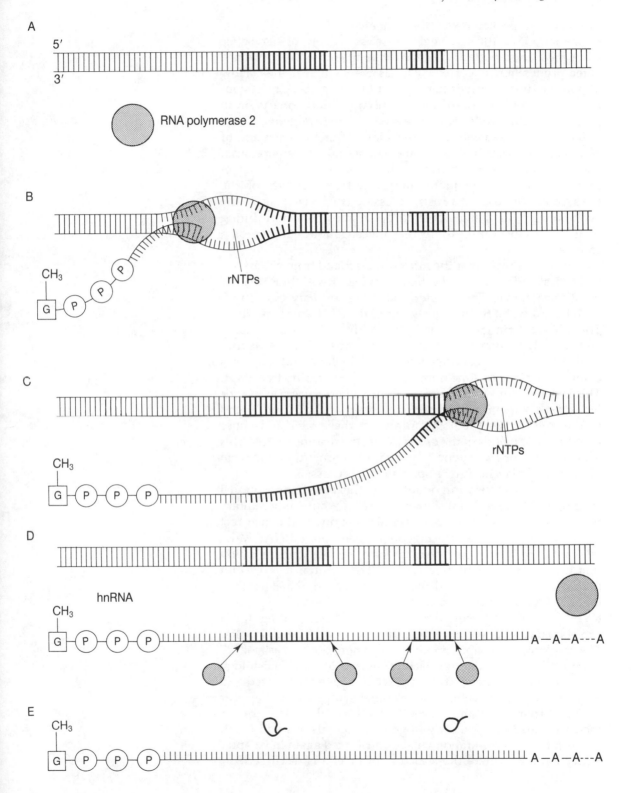

A

5′
3′

RNA polymerase 2

B

CH₃

G — P — P — P — P

rNTPs

C

rNTPs

CH₃

G — P — P — P

D

hnRNA

CH₃

G — P — P — P A—A—A---A

E

CH₃

G — P — P — P A—A—A---A

this allowed prokarocytic DNA time to rid itself of useless segments? Or do the seemingly senseless sections of eukaryotic DNA have an important function? It seems more likely that the latter proposition is correct. For, as we shall see, they allow important post-transcriptional control of gene expression. Different combinations of exon transcripts allow one gene to programme the production of several different proteins. These different proteins may be characteristic of different tissues and/or of different stages in the development of one tissue. Perhaps, also, the more complicated structure of the eukaryotic gene has something to do with the more complicated cytogenetics of the eukaryotes (mitosis, meiosis, crossing-over, etc.) and the evolutionary possibilities opened up by recombination during sexual reproduction. Only further investigation will give us a complete answer.

Figure 3.4 shows that the mRNA transcribed from eukaryotic DNA first of all forms the heteronuclear RNA (hnRNA) we mentioned above. This is often called the 'primary transcript'. Both the exon and the intron regions of the DNA are transcribed. The mRNA chain is modified by the addition of a **cap** to the 5' end (usually a guanine (G) nucleotide) and a lengthy sequence of about 150 to 200 adenosine nucleotides to the 3' end. Enzymes cut out the intron regions from the hnRNA or primary transcript. This is done with great accuracy. The enzymes recognise specific 'consensus sequences' of nucleotide bases at the 5' and 3' end of the introns. They cut the introns at these sites and splice together the cut ends of the exons to give the mature mRNA. This is now ready for translation. The excised introns curl up to form 'lariats' and play no further part in the process.

It is, of course, very important to get this post-transcriptional splicing right. It has been shown that several human hereditary blood diseases known as **thalassaemias** are due to the incorrect intron excision and resplicing of β-globin pre-mRNA. More relevant to molecular neurobiology has been the demonstration that the **jimpy (jp)** mutation which affects **central myelination** in the mouse is also due to defective post-transcriptional processing. It is found that the genetic defect causes the splicing process to omit a 74-base sequence from the mRNA coding for a proteolipid component of central (though not peripheral) myelin. The resulting proteolipid protein, which normally consists of 277 amino acids, consequently lacks residues 208–232. Histology shows that the white matter in the CNS is severely affected and very little myelin develops. Behavioural symptoms first appear as body tremor on the eleventh postnatal day. The tremor increases, leading ultimately to general convulsions and death in week five. This mutation will be considered again in Chapter 6 (Section 6.7), where the structure of myelin is discussed.

The gene for central myelin is carried on the X chromosome in both mouse and man. The jimpy mutation is regarded as analogous to **Pelizaeus–Merzbacher disease**—a sex-linked recessive leucodystrophy (i.e. white matter deficiency)—which affects humans.

3.2.3 Translation

The business of translating the mRNA message into protein structure is even more complicated than the mechanisms of transcription described above. It involves a large and hetero-geneous group of co-operating factors.

The most significant members of this group are **ribosomes**, **tRNAs**, **aminoacyl synthetases**, **mRNA**, **amino acids**, and numerous proteinaceous **initiation** and **elongation** factors.

Again the process is best known in prokaryotic systems such as *E.coli* and again it is believed that the eukaryotic mechanisms are basically similar.

Translation begins by the attachment of the appropriate amino acid to its designated tRNA. This vital step is catalysed by an **aminoacyl synthetase enzyme**. We noted in Chapter 2 that just as there is a specific tRNA molecule for each of the 20 different amino acids so there is a specific aminoacyl synthetase enzyme for each amino acid. These enzymes play a central role in the whole complicated business. It is upon their ability to recognise *both* the specific amino acid and the specific tRNA that the entire operation of translation depends. Energy for the attachment is provided by the hydrolysis of ATP:

amino acid + tRNA + ATP = aminoacyl tRNA + AMP + PP_i

Figure 3.5 shows, schematically (little is as yet known of this vital step), the recognition of tRNA and amino acid by the aminoacyl synthetase enzyme. It is clear that the distinctive conformation of tRNA, which we described in Chapter 2, is of great importance. It is this conformation which the tRNA active site of the synthetase enzyme is designed to recognise. The synthetase enzyme has yet another remarkable property. It is able to 'proof-read'. It recognises any incorrect pairing of tRNA and amino acid and decomposes it back into free tRNA and amino acid. This striking feature highlights once again the crucial importance of uniting an amino acid with its correct tRNA. Alanine is coupled to $tRNA_{ala}$, serine to $tRNA_{ser}$, etc.; any mispairings are eliminated.

The **amino acid–tRNA complex** (or **charged tRNA**) now encounters a ribosome. This occurs by random 'thermal' motion in the cytosol.

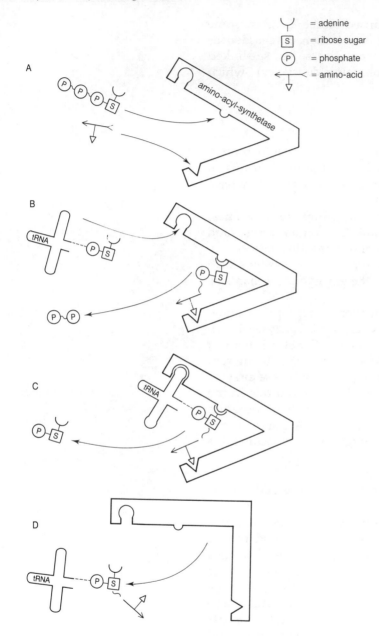

= adenine
S = ribose sugar
P = phosphate
= amino-acid

A

amino-acyl-synthetase

B

tRNA

C

tRNA

D

tRNA

Figure 3.5 Recognition and coupling of tRNA and appropriate amino acid by an aminoacyl synthetase. (A) The aminoacyl synthetase has three complementary surfaces. One of these surfaces fits a specific amino acid (symbolised by an arrow with a triangle representing its side chain). Another surface fits adenine (represented by a semicircular cup). The third complementary surface is designed to accept a specific tRNA (symbolised by the conventional cross-shaped clover leaf). (B) The adenosine triphosphate (ATP) has occupied the adenine site and the amino acid has taken up position in its site. The amino acid is activated to an aminoacyl-adenylate (i.e. amino acid – AMP complex) by displacing pyro-phosphate (P—P) from the ATP. (C) An appropriate tRNA arrives and finds its complementary site in the aminoacyl synthetase. The adenosine which is always present at the end of the amino acid acceptor stem of tRNA displaces AMP's adenine and the 3′ OH of its ribose moiety accepts the energy-rich bond of the amino acid. AMP is released from the enzyme. (D) The amino acid – tRNA complex is released from the aminoacyl synthetase enzyme. The figure is highly schematic. Very little is known of the molecular structure of aminoacyl synthetases

Eukaryotic ribosomes resemble minute cottage loaves. They have a sedimentary coefficient of 80S and easily dissociate into a 60S and a 40S subunit. The larger subunit consists of 28S rRNA, 5.8S rRNA and 5S rRNA and about 45 different proteins, whilst the smaller sub-unit is built of 18S rRNA and about 33 different proteins.

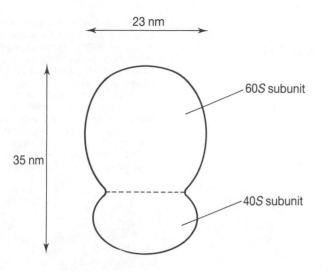

23 nm

35 nm

60S subunit

40S subunit

Figure 3.6 Eukaryotic ribosome. The figure shows the 'cottage-loaf' structure of a eukaryotic ribosome. The 60S and the 40S subunits together constitute an 80S (about 4.3 MDa) organelle with a maximum diameter of about 35 nm

In the cytosol the two subunits of the ribosome exist independently of each other. The coming together of the two subunits and the initiation of translation is a very intricate affair. It requires the interaction of a large number of factors.

First, the smaller ribosomal (40S) subunit comes into contact with the 5′ end of an mRNA strand. An initiation factor (IF3) is also involved at this stage. Next the mRNA–40S complex picks up a **tRNA$_{\overline{met}}$met** complex. This is due to the presence of the initiation signal, AUG, close to the 5′ end of mRNA, and is assisted by another initiation factor (IF2). The anticodon of tRNA$_{met}$ (UAC) recognises AUG by Watson–Crick base-pairing. The 40S initiation complex so formed now binds to the 60S ribosomal subunit with the help of yet another initiation factor (IF1), the energy being provided by GTP. This series of events is schematised in Figure 3.7.

The stage is now set for the translation of the mRNA message into the amino acid sequence of a protein or polypeptide.

The 60S ribosomal subunit contains two sites which can accept charged tRNA molecules. The first site (see Figure 3.8) is called the **'p' site** (polypeptide or protein site), the second the **'a' site** (amino acid site). So far in our account tRNA$_{\overline{met}}$met occupies the 'p' site. Which tRNA can occupy the 'a' site depends on the codon immediately to the right of AUG in the mRNA strand. Suppose (as in Figure 3.8) it is UUC. AAG is the Watson–Crick complement of UUC. The anticodon domain of tRNA$_{\overline{phe}}$phe happens to be AAG. Hence this tRNA–amino acid complex will be able to slot into this site. With the help of a number of other factors, including various 'elongation factors' (EFs), a peptidyl transferase present in the 60S subunit and a further input of

A

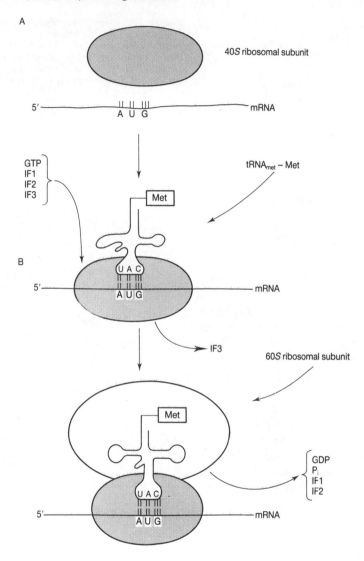

40S ribosomal subunit

5'———————— || || ||| ———————— mRNA
                A U G

GTP
IF1
IF2
IF3

tRNA_met – Met

Met

B

5'————————(U A C)———————— mRNA
                A U G

IF3

60S ribosomal subunit

Met

GDP
P_i
IF1
IF2

5'————————(U A C)———————— mRNA
                A U G

Figure 3.7 Initiation of translation at the ribosome. (A) The 40-*S* ribosome and a length of mRNA approach each other. (B) In the presence of a group of initiation factors (IF1, IF2 and IF3) and GTP the 40*S* ribosome binds to the start signal (AUG) towards the 5' end of mRNA. A tRNA$_{met}$met complex binds through its anticodon to AUG. IF3 is released. (C) The complex is now joined by the 60*S* subunit, GTP is hydrolysed to GDP and P$_i$, IF1 and IF2 are released. The stage is now prepared for chain elongation

energy from GTP, the NH$_2$ group of phe forms a peptide link with the COOH group of met. When this occurs met is released from tRNA$_{met}$ and the latter in turn is released from the ribosome. tRNA$_{phe}$phe now shifts into the 'p' site in the 60*S* subunit as the entire ribosome moves three nucleotides (i.e. one codon) in the 3' direction along the mRNA strand. This brings another codon into the bottom of the 'a' site, specifying another tRNA, and the whole process repeats itself.

The figure shows that a repetition of the sequence of events outlined in the previous paragraph will result in a steadily growing peptide chain. The growth will continue until one of the 'stop' codons (UAA, UGA or UAG) comes under the 'a' site.

A

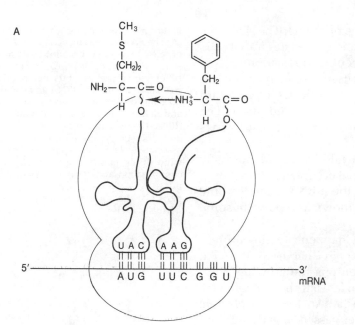

B

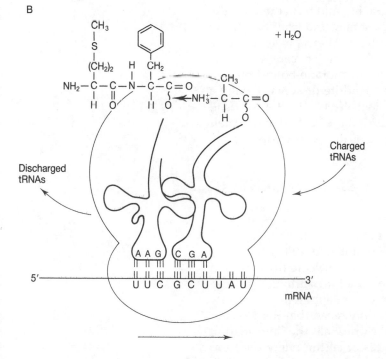

Figure 3.8 Peptide elongation. (A) tRNA$_{met}$–met occupies the 'p' site in the ribosome. The mRNA codon beneath the 'a' site is UCC. This is complementary to AAG. The anticodon of tRNA$_{phe}$ is AAG. Hence this can occupy the 'p' site. When it does so the NH$_3^+$ group of its phe residue is brought into the near neighbourhood of the energy-rich bond attaching met to tRNA$_{met}$. (B) With the help of elongation factors and ribosomal enzymes a peptide bond is formed between phenylalanine and methionine. A complex series of biochemical events now ensures that the tRNA$_{met}$ is released from the 'p' site, that the ribosome moves three bases in the 3' direction along the mRNA and that the tRNA$_{phe}$ comes to occupy the 'p' site. Another tRNA–amino acid complex (in the diagram tRNA$_{ala}$–ala) can now occupy the 'a' site and the cycle begins again

When this happens no tRNA molecule can occupy the 'a' site and instead a release factor (eRF) alters the activity of the peptidyl transferase so that instead of catalysing the formation of peptide links it hydrolyses the final amino acid from its tRNA. The polypeptide chain is thus freed from the ribosome. The ribosome meanwhile detaches from the mRNA and dissociates into its 60*S* and 40*S* subunits ready for another bout of translation.

The freed polypeptide chain twists itself into its more or less complex tertiary structure as its amino acid residues interact with each other and with the environment in which it finds itself. **The genetic code only specifies primary structure**—the rest follows automatically.

Finally, it is worth noting that an mRNA strand normally supports several ribosomes. These are all occupied in translating the genetic message and move down the mRNA strand in line one behind the other. The complex is known as a **polyribosome** or **polysome**.

We shall return to consider what happens to the protein manufactured by this complex machinery in Chapter 14. We shall see that in eukaryotic cells such as neurons the growing poly-peptide chain may suffer one of several fates. If the ribosome (as is the case with the majority) is attached to the endoplasmic reticulum then the polypeptide is either passed directly into the cisterna of the endoplasmic reticulum (ER) and from there via the Golgi apparatus into the axon where it may find itself caught up and carried along in the axoplasmic flow. Alternatively, because of its hydrophobic characteristics, it may be caught in the membrane of the ER and carried as a membrane-bound protein to its final destination in the axon, dendrite or soma. Finally a small number of ribosomes remain 'free' in the cytosol, unattached to ER membranes, and these will deliver their polypeptide directly into the cytosol of the perikaryon.

3.3 CONTROL OF THE EXPRESSION OF GENETIC INFORMATION

It is possible in some amphibia (e.g. the clawed toad, *Xenopus*) to remove the nucleus from a differentiated cell (e.g. a gut epithelial cell) and introduce it into an enucleated oocyte and induce that oocyte to develop into an adult. Although a large number of spontaneous abortions occur, apparently perfectly normal toads often result. This can only mean that the DNA in the epithelial cell's nucleus still carries all the information necessary to programme the features of all the many different types of cell (muscle, neuron, fibroblast, hepatocyte, etc.) which make up an adult's body. Yet, of course, a gut epithelial cell is nothing like a neuron or a muscle fibre. It follows that much of the information in the DNA of an adult differentiated cell must be dormant, switched-off, repressed or in some other way unexpressed. This conclusion has been confirmed by some of the

Figure 3.9 Termination of translation. (A) The ribosome has moved to the 3' end of mRNA, where it encounters a 'stop' signal (UAA, UAG or UGA). The release factor (eRF) ensures that the polypeptide chain falls free from its tRNA and that the ribosome dissociates into its two subunits and detaches from mRNA. (B) mRNA, tRNA, the two subunits of the ribosome and the polypeptide are now dis-associated. The polypeptide begins to wind itself into a three-dimensional conformation and is often subjected to post-translational processing. In particular the N-terminal met residue is normally excised ⟶

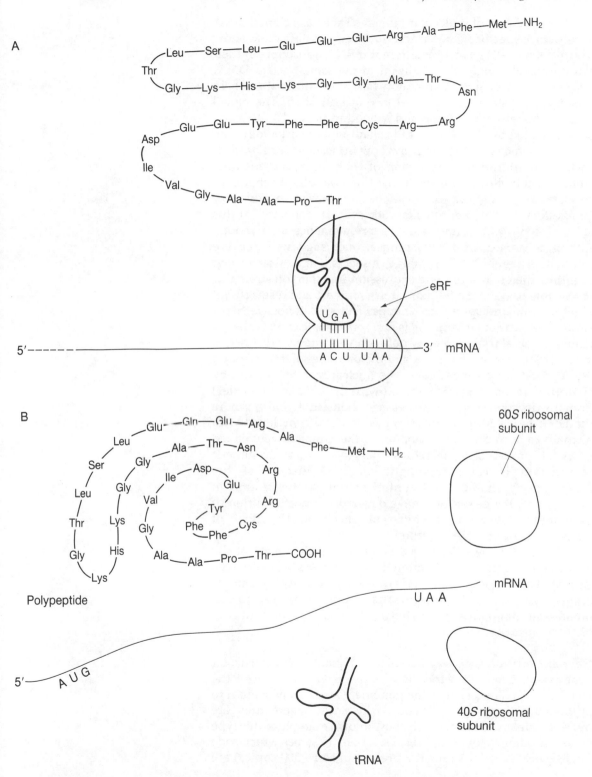

newer techniques of molecular biology. These use cloned DNA to recognise specific mRNA transcripts. It is not difficult to show that different cells have very different mRNA transcripts in their cytoplasms although all contain much the same nuclear DNA.

The control of gene expression has been much studied in prokaryotic systems, especially (once again!) *E.coli*. The Nobel prize-winning work of Jacob and Monod in the early 1960s has been followed by a great deal of brilliant molecular biology, the upshot of which has been to show how intricate molecular feed-back loops control the expression of the prokaryotic genome. Unfortunately it does not seem that the molecular mechanisms at work in prokaryotic cells can be generalised in any very straightforward manner to eukaryotic cells. It seems that at this level of complexity *E.coli* loses its pre-eminence as a model. Although Monod, in a vivid phrase, once suggested that the elephant is merely *E.coli* writ large, it seems that he was wrong!

In fact the control of gene expression in eukaryotes remains at the time of writing a field of intense interest and research but of rather little undisputed knowledge. This should not, perhaps, surprise us. The eukaryotic cell is far more complex and far larger than the typical prokaryote. By definition it contains a distinctive nucleus. This means that DNA and the processes of **transcription** are segregated by a membrane (the nuclear membrane) and by an appreciable distance (compared with the sizes of molecules) from the ribosomes and the processes of **translation**. Furthermore the DNA is coiled in an intricate fashion and complexed with histones to form chromosomes, unlike the comparatively naked DNA of prokaryotes. It seems that the control of genetic information is correspondingly complex. Instead of the comparatively simple direct control of transcription found in prokaryotes, the eukaryotes have developed a host of different mechanisms operating at different stages in the flow of information from DNA to protein.

Figure 3.10 shows the major points at which control of the expression of genetic information in eukaryotes is believed to be exerted. The figure shows that there seem to be at least five major levels: **genomic**; **transcriptional**; **post-transcriptional**; **translational**; and **post-translational**. We shall look briefly at each of these in turn.

Genomic control. One way in which the quantity of a particular gene product may be varied is by loss or amplification of the amount of DNA present in the genome. Genes seem seldom to be lost but there are well-known instances where they are multiplied many times over. The best-known example of this type of amplification is found in *Xenopus*, where the genes which code for 18*S* and 28*S* rRNA (already present in some 500 copies) are

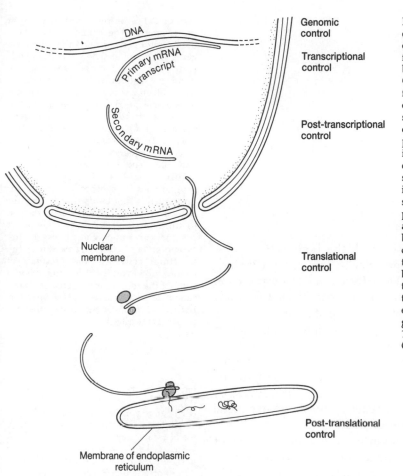

DNA

Primary mRNA transcript

Secondary mRNA

Nuclear membrane

Membrane of endoplasmic reticulum

Genomic control

Transcriptional control

Post-transcriptional control

Translational control

Post-translational control

Figure 3.10 Multilevel control of the expression of genetic information in a eukaryotic cell. The figure distinguishes five levels at which the information held by nuclear DNA may be controlled. **Genomic control** involves loss or amplification of DNA; **transcriptional control** consists of the 'switching' on and off of structural genes; **post-transcriptional control** involves the manipulation of the primary mRNA transcript by excising introns and resplicing exons; **translational control** influences the highly complex sequence of events by which the message in the mRNA determines the primary structure of the protein; and, finally, **post-translational control** allows the alteration of the protein or polypeptide by proteolytic enzymes. This last process commonly occurs within the cisternae of the endoplasmic reticulum and/or Golgi body. It should be borne in mind that these are just some (by no means all) of the control mechanisms available to the eukaryotic cell. Further explanation is given in the text. (Partly after Becker, 1986, *The World of the Cell*, Menlo Park, California: Benjamin/Cummings.)

multiplied some 4000-fold during oogenesis so that the mature oocyte ultimately comes to possess about two million copies. This is apparently necessary to ensure a sufficiency of ribosomes to sustain the intense protein synthesis characteristic of early embryogenesis. However, although some other instances are known, gene amplification does not at present seem to be a major mechanism of gene control in adult eukaryotes.

Transcriptional control. Transcriptional control is (as we shall see below) by far the most important (and well-understood) control mechanism in prokaryocytes. There seems little doubt that it also plays an important role in eukaryotes. It is not difficult to show (as mentioned above) that different cells of a single organism contain very different mRNA transcripts. The brain, furthermore,

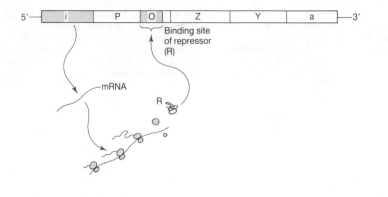

5' i P O Z Y a 3'

Binding site
of repressor
(R)

mRNA

R

Figure 3.11 Control of transcription at
the *lac* operon. The *lac* operon consists of
the operator gene (o) and three structural
genes (z, y and a). The structural genes
code for β-galactosidase, lactose
permease and transacetylase, respectively—all enzymes involved in the metabolism of lactose by the bacterial cell. The
figure shows that the operator gene
consists of a short sequence of nucleotides (21) towards one end of the
promoter sequence. 'Upstream' from the
promoter (p) is another gene, the
regulator gene (i). The regulator gene
programmes the synthesis of a repressor
protein (R). This binds to the operator
sequence. When the repressor is attached
to the operator DNA-dependent RNA
polymerase cannot gain access to the
promoter and start transcribing the
structural genes. In the presence of
lactose, however, the three dimensional
form of the repressor is altered so that it
can no longer attach itself to the operator.
In this circumstance the structural genes
can be transcribed

is the most histologically diverse of all the body's tissues. It
consists of a great variety of different cells. It is not surprising,
therefore, to find that about **125 000 different mRNA transcripts**
are expressed at different times and in different cells in the brain:
three to five times greater than in any other tissue.

Because of the great importance of transcriptional control it will
be useful to outline the well-known mechanisms at work in
prokaryocytes. The widely used distinction between **regulator**,
operator and **structural** gene was first developed in these systems.
An understanding of transcriptional control in prokaryocytes is,
moreover, of importance if some of the techniques used in genetic
engineering (Chapter 5) are to be grasped.

Figure 3.11 shows the best-known of all prokaryotic control
systems—the ***lac*** operon in *E.coli*. The bacterial DNA contains four
relevant regions: a **regulator gene**, a **promoter sequence** (already
discussed), an **operator sequence** (which partially overlaps the
promoter) and a set of **structural genes** (z, y and a). The regulator
gene programmes the synthesis of a tetrameric **repressor protein**
which normally attaches itself to the operator sequence, thus
blocking the insertion of RNA polymerase. In consequence the
structural genes cannot be transcribed—in other words they are
switched off, or **repressed**. In the presence of an **inducer** molecule
(in this case **lactose**) the repressor protein undergoes an allosteric
change in its conformation which makes it unable to stick to its
site on the operator. In consequence the RNA polymerase can
insert itself and transcribe the structural genes. These genes
programme the synthesis of a group of enzymes involved in the
entry of lactose into the cell and its subsequent metabolism: β-
galactosidase, galactoside permease and thiogalactoside acetyltransferase. We shall see in Chapter 5 that if a foreign gene is
spliced into the operon it too will by controlled by the operator.
Hence it can be switched on (induced) by adding lactose to the
medium.

Figure 3.12 Post-transcriptional processing of PPT gene. The preprotachykinin
(PPT) gene consists of seven exons and
six introns (hatched). Two primary
mRNAs are transcribed: α-PPT mRNA
which lacks the substance K (SK) exon
and β-PPT which is a complete transcript.
After polyadenylation and excision of the
introns the two PPT mRNAs are ready for
translation. Two PPT polypeptides are
formed: α-PPT (112 amino acids in
length) and β-PPT (130 amino acids). The
first 20 or so amino acids in both
polypeptides form a 'signal sequence'.
This sequence, as we shall see in Chapter
14, is required to attach the ribosome to
the ER. It is composed of mainly hydrophobic residues so that it can pass
through the membrane into the cisterna
of the ER. It is then excised. In post-
translational processing the substance P
(SP) peptide (11 residues) and the
substance K peptide (10 residues) are
excised from the PPT polypeptides. The
cutting points are marked by basic
residues—Arg, Lys. The end results of all
this processing are two copies of the SP
peptide and one copy of the SK peptide.
(Partly after Karpati, 1984, *Trends in
Neurosciences*, **7**, 57–59; and Nawa,
Kotani and Nakashani, 1984, *Nature*, **312**,
729–734.)

Unfortunately because of the much greater molecular complexity of the eukaryotic chromosome it has not yet been possible to determine the exact molecular mechanisms which control transcription in this system. In some cases it seems likely that a control molecule causes the eukaryotic chromosome to unravel (= **decondense**) so that selective lengths of its DNA become accessible for transcription by DNA-dependent RNA polymerase. It is likely that in this decondensed state control mechanisms analogous to those of the *lac* operon are at work. It seems, however, that eukaryotic transcription is often a more complex affair than the relatively straightforward system of *E.coli lac* operon. It has been shown, for instance, that in many neuro-

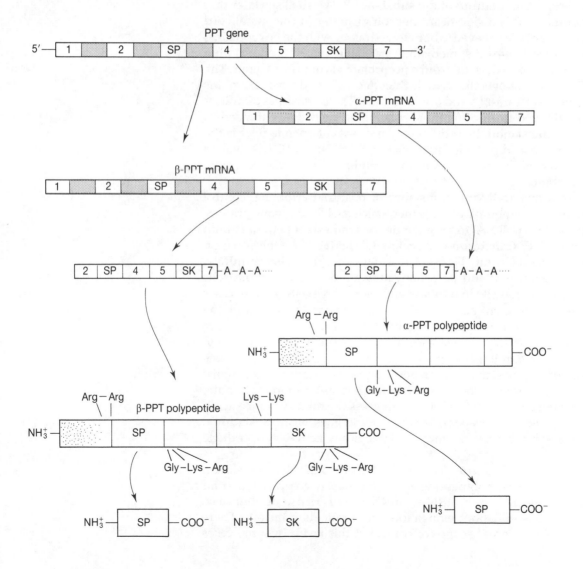

biologically important cases (for instance many of the channel-protein genes) there is more than one promoter region. These different promoter regions are differentially accessible in different tissues. Hence the primary mRNA transcript synthesised in one tissue may differ from the primary transcript synthesised from the same gene in another. It has become customary to refer to these genetic regions as 'transcription units'.

Post-transcriptional control. We have already looked at post-transcriptional processing in Section 3.2.2. It is appropriate here, therefore, to look at some instances of post-transcriptional processing relevant to neurobiology. First let us consider the post-transcriptional processing which occurs during the synthesis of an important neuropeptide: **substance P**. We shall see later that substance P is a significant neurotransmitter in the spinal cord and brain. It is believed to be involved (along with the enkephalins) in nerve pathways mediating pain. Figure 3.12 shows that substance P is derived from a **preprotachykinin (PPT)** gene. The figure also shows that two distinct mRNAs are derived from this gene: α-PPT mRNA and β-PPT mRNA. These two types of mRNA are derived from differential splicing of the primary transcript. After translation the α-PPT polypeptide is cut open to release the 11 amino acid peptide, substance P, whilst the β-PPT is cleaved to give both substance P and another neuroactive peptide, **substance K**.

Another well-known instance of post-transcriptional control in molecular neurobiology is that which enables the same primary transcript (hnRNA) to programme the synthesis of both **calcitonin** and **CGRP (calcitonin-gene-related peptide)**. Here the situation is a little different. Figure 3.13 shows that the primary mRNA transcript is cut and polyadenylated at one site in thyroid cells and at another site in pituitary and some nerve cells. In both cases the resulting mRNA strand has its introns cut out and the remaining exons spliced together to form the final strand from which translation takes place. Whilst calcitonin is a well-known calcium-controlling hormone, the function of CGRP is, at the time of writing, obscure: it is an addition to the steadily growing list of neuropeptides found in the brain. It is also important to note, as Figure 3.13 shows, that in both cases the mRNA is once again translated as a prepeptide which undergoes **post-translational** processing before yielding the biologically active end-product.

Translational control. We saw in Section 3.2.3 that translation of mRNA into polypeptide is an enormously complicated affair involving not only tRNA, mRNA and ribosome but also numerous initiation, elongation and termination factors. There is evidently great scope for control at this level. In some cases

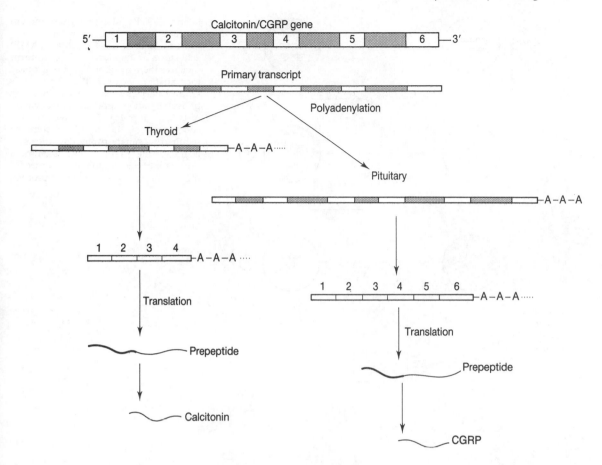

Figure 3.13 Differential post-transcriptional processing to yield calcitonin and CGRP. The calcitonin/CGRP gene has six exons separated from each other by introns. The primary mRNA transcript is cut and polyadenylated at different places in the thyroid and the pituitary. After excision of the introns translation yields two different prepeptides. These, in turn, are further processed to give calcitonin and CGRP. See text for further details

(e.g. sea-urchin oocyte) it can be shown that although all the necessary mRNA is present in the cytoplasm very little, if any, translation occurs until the egg is fertilised. Presumably some triggering factor is released by sperm entry. In other cases the **stability** of the mRNA strand may be affected so that it persists for a longer or shorter time in the cytoplasm and hence programmes the synthesis of more or less polypeptide. In yet other cases it has been shown that control of the synthesis of a protein is effected by control of the activity of an **initiation factor**. In erythrocytes, for instance, it appears that the synthesis of globin is controlled through the **phosphorylation** (and hence **inactivation**) of one of the initiation factors. This phosphorylation in turn depends on the activation (by phosphorylation) of an initiation factor **kinase** which then catalyses the phosphorylation of the IF. Because second messenger systems in neurons often control protein kinases this erythrocyte mechanism may be of general relevance. It is schematised in Figure 3.14.

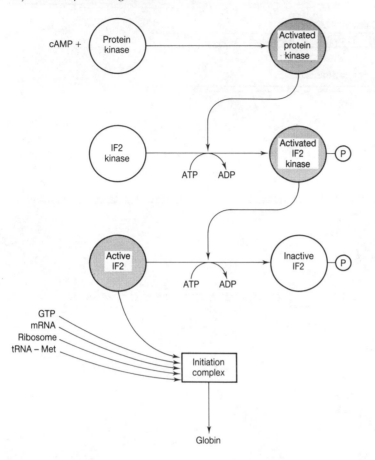

Figure 3.14 Regulation of translation in erythrocytes by phosphorylation of a protein kinase. Cyclic AMP (cAMP) activates a protein kinase. This, in turn, catalyses the phosphorylation of a kinase for initiation factor 2 (IF2). Lastly this kinase catalyses a reaction leading to the phosphorylation-dependent inactivation of IF2. IF2 (see Fig. 3.7) is an essential component of the initiation complex required to initiate protein synthesis. It is interesting to note that haemin, a precursor of haemoglobin, is required if the first step in the cascade is to proceed

Post-translational control. Many proteins are released from the ribosome as precursors requiring further biochemical change before they assume their mature and biologically active form. One well-known example is provided by insulin. This is synthesised as preproinsulin—a single continuous amino acid chain of 108 residues. The 24 N-terminal residues constitute a 'signal sequence'. They are necessary for the attachment of a ribosome to the ER membrane and for the initial insertion of the protein into the lumen of the ER (see Chapter 14). Once inside the ER the signal sequence is cut away, leaving the 84-residue proinsulin. After folding into a specific shape proinsulin is stabilised by the formation of disulphide linkages. A protease then removes a large run of the amino acid chain (33 residues) leaving the mature insulin as two separate chains joined together by disulphide linkages (Figure 3.15).

An interesting neurobiological instance of post-translational control is provided by the so-called '**natural opioids**': the

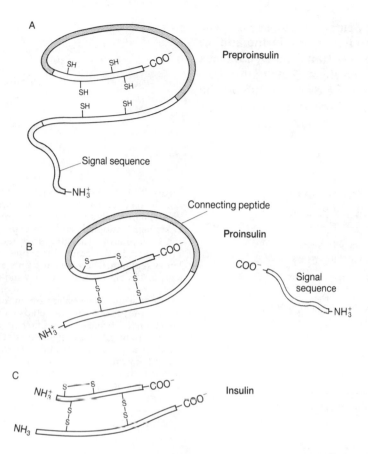

Figure 3.15 Post-translational modification of insulin. (A) The ribosome initially translates the insulin mRNA to form 'preproinsulin'. The 24 amino acids at the N-terminal end of this molecule constitute a hydrophobic 'signal sequence' which (as we noted in Fig. 3.12) enables the ribosome to attach to an ER membrane and for the protein to be inserted into the ER lumen. (B) Once inside the ER the signal sequence is excised, leaving the 84-residue 'proinsulin'. This orientates itself so that the correct disulphide linkages are formed. (C) The 33-residue connecting or C peptide is excised, leaving the familiar disulphide-linked α- and β-chain structure of insulin. The α-chain consists of 21 amino acid residues, the β-chain of 30 residues

enkephalins and **endorphins**. There are two enkephalins—**met-enkephalin** and **leu-enkephalin**. Both consist of five amino acids.

leu-enkephalin: tyr-gly-gly-phe-leu-OH

met-enkephalin: tyr-gly-gly-phe-met-OH

The enkephalins have been dubbed natural opioids because they seem able to inhibit the synaptic transmission of impulses in the brain's pain pathways. Their action will be discussed in more detail in Chapter 15.

It is relevant to note in this section, however, that the two enkephalins arise from two much larger precursor peptides—**preproenkephalin A** and **preproenkephalin B**. It is found that preproenkephalin A contains six copies of met-enkephalin and one of leu-enkephalin, whilst preproenkephalin B contains three copies of leu-enkephalin and none of met-enkephalin. In addition it has been shown that the enkephalin sequences hidden in the precursors are marked at each end by signal amino acids. These may be either two lysines or two arginines or a lysine and an arginine. These signals mark where post-translational enzymes can cut the precursor. The first enzyme always cuts to the right of the signal residue. The second cuts the extra residue off the right-hand end to give the final enkephalin structure. These steps are shown in Figure 3.16.

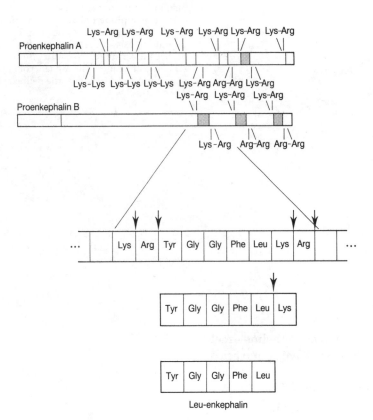

Figure 3.16 Post-translational production of met- and leu-enkephalin. Pro-enkephalin A contains six copies of met-enkephalin (stippled) and one copy of leu-enkephalin (darkly stippled). Proenkephalin B contains three copies of leu-enkephalin. The excision points are signalled by basic amino acids (lys and/or arg). The bottom part of the diagram shows that the enkephalins are cut out of the propeptide in two steps. The arrows indicate that enzymes first attack to the right of each signal residue, yielding a six-residue peptide. Then a second enzyme cuts to the left of the C-terminal residue, leaving the penta-peptide leu-enkephalin

The other natural opioids—the endorphins—are produced by a similarly complicated post-translational processing of a large (265-residue) precursor known as **pro-opiomelanocortin (POMC)**. It is interesting to note that this large precursor contains within it both β-endorphin and α-endorphin and also several pituitary hormones e.g. ACTH, α-MSH and β-MSH. It is clear that the informational machinery within cells economises wherever possible. A large and sometimes diverse assemblage of protein and polypeptide end-products may be derived form a single hnRNA primary transcript. These new insights into the relatedness of neuropeptides and peptide hormones also have evolutionary implications. Molecular evolution forms the subject matter of the next chapter and we shall consider these peptides again there.

Thus, in conclusion, we can see that there are many different ways in which the expression of the genetic information held in the DNA can be controlled. The nervous system is, as we have already noted, the most heterogeneous of the body's tissues. Its cells assume a great variety of shapes and sizes. It is not difficult to see that the ability to control gene expression is of great importance. We shall return to it in later chapters when, for instance, we discuss the embryology of the brain and the formation of nerve pathways.

Chapter 4
Molecular evolution

On first consideration it seems almost impossible to believe that the remarkable molecules and mechanisms described in the last two chapters could conceivably have originated by, as Jacques Monod put it, 'chance and necessity': blind variation and selective retention. We feel an awe similar to that felt by the natural theologians of the nineteenth century who considered that the superb design, the exact fitness for purpose, of living organisms could not but imply a designer, a creator. Yet since 1859, the publication date of *The Origin of Species*, all orthodox biologists have worked on the assumption that the living world did in fact come to be by the Darwinian mechanism of **random variation** and **environmental (both abiotic and biotic) selection**.

One of the most valuable contributions of molecular biology has been to support the neo-Darwinian synthesis. It has enabled us for the first time to quantify evolutionary change. Vice versa, the evolutionary approach is beginning to illuminate relationships between molecules which otherwise seem very dissimilar. The recognition that biological molecules have evolutionary relationships is, indeed, beginning to provide us with a classificatory scheme, just as the evolutionary insights of the late nineteenth century led to improved (so-called 'natural') classifications of the animal and plant kingdoms. Furthermore just as nineteenth-century evolutionary thought changed our perception of the living world and suggested new questions to ask, so the viewing of biomolecules in an evolutionary context suggests a variety of new possibilities and questions. Are there molecular fossils within us dating back to the beginning of life? Are there vestigial molecules which have no function in modern cells? Are evolutionary 'advances' at first 'reactionary' as Romer suggested? Does the distinction between 'analogy' and 'homology' apply at the molecular level in the same way as it does at the organismic level? Can we, by making reasonable assumptions about the rate of molecular evolution, propose a date for the common ancestor of two dissimilar but evolutionarily related molecules? And so on and so forth.

The study of molecular evolution has become possible because of our rapidly increasing understanding of the primary and higher structures of proteins, of the structure of DNA and its organisation to form the genetic material, and finally of the interrelationship between DNA and proteins. Because these insights have been revolutionised in recent years, our understanding of molecular evolution has accelerated at a phenomenal pace. Our knowledge of gene structure has, for instance, leapt ahead owing to new methods of DNA sequencing. This, in turn, owing to the discovery of 'reverse transcriptases', has led to a great increase in our knowledge of protein primary structure. We noted in Chapter 2 that protein tertiary structure very often consists of 'domains' which reappear in different combinations in different proteins. We saw in Chapter 3 that eukaryotic DNA consists of meaningful 'exons' separated by apparently unmeaningful 'introns'. In this chapter we shall see that there is good evidence that some genes (transposons) can be moved from one site to another in the eukaryotic genome. All of these recent developments are beginning to coalesce to greatly increase our understanding of molecular evolution.

It may perhaps be asked: what has all this molecular biology to do with neurobiology? A few years ago that might have been a somewhat difficult question to answer. Not now. Profound interconnections between molecular and neurobiology are becoming more and more apparent. It is now not only possible to understand the relatedness of some of the most important of the proteins of which the nervous system consists or which it uses but also, as we shall see in subsequent chapters, to use some of the central techniques in genetic engineering to investigate and understand the structures and functions of crucial neurobiological molecules: membrane receptors, ion channels, neurotransmitters and modulators, cytoskeletal proteins, etc.

In this chapter we shall proceed as follows. First we shall look at the molecular basis of mutation and the vital process of gene duplication. Then we shall briefly consider the phenomenon of gene transposition. Finally we shall consider the evolution of some important neurobiological polypeptides and proteins.

4.1 MUTATION

Mutations may be divided into two large categories: **point mutations** and **chromosomal mutations**. Point mutations are changes in single base pairs; chromosomal mutations are changes in large stretches of DNA including, most importantly, the deletion and/or duplication of entire genes. Let us examine point mutations first.

4.1.1 Point mutations

Point mutations may be caused by a large number of agents: some **chemical** (e.g. nitrous acid, 5-bromouracil), some **physical** (ultraviolet irradiation, X-rays, radioactive emissions). Furthermore the DNA molecule itself has an inherent tendency to mutate. This is yet another feature which makes it a good genetic molecule. Without mutation living forms could not be selected to fit their environments: evolution could not have occurred. Indeed DNA's mutability is perhaps too great for its own good. It has to be held in check (as we shall see) by repair mechanisms.

Let us look first at DNA's spontaneous mutability. Consider the cytosine/guanine pair:

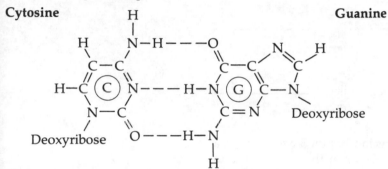

In about one case in every 10^4 or 10^5 cytosine rearranges into another **tautomeric** form:

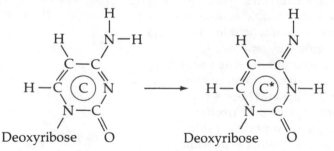

This clearly can no longer pair with guanine. It can, however, pair with adenine:

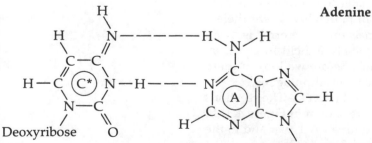

Hence, at replication, A is specified instead of G. At a subsequent replication cytosine is likely to return to its more stable tautomer, but A will remain to pick up T. Hence an **A/T pair** is substituted for a **G/C pair**:

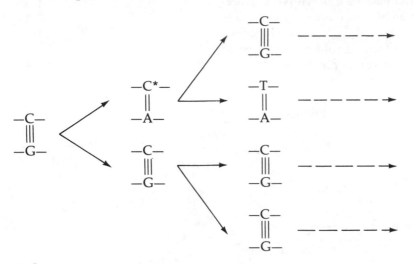

Reference back to the table of codons in Chapter 3 will show that such a substitution, especially if it occurs in the first or second position of a triplet, could have a profound effect on the amino acid specified. In some cases the amino acid newcomer will not vary greatly in its physico-chemical characteristics from the residue it replaced (see Table 2.1). If a hydrophobic residue is replaced by another hydrophobic residue, an aromatic side chain by a similar bulky side chain, a basic group by another basic group, an acidic by another acidic, or a hydrophilic side chain by another hydrophilic side chain the three dimensional conformation of the protein may not be too greatly upset. These acceptable newcomers are referred to as **conservative substitutions**. Radical substitutions where, for instance, a hydrophobic residue is replaced by a hydrophilic residue, or a basic group by an acidic group, are, however, much more difficult to accept.

We noted in Chapter 2 that all the classical Watson–Crick bases are conjugated structures and hence liable to tautomeric change. Hence the DNA molecule has built-in mutability. Nevertheless it has been calculated that in mammals only one error is made in every 10^9 base pairs. DNA's mutability is held in check by **proof-reading** and **repair** mechanisms. Before we look at these let us briefly consider the effect of chemical mutagens.

As an example let us take **nitrous acid (HNO$_2$)**. The reactions of HNO$_2$ with adenine and cytosine are shown in Figure 4.1. In the first case a C/G pair is substituted for an A/T pair and in the second case an A/T pair is substituted for a C/G pair.

A

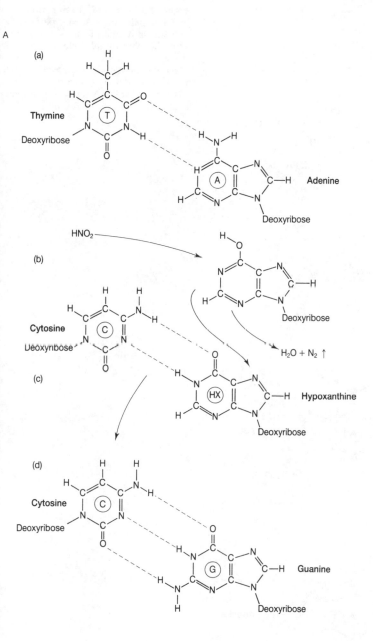

(a)

Thymine

Deoxyribose

Adenine

Deoxyribose

HNO₂

(b)

Cytosine

Deoxyribose

Deoxyribose

H₂O + N₂ ↑

(c)

Hypoxanthine

Deoxyribose

(d)

Cytosine

Deoxyribose

Guanine

Deoxyribose

Figure 4.1 The mutagenic effect of nitrous acid (HNO₂). (A) Substitution of a C≡G pair for a T=A pair. In (a) thymine and adenine are shown paired as in the DNA double helix; (b) HNO₂ is shown to deaminate adenine, which after rearrangement of the hydroxyl group forms (c) hypoxanthine (HX), which partners cytosine; (d) at the next DNA replication cytosine acts as a template for guanine. (*Continued overleaf*)

B

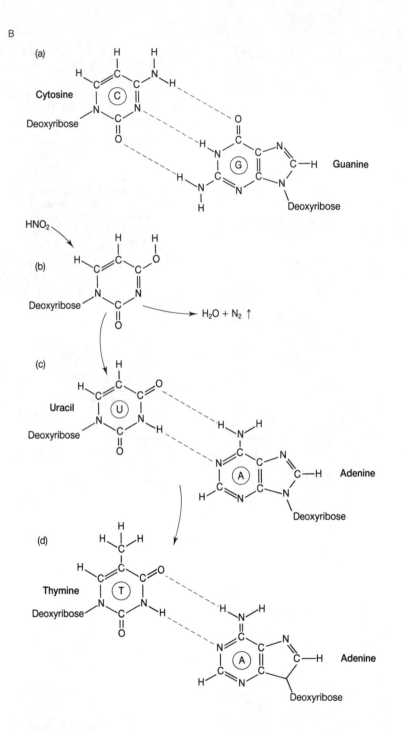

Figure 4.1 (*continued*) (B) Substitution of a T=A pair for a C≡G pair. In (a) cytosine and guanine are shown paired as in the DNA double helix; in (b) HNO₂ deaminates cytosine, which after rearrangement of the hydroxyl group (c) forms uracil (U), which partners adenine; (d) at the next DNA replication adenine acts as a template for thymine

It is worth noting that in all the cases considered so far a **pyrimidine** has been exchanged for another **pyrimidine** or a **purine** by a **purine**. This type of point mutation is known as a **transition**. The exchange of a purine for a pyrimidine or vice versa is much rarer but may occur very occasionally by mispairing during replication. This second (very unusual) type of point mutation is called a **transversion**.

Before leaving the topic of point mutations it is worth noting that if they should occur at a splice junction between an exon and an intron or on a **regulator** rather than a structural gene the consequences can be far more dramatic. It has been suggested that such mutations might well account for 'sudden' evolutionary changes.

4.1.2 Proof-reading and repair mechanisms

It was emphasised above that although DNA is very mutable, replication is nevertheless normally carried out with extremely high fidelity. This is because (at least in prokaryocytes) one of the DNA polymerase enzymes (polymerase 3) responsible for laying down a daughter polynucleotide strand alongside the parent polynucleotide template eliminates errors by 'proof-reading' the new strand.

Three **DNA polymerases** (do not confuse with the DNA-dependent **RNA** polymerases of Chapter 3) have been isolated, all of which act in the 5' to 3' direction. In prokaryocytes these are classified as **polymerase 1, 2 and 3**; in eukaryocytes they are referred to as α, β, and γ. Eukaryotic **polymerase** α is equivalent to prokaryotic **polymerase 3** in being the most important in the synthesis of new polynucleotide strands. The DNA polymerases also have **exonuclease** activity. Polymerases 1 and 3 show this activity in both the 3' to 5' and the 5' to 3' direction; polymerase 2 is only able to act in the 3' to 5' direction. In bacterial systems it has been shown that polymerases 1 and 3 cannot join a new deoxribonucleotide to the 3' end of the preceding deoxribonucleotide if the latter is not **securely base-paired** to its parent polynucleotide template. Their 3' to 5' exonuclease activity is switched on when they discover an incorrectly matched base pair. The offending nucleotide is clipped off. Thus polymerases 1 and 3 act as **self-correcting enzymes** and '**proof-read**' out errors as they go along. A similar process is believed to occur with polymerase α in eukarocytes. The prokaryotic process (which is much better known) is shown diagrammatically in Figure 4.2. In parenthesis here it worth noting that the dual polymerase/exonuclease activity of bacterial DNA polymerase 1 has been made use of in the technique of '**nick translation**'. A deoxyribonuclease (DNase 1) enzyme derived from the pancreas is used

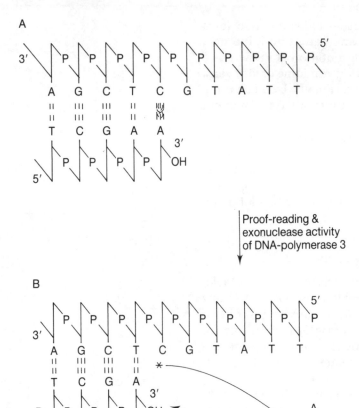

Figure 4.2 Proof-reading activity of DNA polymerase 1. (A) An incorrect adenosine has been added to the 3' end of the growing chain. (B) DNA polymerase 1 detects the faulty base pairing, excises the incorrect residue and replaces it by a correct deoxyribonucleotide

to break open (i.e. 'nick') a DNA double helix at random points. This leaves free 3'-hydroxyl and 5'-phosphate groups. DNA polymerase 1 is simultaneously used to progressively remove nucleotides from the free 5' end and to add fresh nucleotides to the 3' end of the nicked chain. In other words the polynucleotide strand is 'chewed' back in the 5' to 3' direction and fresh nucleotides added in the same direction. If one or more of the the nucleoside triphosphates being added is radiolabelled or biotinylated the DNA can be effectively tagged.

It is also worth noting at this stage that the necessity for high-fidelity DNA replication explains the existence of **thymine** in DNA but **uracil** in RNA. Thymine, as we noted in Chapter 2, possesses a methyl group at a position where uracil only has a hydrogen atom. In consequence it requires appreciably more energy to synthesise than uracil. It turns out, however, that cytosine is not only open to nitrous acid deamination to uracil (Figure 4.1) but that this may happen spontaneously by hydrolytic reaction with ambient water molecules. Such deaminated bases (Figure 4.1 shows that cytosine is not the only possibility) are recognised by specific enzymes—**DNA glycosidases**—which remove the base from the nucleotide by cleaving the glycosidic bond which links it to the deoxyribose. This leaves a hole in the base sequence usually known as an **AP** (i.e. apurinic or apyrimidinic) site. Another enzyme, a **repair or AP endonuclease**, detects the defective nucleotide and removes it entirely from the poly-nucleotide strand, leaving a **'nick'** in the phosphodiester backbone. DNA polymerase 1 now comes into play. It detects the nick and its endonuclease activity works back in the 5' to 3' direction, removing a short run of nucleotides and replacing them with fresh nucleotides. Finally the phosphodiester bond is sealed again by **DNA ligase**.

This complicated set of events is shown in Figure 4.3. We shall refer to some of these enzymes and processes again in Chapter 5 when we look at some of the techniques and enzymes involved in genetic engineering. But, returning to the topic of this section, it is clear that if uracil were anyway present in DNA in the first place, it would be impossible for a DNA glycosidase to distinguish between what should be present and what should not: between correct uracils and those due to the deamination of cytosine.

Nonetheless, in spite of all this ingenious molecular machinery to ensure that the genetic message is not degraded, in spite of a fidelity of **one part in a billion**, point mutations, especially transitions, are bound to creep in during the countless generations of geological time and in the vast number of DNA replications occurring in biological populations.

4.1.3 Chromosomal mutations.

The most important types of chromosomal mutation from the standpoint of molecular evolution are **gene duplications**.

These occur by incorrect crossing over at meiosis. Several instances of this have been thoroughly studied in *Drosophila*. If two non-sister chromatids line up somewhat imprecisely at the beginning of meiotic division, chiasmata may occur in such a way that one of the daughter nuclei resulting from the division contains two copies of a gene and the other daughter nucleus does not contain the gene at all. The latter will probably not survive, but the former, as we shall see, has great evolutionary possibilities ahead of it.

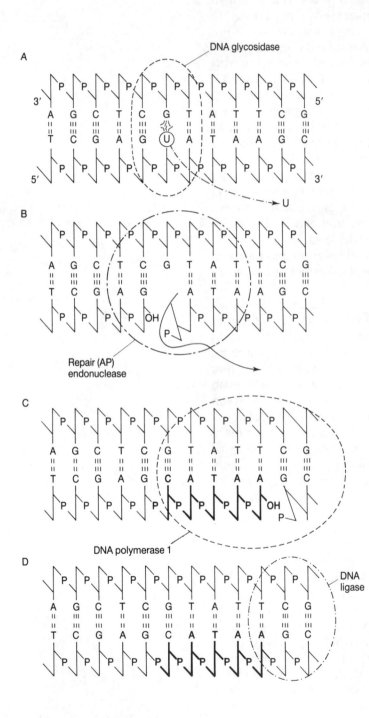

Figure 4.3   Repair of deaminative point mutations. (A) Portion of a DNA double helix in which cytosine has been deaminated to uracil (see Fig. 4.1). DNA glycosidase recognises the deaminated base and removes it by cleaving its glycosidic linkage to deoxyribose. (B) A repair or AP endonuclease recognises the AP (i.e. apurinic or apyrimidinic) site and cuts the phosphodiester backbone. (C) DNA polymerase 1 now cuts back a few nucleotides from the 'nick' in the phosphodiester backbone and fills in the gap so created with fresh nucleotides. This important activity is known as 'nick translation'. (D) Finally DNA ligase seals the 'nick' by re-forming the phosphodiester linkage

A

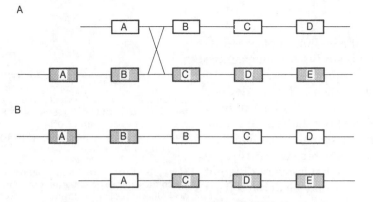

Figure 4.4 Imprecise alignment of chromatids leading to gene duplication at cross-over. (A) Chromatids misalign themselves at the commencement of meiotic division. (B) Recombination leads to gene duplication in one chromatid and gene deletion in the other

We shall return to consider the consequences for molecular evolution of gene duplication in Section 4.3.

4.2 TRANSPOSONS

Evidence for the existence of **'jumping genes'** was first published by Barbara McClintock in the 1940s, although she had to wait until the 1980s to receive recognition for her work by the award of a Nobel prize. This long wait was partly because the molecular methods required to establish her interpretation were not available until fairly recently.

There is, however, overwhelming evidence today that the genomes of microbial, plant and animal organisms are not as unchanging as classical geneticists thought. Two types of movable elements are nowadays believed to exist: **insertion sequences (IS)** and **transposons (Tn)**. The insertion sequences are fairly short stretches of DNA which are only involved in movement from one part to another of a genome; transposons are longer (up to 40 kbp) and much more interesting DNA sequences. Not only are they capable of moving about from one part of a genome to another but they also carry with them a structural gene or genes. Figure 4.5 shows that in addition to the structural gene(s) a typical transposon also includes a **transposase** and **resolvase** gene. The latter genes are both involved in the excision and reinsertion of the transposon. At each end of the transposon are near-identical nucleotide sequences (20–40 base pairs), running in the opposite sense to each other, which are presumably involved in excision and reinsertion.

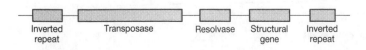

Inverted repeat   Transposase   Resolvase   Structural gene   Inverted repeat

Figure 4.5 Transposon. The main structural features of a typical transposon are shown. At each end of the transposon is a a nearly identical sequence of bases which are orientated in the opposite sense to each other. Further explanation in given in the text

4.3 PROTEIN EVOLUTION

We are now in a position to consider the evolution of proteins. There are several different aspects to this study. We can examine the amino acid sequences of the 'same' protein in a variety of organisms and by noting degrees of similarity deduce **phylogenetic relationships**. Or, secondly, we can take note of the fact that proteins which have different functions in the same organism have marked sequence and/or structural similarities. This again suggests an evolutionary relationship. Or, finally, we can observe that proteins (or polypeptides) having very different primary sequences and different functions may be derived from the same mRNA transcript by differential post-transcriptional or post-translational processing.

We touched on the last of these aspects in Chapter 3, where we considered the generation of the enkephalin and endorphin neurotransmitters and some of the pituitary hormones from single 'mother' primary transcripts. We shall return to this topic at the end of this chapter. To begin with, however, let us consider the first two aspects of protein evolution listed above.

4.3.1 Evolutionary development of protein molecules and phylogenetic relationships

The respiratory co-enzyme **cytochrome c**, whose primary structure has been determined in more than 80 different species,

Figure 4.6 Phylogenetic tree for cytochrome c. The respiratory haem-containing coenzyme, cytochrome c, is found throughout the living world from prokaryotes to man. Although the number of amino acids in its primary structure varies considerably (e.g. 134 in *Paracoccus*, 82 in *Pseudomonas*, 122 in *Homo*) its tertiary structure remains very much the same. By comparing the amino acid differences in cytochromes c derived from a wide variety of organisms, relating them to the underlying nucleotide changes in the codons, and incorporating data on the observed rates at which different nucleotides change, it is possible to construct an evolutionary tree. This tree is shown in the figure. The numbers on its branches indicate the number of nucleotide substitutions required to join one branch point to another. As it has been estimated that in cytochrome c a 1% change in amino acid sequence takes about 20 million years it is possible to gain a rough idea of the evolutionary time elapsing between the branch points. (From Avers, 1986, *Molecular Cell Biology*, Menlo Park, California: Benjamin/Cummings; with permission.)

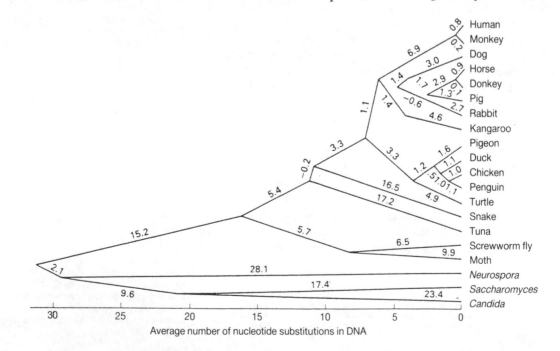

from *Neurospora* to man, is often taken as an example of the use of sequence data to suggest phylogenetic relationships. Another favourite example is provided by the **globins**: the α and β chains of haemoglobin and the single globin chain of myoglobin.

An initial question which requires an answer is whether change in amino acid sequence is related to number of generations or simply to elapsed time. Clearly this is crucial to any phylogenetic interpretation. It turns out that sequence changes are related straightforwardly to **elapsed time**, not to number of replicative events, and, furthermore, that changes occur fairly steadily with time. This, of course, is not to say that all proteins and poly-peptides evolve at the same rate. On the contrary there is good evidence that **different proteins evolve at different rates**: fibrino-peptides, for instance, comparatively rapidly, the histones comparatively slowly. This, of course, has to do with the importance of the exact primary sequence for biological function. Knowing the rate at which amino acid residues change for a given protein it is possible to calculate how far back in time a common ancestor must have existed. An example of this molecular phylogeny is given in Figure 4.6 for cytochrome c.

Another very important 'model' for molecular evolution is provided by the globins: haemoglobin and myoglobin. Probably more is known about the molecular biology of the globins than any other protein. The globin gene may be traced back 600 million years to its origin in the earliest invertebrates. Unlike the cytochrome c gene its evolution is marked by a number of **duplications**. A phylogeny is shown in Figure 4.7.

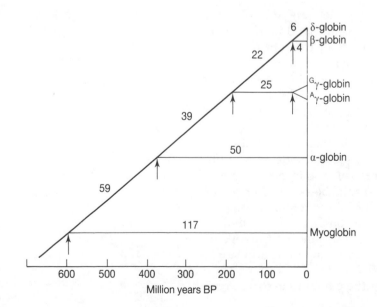

Figure 4.7 Phylogeny of human globins. Duplications are represented by arrows. The figures indicate the number of base substitutions required to transform one globin into another. Further explanation is given in the text

Figure 4.7 shows that the earliest globin is believed to have been a single unit, such as myoglobin is now. The earliest duplication, occurring some 600 Ma ago, freed one gene from severe selection pressure. This is an example of the great importance of gene duplication in molecular evolution. **So long as one gene continues to programme the synthesis of a viable protein the other can 'experiment' creatively**. Many instances of this trick have occurred in protein evolution. In the case of the globin gene another duplication occurred, as Figure 4.7 shows, some 400 Ma ago, producing the precursors of the α- and β-**globin** genes. More recently, the β-globin gene has duplicated several times (as indicated) producing genes coding for ϵ-**globin (embryonic)**, γ-**globin (fetal)** and, most recently, δ-**globin**. The γ-globin gene, furthermore, has duplicated (perhaps about 25 Ma ago) into $^G\gamma$ and $^A\gamma$ genes, differing by only one nucleotide.

It is clear from the foregoing that the genetic representation of the globins is rather complicated. A whole **cluster** of genes— α, β, ϵ, δ, $^G\gamma$ and $^A\gamma$—is involved. In addition there are a number of **pseudogenes**, i.e. inactive duplicates of functional genes. Pseudogenes are symbolised by the prefix ψ, e.g. $\psi\beta$. The β-like cluster is carried on human chromosome 11. It is spread over a length of about 60 000 base pairs (60 kbp). About 95% of this length consists, however, of non-coding DNA. The gene programming for α-globin along with some pseudogenes is carried on chromosome 16.

Can we relate the globin gene structure to the **exon/intron** organisation of the genome which we discussed in Chapter 3? Interestingly it does seem that the exon/intron organisation of all the globin genes is very similar (Figure 4.8). It is particularly interesting to note that even though they are on different chromosomes the organisation of the α- and β-globin genes is almost identical (although the magnitude of the introns in the β-globin cluster is much greater than the magnitude of those in the α-globin gene). The 'splice' junctions (where the exon is joined to the intron) are, moreover, virtually identical throughout the β-cluster. This observation adds weight to the argument that the presence of introns in eukaryotic genomes has something to do with crossing over, gene duplication and molecular evolution.

It is beginning to seem likely that the globin model may apply to many of the receptor proteins which play so important a role in animal nervous systems. At present the best-characterised of these protein complexes is the nicotinic acetylcholine receptor (nAChR). We have already seen that it consists of five subunits (Chapter 2). At the vertebrate neuromuscular junction the nAChR has been found to consist of two identical α-subunits and single copies of β-, γ- and δ-subunits (see Chapter 9). Although the precise nature of the subunits varies the pentameric structure is

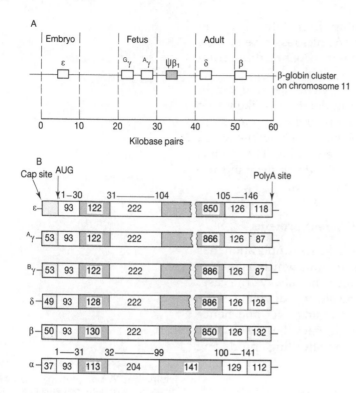

Figure 4.8 Exon/intron organisation of the human globin genes. (A) The β-globin cluster on chromosome 11. Functional genes are unshaded; the pseudogene is hatched. (B) Exon/intron organisation of human globin genes. The transcribed sequences are compared beginning with the 5' cap site. The numbers in the boxes indicate the number of nucleotides present in each region whilst the numbers above the boxes indicate the amino acid residues in the resulting polypeptide. The stippled boxes at the beginnings and ends of the sequences show regions which are transcribed but not translated. The second introns in the β-cluster globins are broken to align them with the much shorter intron in the α-globin gene. Exons unshaded, introns hatched. (Modified from Darnell, Lodish and Baltimore, 1986, *Molecular Cell Biology*, New York: Scientific American Books.)

believed to occur throughout the vertebrates and in those invertebrates which have been examined.

It is important to note, however, that, like the globins, the amino acid sequences of nAChR subunits, and hence the pharmacological properties of the receptor, differ from species to species and indeed vary from one part (e.g. central nervous system) of an organism to another (e.g. peripheral nervous system). It seems likely that the original gene coded for an ancestral α-subunit and that, as with the globins, gene duplication brought about the subsequent appearance of β-, γ- and δ-subunits. Additionally, early in the evolutionary development of vertebrates, the gene clusters coding for peripheral nAChRs began to diverge from those coding for central nAChRs. Indeed there is evidence that brain nAChR pentamers consist of only two types of subunit. This developing insight into the evolution of nicotinic acetylcholine receptors is strengthened by the finding that nAChRs isolated from insect nervous systems resemble in size and complexity vertebrate brain nAChRs. Breer, furthermore, has isolated a pentameric nAChR from the cockroach *Periplaneta americana* which he believes to consist of just one type of subunit. He suggests that this homo-oligomer of units resembling the vertebrate α-subunit may resemble the ancestral nAChR from which all the others have evolved. Finally, turning from phylogeny to ontogeny, it is interesting to note that nAChRs resemble globins in yet another respect: the subunits of fetal nAChRs differ from those of the mature pentamer.

We shall return to the nicotinic acetylcholine receptor in Chapter 9, where we shall examine it in detail. It is likely that many of the other receptors with which neural membranes are studded have complex evolutionary biologies similar to that which is just beginning to be worked out for the nAChR. The globins may thus form a useful model with which to understand the molecular biology of neural receptor molecules.

4.3.2 Evolutionary relationships of different proteins

In the case of the globin and nAChR genes duplication has resulted in the production of separate subunits which have then undergone independent evolution. This is not always the case. In many instances duplication simply results in a doubling of the original protein's size. In other cases crossing over and hence duplication may occur within an exon. In yet other cases there is evidence of what Doolittle calls 'exon shuffling' producing

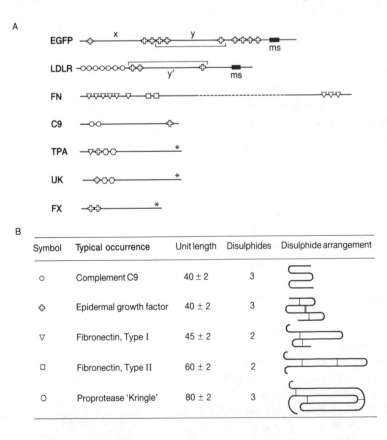

Figure 4.9   Mosaic proteins. (A) Seven disparate vertebrate proteins possessing homologous 'modules'. (B) The nature of the modules represented by symbols in (A). The nature of the disulphide arrangement in the C9-type unit is unknown. EGPF = epidermal growth factor; LDLR = low-density lipoprotein receptor; FN = fibronectin; C9 = complement component 9; TPA = tissue plasminogen activator; UK = urokinase; FX = blood clotting factor X; * = active site of serine proteases; x,y and y' = homologous sequences; black rectangles labelled ms represent membrane spanning segments of the proteins. (From Doolittle, 1985, *Trends in Biochemical Sciences*, **10**, 233–237; with permission.)

'**mosaic proteins**'. Such proteins show evidence of the combination and recombination of exons coding for valuable 'domains' (see Chapter 2). Doolittle gives an example of an otherwise apparently unrelated group of vertebrate proteins which appear to consist of just such combinations of well-tried domains. These are shown in Figure 4.9.

But, more interesting to the neurobiologist, are the numerous hints which are beginning to emerge which suggest that groups of neurobiologically important proteins may be evolutionarily related to each other. We shall note several of these interesting relationships in Chapters 6–10. We shall see in Chapter 6 that the **gap junction protein** shows considerable resemblance to the **nicotinic acetylcholine receptor** whilst the latter is related to the **GABA$_A$ and glycine** receptors. The latter three receptors are discussed in in Chapter 9. In Chapter 7 we shall note the similarities between the **β-adrenergic receptor**, the **muscarinic acetylcholine receptor**, the **substance K receptor** and the photopigment protein, **opsin**. In this case the evolutionary relationship is made more obvious by all four proteins acting through a similar 'collison-coupling' mechanism. In Chapter 8 we shall see that the vital membrane-embedded pump proteins, the **Na$^+$ + K$^+$-ATPase** and the **Mg^{2+}-dependent Ca^{2+}-ATPase** show striking homologies and, finally, in Chapter 10 we shall look at the molecular similarities of the **sodium, potassium** and **calcium voltage-gated channels**. These are far from all the evolutionary relationships which molecular neurobiology is revealing. It seems that the evolutionary process here, as elswhere, has modified a number of basic structures to serve somewhat different functions. It seems that many of the molecules at the basis of neurobiology fall into a small number of 'superfamilies'.

A superfamily of proteins is conventionally defined as a group whose primary sequences resemble each other with greater than chance probability and whose tertiary structure is obviously similar. The members of a superfamily are often themselves families of proteins. It has turned out to be an error to suppose that there is, for instance, *a* muscarinic acetylcholine receptor or *a* Na$^+$ + K$^+$-ATPase. Instead these names denote groups of proteins having a similar (not identical) function and resembling each other in 50% or more of their amino acid residues. At the level of these great protein molecules we leave behind the simplicities of small molecule biochemistry where, for example, the names glucose or phenylalanine always denote the same chemical structure. The further research proceeds the more heterogeneous do neurobiological proteins turn out to be. Different cells express subtly different subtypes of a protein family. The brain retains its complexity and functional differentiation all the way down to the molecular level.

4.3.3 Evolution by differential post-transcriptional and post-translational processing: the opioids and other neuroactive peptides

We have already met some of the opioids when we discussed post-translational control in Section 3.3. They are found throughout the living world, from *Tetrahymena* to man. What are their evolutionary relationships?

It will be recalled that the opioids are a group of peptide neurotransmitters and hormones which are involved in responses to stress. In Section 3.3 we concentrated on the two enkephalins—**met-** and **leu-enkephalin**. There are, however, a number of other related peptides: **substance P, α-, β-** and **γ-melanocyte-stimulating hormone (MSH), α-** and **β-endorphin, adrenocorticotrophic hormone (ACTH)** and **cortico-releasing factor (CRF)**. In addition there is a long list of other peptides which show opioid activity. These turn out to be amino acid extensions of the carboxyterminal of met- or leu-enkephalin. Many members of this great collection of neuroactive peptides can be shown to be derived from just three different precursors: pro-opiomelanocortin (POMC) (265 amino acid residues); pre-proenkephalin A (263 amino acid residues); and preproenkephalin B (256 amino acid residues). These three precursor proteins are schematised in Figure 4.10.

Figure 4.10 Precursor proteins of the opioid peptides. (A) Pro-opiomelano-cortin (POMC) (263 amino acid residues). This precursor protein contains amino acid sequences for γ-MSH, ACTH and β-LPH. It is processed differently in different lobes of the pituitary. In the intermediate lobe ACTH is cleaved into α-MSH and CLIP (corticotropin-like intermediate lobe protein), whilst β-LPH (β-lipotropic hormone) is divided into another molecule of γ-MSH and β-endorphin. A different post-translational processing occurs in the anterior lobe. The cleavage sites are marked by pairs of basic amino acids. (B) Proenkephalin A (263 amino acid residues). This precursor contains six copies of met-enkephalin (ME) and one of leu-enkephalin (LE). Cleavage sites are again marked by basic amino acids. The initial processing releases peptide F, peptide E and peptide B. Subsequently the enkephalins are cut free from these larger peptides. (C) Proenkephalin B (256 amino acid residues). This slightly smaller precursor contains three copies of leu-enkephalin (LE). Cleavage sites are signalled by basic amino acids. Again initial post-translational processing releases two larger peptides—neo-endorphin and dynorphin—and leu-enkephalin pentapeptides are cut from these. All three precursor proteins have N-terminal signal sequences which allow secretion from the ribosome through the ER membrane into the ER cisterna. (After Douglass, Civelli and Herbert, 1984, *Annual Review of Biochemistry*, **53**, 665–715; and Lynch and Snyder, 1986, *Advances in Biochemistry*, **55**, 773–799.)

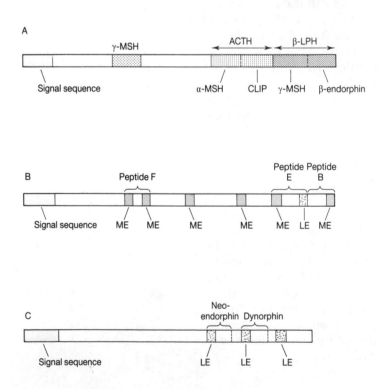

It is clear that the three precursors are all nearly the same length. They are examples of a class of proteins sometimes called **polyfunctional** proteins or **polyproteins** because they contain two or more copies of a bioactive protein or polypeptide, or perhaps copies of more than one type of bioactive protein or polypeptide.

Figure 4.10 shows that the neuroactive peptides are mostly found towards the carboxyterminal end of the polyprotein precursor. Furthermore it has been shown that the neuroactive 'domains' of the precursors are marked by pairs of basic amino acid residues (see Section 3.3) which form potential cleavage sites for trypsin-like enzymes.

It is found that the same precursor protein occurs in several different tissues (for instance anterior and intermediate lobes of the pituitary, hypothalamus, placenta, intestine) but undergoes different post-translational processing. This is evidently a neat way of achieving adaptive variety from a single transcript. The interesting question in this chapter, however, is whether the three precursors are evolutionarily related.

It seems likely that the differences in the three precursor proteins—**POMC**, **preproenkephalin A** and **preproenkephalin B**—arise from differences in the splicing of the mRNA chains after the excision of introns. That POMC and preproenkephalin A are evolutionarily related is shown by the similarity of their exon/intron structure (Figure 4.11). The preproenkephalin gene, however, is located on human chromosome 12 whilst the POMC gene is on chromosome 2. Is this (like the similar situation obtaining for the α- and β-globins) a relic of some past episode involving transposon shuffling?

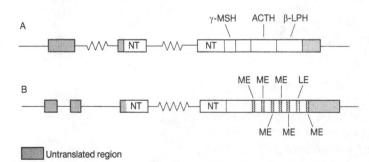

Figure 4.11 Exon/intron structure of (A) human POMC and (B)preproenkephalin genes. The exons are represented by boxes, the introns by lines. NT = N-terminal end; other abbreviations as in Fig. 4.10. (After Douglass, Civelli and Herbert, 1984, *Annual Review of Biochemistry*, **53**, 665–715.)

If human, rat and mouse POMC genes are compared, the sequences are found to be highly conserved. Taking an evolutionarily greater jump to the preproenkephalin gene of the clawed toad, *Xenopus*, sharing a common ancestor with man some 350 Ma ago, we find that the exon/intron structure remains very similar although the nucleotide homology in the spacer sequences is sometimes quite dissimilar, ranging from 36 to 91%. It is interesting to note, furthermore, that although met-enkephalin is represented there is no leu-enkephalin sequence at the carboxy-terminal end. Perhaps leu-enkephalin has evolved more recently.

We can perhaps conclude that the met-enkephalin gene is the primordial unit and that this has been duplicated and rearranged numerous times during evolution.

The opioids are far from being the only neuroactive peptides which have evolved through differential post-transcriptional and post-translational processing. The **procholecystokinin (PCCK)** polyprotein is also subject to tissue-specific processing. In the intestine a large 33-residue polypeptide (CCK 33) is excised from the 115-unit precursor, in the brain an eight-residue unit (CCK 8) is cut out, whilst in the nerves innervating the pancreas a yet smaller fragment is used (CCK 4).

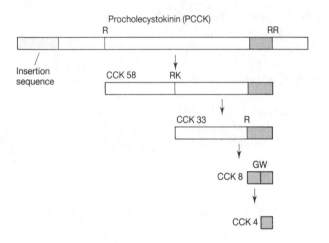

Figure 4.12   Processing the PCCK polyprotein. The 115-residue PCCK precursor is cut first to a 58-residue unit and then to the 33-residue CCK which is found in the intestine. In the brain CCK is further cut first to CCK 8 and finally, in the nerves innervating the pancreas, to CCK 4. R, K, G and W symbolise the amino acids arginine, lysine, glycine and tryptophan which mark cleavage sites. (After Lynch and Snyder, 1986, *Advances in Biochemistry*, **55**, 773–799.)

Another interesting case of differential processing is provided by the **preprotachykinin (PPT)** gene. This gene consists of seven exons, of which six code for preprotachykinin. We saw in Chapter 3 (Figure 3.12) that differential splicing of the primary hnRNA transcript leads to two mRNAs: α-PPT mRNA and β-PPT mRNA. Translation then occurs in the usual way but the resulting polypeptides are then subject to further processing. The α-PPT polypeptide is processed to give substance P (SP) whilst the β-PPT is differentially processed to give both SP and substance K (SK).

It can be seen in these peptide examples that the evolutionary process is as parsimonious at the molecular level as it is at the organismic level. Just as at the organismic level gill arches become jaws and auditory ossicles, so at the molecular level the same precursor protein is modified to carry out different functions. The evolutionary process works always by modifying existing structures, never by creating entirely new ones. Slight variations on what exists are seized upon by natural selection and over the generations diverge ever further from their ancestral form.

4.4 CONCLUSION

This chapter and the two which preceded it have outlined the mechanisms of, and evidence for, evolution at the molecular level. We shall meet many more examples and suggestive hints of this important theme as we proceed through the pages of this book. But we can already see that molecular biology provides a host of means by which molecules can change their structure and consequently alter their biological function. Beyond the molecular level other structures and functional complexes supervene before the integrated organism presents itself to the processes of Darwinian selection. The nervous system is arguably the most intricate of these higher-level complexes. Variations in the molecular basis of the nervous system can work through the levels of structure to induce momentous consequences. Some of these consequences, and we shall look at some in Chapter 19, are totally disabling. Infrahuman organisms could not survive. Other consequences are more subtle. Nonetheless even slight variations in behaviour can have profound selective consequences. The nervous system, as much if not more than any other part of the organism, is under Darwinian control.

Chapter 5
Manipulating biomolecules

Francis Bacon said, long ago, that knowledge is power. The recent vast increase in our understanding of molecular biology is beginning to give us the power to manipulate living processes. As with every field of scientifico-technological endeavour this is a two-way process. As we begin to be able to engineer organisms and biochemicals we achieve new insights into their structure and activity. These new insights, in their turn, feed back into the design of yet more powerful manipulative techniques. We are at the beginning of a rising spiral of biotechnological expertise.

The nervous system as much as any other part of biology is open to these new approaches. Already fundamental new understandings have been reached or are on the horizon. In this chapter a brief account of the more important and relevant of these new techniques will be presented.

Chapters 2–4 have already laid the groundwork for the subject matter of this chapter. The manipulations of the modern molecular engineer depend essentially on an understanding of the structure and activity of the informational macromolecules we have been considering. They have to do essentially with molecular recognition, with the transfer of sequence information, with the multiplication of specific molecular structures by the cellular mechanisms we have discussed and, most important of all, with the expression of information held in nucleotide sequences where the scientist rather than the cell wants to find it. The molecular biologist is beginning to be able to reach into the information-processing machinery which organisms have evolved over thousands of millions of years and tweak it towards his own ulterior purpose.

The key operations of genetic engineering, so far as molecular neurobiology is concerned, are the isolation of the nucleic acid stretches (i.e. genes) which code for proteins and polypeptides of neurobiological interest and the elucidation of their base sequences. A knowledge of the relevant base sequences enables the primary structure of the resultant protein or polypeptide to be deduced. This knowledge, in turn, can be used to predict the conformation and function of the molecule. If the molecule is embedded in a membrane (as are so many of the most important neurobiological proteins) a knowledge of the distribution of hydrophobic and hydrophilic residues allows its disposition in the lipid bilayer to be predicted.

The methods used combine genetics and biochemistry in complex and intricate ways. The first step is often to break up DNA molecules into more manageable fragments. These fragments may then be 'cloned' to create a 'gene library'. The library has then to be screened and the gene of interest 'fished' out. It may then be sequenced and/or set to work in an 'expression vector' to produce the protein for which it codes. Alternatively a reverse transcriptase may be used to create a cDNA library from neuronal mRNA. This library must again be screened to find the gene of interest. There are numerous other side-lines to this powerful and rapidly expanding technique. In what follows we shall merely look at the essentials.

5.1 RESTRICTION ENDONUCLEASES

DNA molecules, especially eukaryotic DNA molecules, although comparatively simple in structure (as we have seen) are horrendously lengthy: the haploid human genome is computed to consist of three thousand million base pairs. For many years after the Watson–Crick breakthrough it seemed almost an impossible dream to hope to home in on an interesting gene and establish its base sequence. All this changed with the discovery in the late 1960s of **restriction endonucleases**, which cut the DNA strand at specific points into smaller, manageable, fragments. Nowadays well over 100 different restriction endonucleases are known and commercially available. Let us look at a few examples.

EcoR1: this is one of the best known and most used restriction endonucleases. It is found in *E.coli* RY13: hence the name. This endonuclease recognises a portion of the double helix which reads:

> polynucleotide-G-A-A-T-T-C-polynucleotide
> polynucleotide-C-T-T-A-A-G-polynucleotide

It then makes a very precise cut in the helix between the G and the A in each strand to give:

> polynucleotide-G

polynucleotide-C-T-T-A-A

and

A-A-T-T-C-polynucleotide

G-polynucleotide

EcoR1 will cut DNA wherever this particular base sequence turns up. It can be calculated that if the four nucleotide bases appear in random order in the double helix then this particular sextuplet will occur once every 4096 base pairs (i.e. 4^6). EcoR1 is thus likely (left long enough) to cut the millions or hundreds of millions of base pairs in a eukaryotic DNA strand into much more manageable 4000–5000 bp segments.

There are a couple of other points to note about the action of EcoR1. First, the sequence which it recognises is **palindromic**, that is, like the words 'radar' and 'refer', it makes the same sense read forwards or backwards. It turns out that this is a general feature applying to all restriction endonucleases. The sites on the DNA double helix which they recognise are invariably palindromic. The second important feature to note is that the polynucleotide fragments resulting from the enzyme's action have **'sticky ends'**. The A-A-T-T-end projecting from the DNA fragment will very readily join with its Watson–Crick partner.

Far from all restriction endonucleases produce fragments with 'sticky ends'. An endonculease derived from another bacterium, *Haemophilus parainfluenzae*, known as **Hpa1**, recognises the following DNA sequence:

polynucleotide-G-T-T-A-A-C-polynucleotide

polynucleotide-C-A-A-T-T-G-polynucleotide

and cuts it in the position shown by the arrows into

polynucleotide-G-T-T

polynucleotide-C-A-A

and

A-A-C-polynucleotide

T-T-G-polynucleotide

We shall see later that these so-called **'blunt-ended'** restriction fragments have their own uses.

Finally, many restriction endonucleases recognise not a sequence of six but a sequence of **four** nucleotides. An example of this is an endonuclease derived from *Haemophilus haemolyticus*, **Hha1**. This recognises the sequence:

$$\downarrow$$

-G-C-G-C-

-C-G-C-G-

$$\uparrow$$

Elementary statistics tells us that groups of four nucleotides are much more likely to turn up by chance than groups of six. They should indeed appear every 4^4, i.e. 256, nucleotides. Hence the application of these restriction enzymes results in much shorter fragments than those obtained with endonucleases recognising sextuplets.

The length of time the restriction endonuclease is allowed to act on the DNA double helix materially affects the number of fragments obtained. Only by allowing an endonuclease such as Hha1 to act on a DNA strand for a very long time will **all** the appropriate -G-C-G-C- sites be found. Only then will fragments of about 250 bp result.

5.2 SEPARATION OF RESTRICTION FRAGMENTS

Having broken up the DNA strands into smaller, more manage-able fragments it is then necessary to separate the mixture. This can be done by a number of methods, of which **electrophoresis on agarose gels** is the favourite. The restriction fragments travel unharmed (still double-helical) through the agarose gel at different rates according to their size. They can be visualised on the gel by staining and can then be eluted and sequenced. Techniques have now been developed which allow the routine determination of sequences of up to and beyond 5000 bp in length (see Section 5.12 below).

5.3 RESTRICTION MAPS

By subjecting DNA to different restriction endonucleases, or the same endonuclease for different durations, assortments of frag-ments of different lengths are obtained. By carefully examining

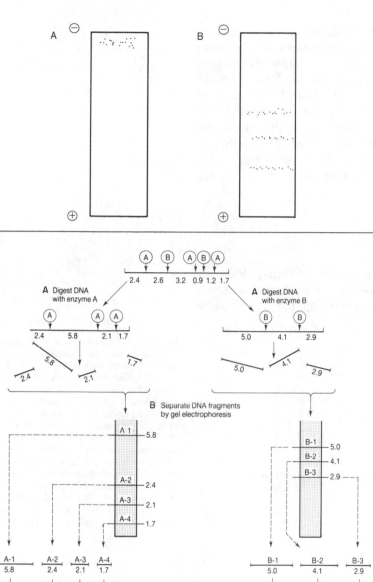

Figure 5.1 Separation of restriction fragments by electrophoresis. A suspension of restriction fragments is placed at the top of an agarose or polyacrylamide gel column (A). Application of a voltage causes the fragments to move through the gel towards the anode. The smaller fragments move faster than the larger (B). After staining for visualisation they can be eluted and analysed

Figure 5.2 Construction of a restriction map. The DNA molecule in the figure contains 12 000 nuclotide base pairs (i.e. (2.4 + 2.6 + 3.2 + 0.9 + 1.2 + 1.7) kbp). It contains three recognition sites for endonuclease A and two for endonuclease B. The numbers between the recognition sites indicate kilobase pairs but these are, of course, initially unknown. (A) Digestion with endonuclease A yields four restriction fragments and digestion with endonuclease B yields three. (B) The restriction fragments are separated by agarose or polyacrylamide gel electrophoresis. The fragments are conventionally numbered from largest to smallest. (C) Each fragment is eluted from the gel and digested with the other restriction enzyme. In some cases, e.g. A1 and A3 and all three B fragments this results in further cleavage as they contain restriction sites for the other endonuclease. (D) The two sets of fragments can now be examined for overlapping sequences and the best fit determined. The result is a restriction map which shows the sites at which the two endonucleases attack. (From Becker, 1986, *The World of the Cell*, Menlo Park, California: Benjamin/Cummings; with permission.)

the fragments it is possible to find overlapping sequences and hence determine the order in which the fragments were present in the original DNA (see Figure 5.2). As the fragments themselves can be sequenced (as mentioned above) one can begin to build up a nucleotide analysis of the entire DNA strand. Alternatively (and more usually) one is able to determine on which restriction fragment a gene of interest is located. We shall outline the techniques by which this can be achieved later. The upshot of this work is a **'restriction map'** of the DNA, showing where different endonucleases attack and where genes of interest are located.

5.4 RECOMBINATION

The construction of restriction maps is not, of course, the only consequence of the discovery of restriction endonucleases. Of even greater importance is the opportunity the use of such

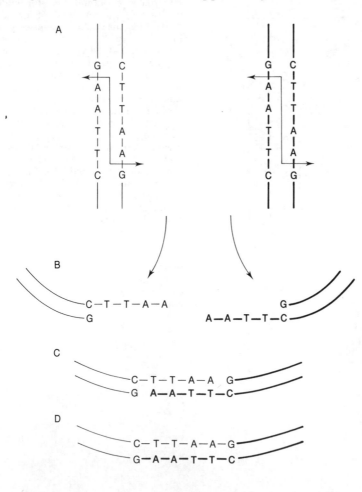

Figure 5.3 Production of recombinant DNA molecules. (A) A restriction enzyme (in the example EcoR1) cleaves DNA from two different sources. The cleavage is shown by the arrow. (B) A mixture of fragments with complementary 'sticky ends' is generated. (C) Mixing the two sets of cleaved fragments allows recombinant DNA strands to form by complementary base pairing. (D) The phosphodiester link between G and C is formed by incubation with DNA ligase. The recombinant DNA fragments will be separated from the homologous fragments which will also have been generated by subsequent cloning procedures

enzymes provides for combining DNA fragments from different sources. In order to do this it is of course necessary that the various DNA fragments have matching 'sticky ends'. This will be the case if the DNA obtained from different sources has been digested with the same restriction endonuclease. If this is the case the sticky ends will find each other by the usual processes of complementary base pairing, and addition of the enzyme **DNA ligase** (Section 4.1.2) will seal the union by covalent bonding.

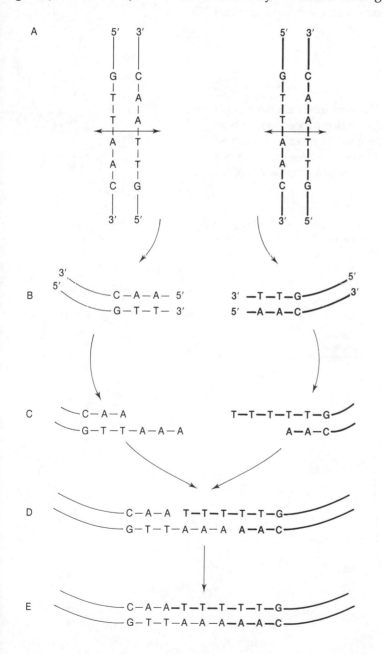

Figure 5.4 Recombination by homopolymer tailing. (A) A restriction enzyme such as Hpa1 cleaves the DNA from two different sources in the position indicated by the arrow. (B) Blunt-ended fragments are generated. (C) Incubation with terminal transferase and either dATP or dTTP adds A or T to the 3′ terminal end of the fragments. (D) The two sets of fragments are mixed and recombination occurs by complementary base pairing. (E) Addition of DNA-ligase forms the missing phosphodiester bond between T and A and A and A

An alternative approach is to use 'blunt-ended' restriction fragments. On their own these of course have no complementary base-pairing properties. However, an enzyme—**terminal transferase**—is known which is able to add nucleotides to the 3' end of such fragments. Thus if a sequence -A-A-A-A-A—— is added to one group of fragments and a sequence of -T-T-T-T-T—— to the other then, once again, the helices will find each other and stick by complementary base pairing. Once again DNA ligase is used to seal the union. For obvious reasons this technique is called **'homopolymer tailing'**.

5.5 CLONING

We are now in a position to consider the way in which genes and their products may by multiplied. This is the process known as **cloning**. In essence it requires that the gene of interest is spliced into a replication or **cloning vector**. There are three major types of cloning vector: **plasmid**, **phage** and **cosmid**. Let us consider each in turn.

Plasmids. Plasmids are tiny circlets of DNA, seldom more than 2000 bp in length, present in many bacteria and yeasts. They replicate independently of the bacterium's major DNA strand—

Figure 5.5   Plasmids within a bacterium

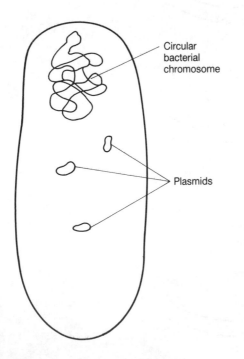

Circular
bacterial
chromosome

Plasmids

forming anything up to 200 copies. The reason for this is that they often carry the genes which confer antibiotic resistance on the bacterium. They provide excellent cloning vectors for the genetic engineer as not only do they replicate within the bacterium but they are also replicated each time the bacterium itself replicates.

Because plasmid DNA is so much smaller than the chromosomal DNA it is easily separated and purified. In the presence of Ca^{2+} plasmids are readily taken up by plasmid-free bacteria and replicated. It is clear that such an organelle provides enormous opportunity for gene cloning.

All the cloner has to do is rupture a bacterium and obtain a plasmid circlet, break it open with a restriction endonuclease leaving sticky ends, provide a length of the DNA he wishes to clone prepared with complementary sticky ends, add DNA ligase, and reintroduce to a population of bacteria in the presence of Ca^{2+}.

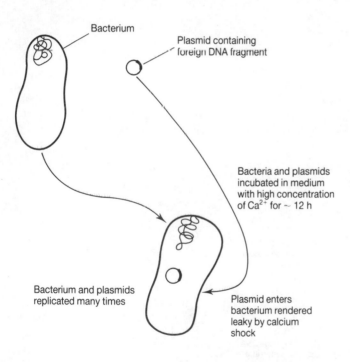

Bacterium

Plasmid containing foreign DNA fragment

Bacteria and plasmids incubated in medium with high concentration of Ca^{2+} for ~ 12 h

Bacterium and plasmids replicated many times

Plasmid enters bacterium rendered leaky by calcium shock

Figure 5.6 Cloning DNA using a plasmid vector

Phage. Bacteriophages (= bacterial viruses) or phage provide alternative vectors which, as we shall see, have some advantages. The phage injects its DNA into its bacterial host much as if it were a tiny syringe. Some of this DNA is copied by the host cell's mRNA and translated into protein in the usual way, whilst other copies of the phage DNA are incorporated into the host's DNA

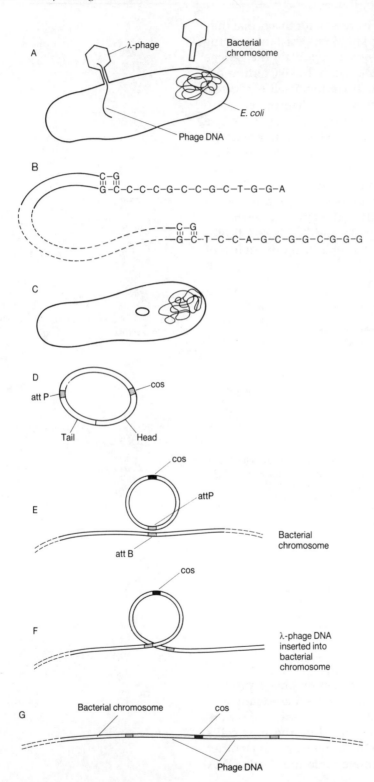

Figure 5.7 Insertion of λ-phage DNA into *E.coli* chromosome. (A) λ-phage is shown injecting its DNA into *E.coli*. (B) λ-phage DNA has two 'sticky' or 'cohesive' (cos) ends. (C) The cos ends ensure that λ-phage DNA circularises in *E.coli*. (D) Enlarged view of plasmid-like λ-phage DNA. The cos site is marked. This is followed by a sequence of genes programming the structure of the head and tail regions of the phage. Lastly there is a region labelled attP which is able to attach to a region (attB) of the bacterial chromosome. (E) attP of the phage DNA finds attB on the bacterial chromosome. (F) Union between the bacterial and phage DNA occurs. (G) The loop straightens out leaving λ-phage incorporated in *E.coli* chromosome as a 'provirus'

by its own DNA polymerase enzymes. In the case of the phage most used for cloning (**λ-phage**) the injected DNA first circularises and is then inserted into the host's chromosome.

The great advantage of phage as a vector for cloning is that it is able to carry far longer stretches of DNA than a bacterial plasmid. Plasmids, being very small, generally become unstable if DNA lengths of more than 1000 or so base pairs (bp) are spliced in. The DNA of phage vectors, such as λ-phage, on the other hand, being much lengthier (48 513 bp), can carry fragments up to 15 000 bp (15 kbp) with ease. Still larger fragments (35–45 kbp) can be cloned using a specially modified λ-phage known as a cosmid.

Cosmids. The preparation of a cosmid is a somewhat complex affair. In essence what is done is to make use of the discovery that λ-phage first makes its 'head' capsid and then has to find a way to package its 48.5 kbp DNA within it. A length of λ-phage DNA consists of a 35 or 45 kbp coding sequence spliced between two short stretches of 'sticky' single-stranded polynucleotide. Because these two ends are complementary they join so that the DNA forms a circle when injected into a bacterium. The join is referred to as the ***cos*** site. During the lytic stage of the phage's life cycle hundreds of copies of λ-DNA are synthesised and their *cos* sites join together end to end to form a long chain or **concatamer**. In the assembly of the next generation of λ-phage a group of enzymes, the **λ-packaging enzymes**, recognise the *cos* sites and break the λ-DNA up into appropriate segments for packaging into the phage heads. It is this feature of λ-phage's biology which is used by the gene cloner. As long as the *cos* sites are untouched the λ-packaging enzymes will unconcernedly do their packaging job no matter what lies between the sites.

The trick used by the genetic engineer is to cut off the *cos* sites from the λ-DNA and clone them in a plasmid. He then breaks open the plasmid with an appropriate restriction endonuclease and inserts a stretch of eukaryotic DNA prepared with a similar endonuclease. It is vital that the eukaryotic DNA is of the correct length: 35–45 kbp. The λ-packaging enzymes are now added and any stretches of eukaryotic DNA of the right length with *cos* sites at each end will be packaged into λ-phage. The phage is now used to infect *E.coli*. When the eukaryotic DNA–*cos* hybrid reaches the interior of the bacterium it exists and replicates as a plasmid.

This rather complicated procedure is, as might be expected, rather less efficient than using straightforward phage or plasmid cloning. Nevertheless it is invaluable if long stretches of DNA such as make up many mammalian genes or *a fortiori* two or more linked genes are to be analysed.

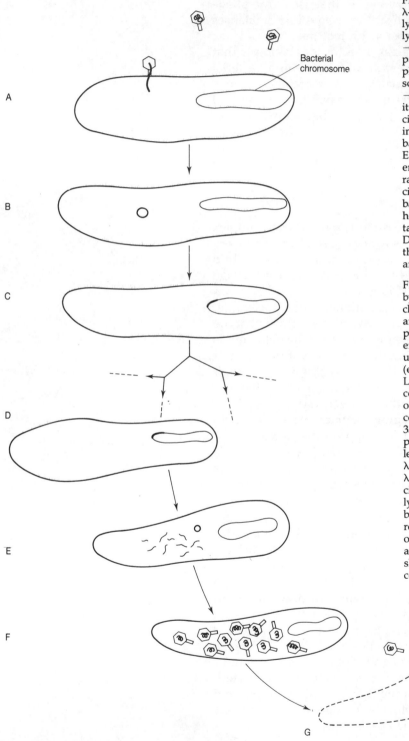

Figure 5.8. Life-cycle of λ-phage. λ-phage life cycle can take two paths: the lysogenic and the lytic. Usually only the lytic path is taken (i.e. (A) → (B) → (E) → (F) → (G)); more rarely the lysogenic pathway involving incorporation of the phage DNA with the bacterial chromosome occurs (i.e. (A) → (B) → (C) → (D) → (E) → (F) → (G)). (A) λ-phage injects its DNA into *E.coli*. (B) λ-phage DNA circularises. (C) λ-phage DNA integrates into the host chromosome and the bacterium multiplies many times. (D) Exposure of the bacterium to some environmental insult (e.g. UV or ionising radiation) releases the phage DNA which circularises. (E) The phage DNA uses the bacterial enzymes to synthesise fresh viral head and tail units. (F) The viral head and tail units are assembled and the phage DNA circle is broken and packaged into the head. (G) λ-phage lyses the bacteria and escapes to begin a new life cycle

Figure 5.9 Cloning of eukaryotic genes by the cosmid technique. The cos sites are cloned in a plasmid vector which contains an antibiotic resistance gene (R). The plasmid is digested with a restriction enzyme and the same endonuclease is used to cleave the eukaryotic DNA (eDNA) which it is desired to clone. Ligase is added to the mixture and a complex set of fragments results. Some of these fragments will, however, consists of two cos sites separated by 35–45 kbp of eukaryotic DNA. The λ-packaging enzymes recognise such lengths and proceed to package them into λ-phage heads. These then infect *E.coli*. λ-phage–eukaryote recombinant DNA circularises through its cos sites (as in the lytic phase shown in Fig. 5.8) and the bacterium divides many times. The recombinant DNA circle consists mostly of eukaryotic DNA but also possesses the antibiotic resistance gene. This, as we shall see, is vital for selecting the bacteria containing the recombinant DNA ⟶

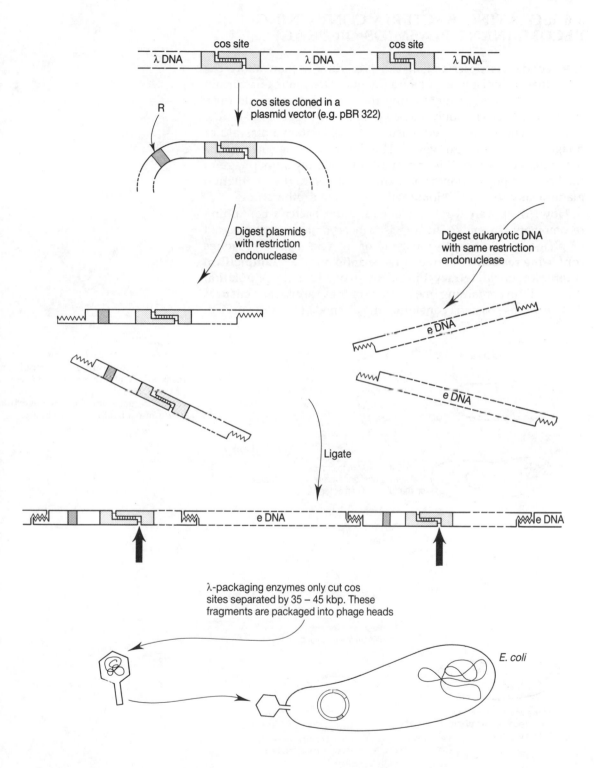

5.6 ISOLATING BACTERIA CONTAINING RECOMBINANT PLASMIDS OR PHAGE

The techniques described in the preceding section allow the molecular biologist to insert a fragment of DNA into a bacterium such as *E.coli* and (remembering that bacteria can divide once every 20 minutes) multiply it a billion-fold in the space of 24 hours.

But, of course, not every bacterium will contain a plasmid or phage with a foreign gene. The insertion step, it will be remembered, is very 'hit and miss'. One simply adds phage to the bacterial population or, if using plasmids, to the population made 'leaky' by Ca^{2+}. Some will be infected, others not.

How, then, can we select out only the bacteria containing recombinant plasmids? The trick is to incorporate into the plasmid or phage in addition to the gene of interest a gene or genes conferring **resistance** to one or more antibiotics, e.g. **ampicillin**, **chloramphenicol**, **tetracycline**. Growth of a bacterial population on a medium containing one or more of these antibiotics ensures that only those bacteria containing the plasmid of interest survive.

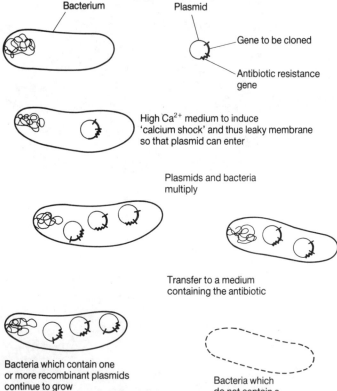

Figure 5.10 Procedure for selecting bacteria containing recombinant plasmids. Only those bacteria which possess plasmids expressing an antibiotic resistance gene survive challenge by a medium containing the antibiotic

5.7 THE 'SHOTGUN' CONSTRUCTION OF 'GENOMIC' GENE LIBRARIES

If a eukaryotic genome is cleaved by a number of restriction endo-nucleases and inserted into plasmids or phage and these are in turn grown up inside bacteria as described above we end up with what has been termed a '**genomic DNA library**'. This is often called the 'shotgun approach'. It is as if we attacked a colony of bacteria with a shot-gun full of genes and fragments of genes—very much a hit and miss affair. All the eukaryotic genes should be present in the bacterial population. But if we are interested in a particular gene, and in practical circumstances we always are, there is a horrific 'needle-in-the-haystack' problem. How can we possibly find the gene of interest amongst the tens of millions of others? It has been remarked that although we may have a library, we lack an index. Indeed its much worse—we do not really

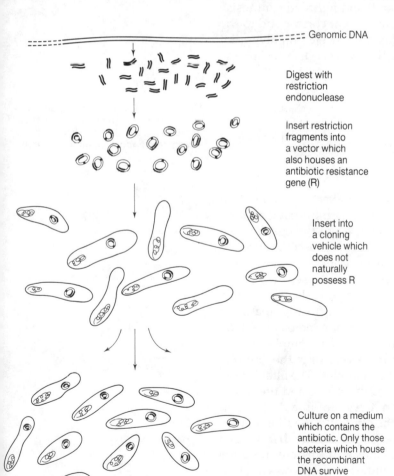

Genomic DNA

Digest with restriction endonuclease

Insert restriction fragments into a vector which also houses an antibiotic resistance gene (R)

Insert into a cloning vehicle which does not naturally possess R

Culture on a medium which contains the antibiotic. Only those bacteria which house the recombinant DNA survive

Figure 5.11 'Shotgun' construction of a 'genomic' gene library have a library at all, just a higgledy-piggledy heap of books! Even worse still the genes (books) may be in fragments, some parts in one plasmid, others in another, and some of the material may be just so much meaningless scribbling, not a book or part of a book at all, in other words it may be an intron or part of an intron.

5.8 A TECHNIQUE FOR FINDING A GENE IN THE LIBRARY

Let us look at a way by which we may fish out the DNA we are interested in. Suppose that we know the **amino acid sequence**, or even a short stretch of the amino acid sequence, of the protein we are interested in. It will then be possible, knowing the genetic code, to synthesise a short stretch of RNA which corresponds to that sequence. It is, of course, important to bear in mind the degeneracy of the code (see Chapter 2) and hence to synthesise **all the possible RNA sequences** which might correspond to the amino acid chain. Next we make this RNA stretch highly radioactive. We now have a **probe** by which we can fish for a gene in the library.

NH_2 --------- Tyr — Trp —Cys — Arg ----------- COOH   Polypeptide

$5'$—UA^U_C—UGC—UG^U_C—AG^A_G—$3'$ mRNA coding sequence incorporating a radioisotope label

Figure 5.12 Construction of an oligo-nucleotide probe from a short amino acid sequence. The longer the oligonucleotide sequence the more accurate the probe

The next step depends on replicating the **exact spatial** location of the bacterial colonies in the culture dish on a nitrocellulose filter. This is done by pressing the filter down on to the culture dish when some members of each of the colonies will become attached (see Figure 5.13). When this has been done we subject the replicated colonies to **alkali digestion**, which releases their DNA, binds it to the filter and, finally, opens up the double helices, thus exposing their complementary surfaces. After further treatment to remove proteins and other contaminants the radioactive RNA probe is added. Given time the probe will find its complementary surface. The longer the probe the more certain is the complementarity and the firmer the DNA–RNA duplex. The filter is now thoroughly washed to get rid of unbound probe and the radioactivity localised by placing it on an X-ray film in a dark room. **If the geography of the colonies on the nitrocellulose filter exactly copies the geography of the colonies in the culture dish** we can go back to the latter and pick out the culture which holds the gene of interest. This colony is replated and grown up knowing that it contains the gene of interest. In practice this procedure is repeated several times to eliminate 'false positive' results. In the end, however, one can be reasonably certain that the one has found the plasmid containing the gene one is looking for. This sequence of operations is shown in Figure 5.13.

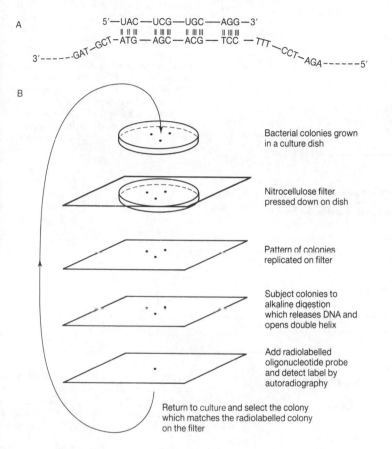

Bacterial colonies grown in a culture dish

Nitrocellulose filter pressed down on dish

Pattern of colonies replicated on filter

Subject colonies to alkaline digestion which releases DNA and opens double helix

Add radiolabelled oligonucleotide probe and detect label by autoradiography

Return to culture and select the colony which matches the radiolabelled colony on the filter

Figure 5.13 Using an oligonucleotide probe to 'fish' for a gene in a gene library

(A) The short oligonucleotide probe synthesised in Fig. 5.12 is shown hybridising with a complementary stretch of single stranded DNA. (B) The figure shows the sequence of steps used to detect which bacterial colony contains plasmids incorporating the gene coding for the polypeptide of interest

5.9 CONSTRUCTION OF A 'cDNA' GENE LIBRARY

An alternative method by which to construct a gene library involves the use of of an enzyme obtained from some RNA tumour viruses—**reverse transcriptase**. As its name indicates this enzyme is able to reverse the transcription step in protein biosynthesis and synthesise DNA alongside an mRNA template. This process is shown in Figure 5.14. The result is first a **single-stranded complementary DNA ((ss) cDNA)** which can be converted by DNA polymerase 1 into **double-stranded cDNA ((ds) cDNA))**, the two strands of which are connected by a hairpin loop; finally an **S1 nuclease** is used to remove this loop and produce a true double-stranded cDNA.

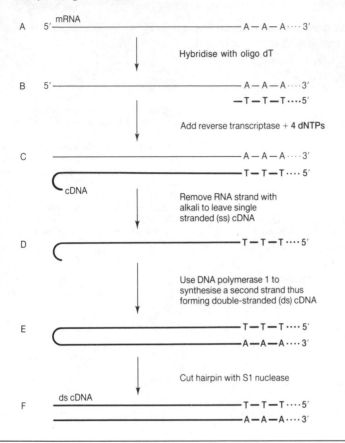

Figure 5.14 Action of reverse transcriptase in synthesising cDNA complementary to an mRNA strand. We noted in Chapter 3 that mRNA usually possesses a lengthy polyA tail. This is made use of in synthesising a primer for reverse transcriptase activity. It is base paired with a length of deoxythymidines (dTs). The reverse transcriptase enzyme makes use of this primer to synthesise a DNA strand alongside the mRNA. The latter is removed by alkali digestion. The remaining (ss)cDNA has a hairpin loop at its 3′ end. This acts as a primer for the synthesis of a complementary strand by DNA polymerase 1. The hairpin loop is cut away by S1 nuclease leaving double-stranded (ds) cDNA. RNA is shown light and DNA bold

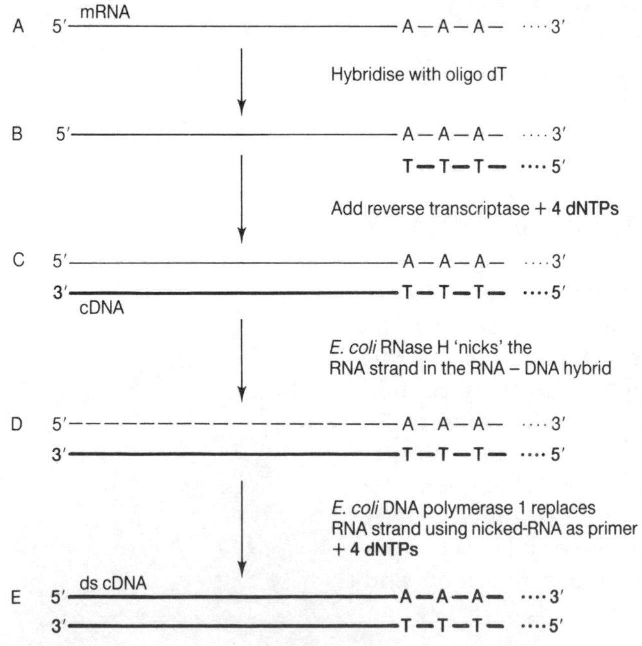

Figure 5.15 Preparation of cDNA using a nick translation technique. The first three steps ((A), (B) and (C)) in the synthesis are the same as in the previous figure. In step (D) *E.coli* RNase H is used to 'nick' the mRNA strand and in step (E) DNA polymerase 1 makes use of the RNA fragments as primers, the ss cDNA as template and the four dNTPs to synthesise ds cDNA. RNA is shown light and DNA bold

Another and somewhat more efficient means of constructing a cDNA library is to make use of a variant of the nick translation mechanism touched on in Section 4.1.2. This technique eliminates the necessity to use S1 nuclease to digest away the hairpin loop which acted as primer in the previous technique and consequently does not risk the loss of significant sequences of cDNA. The main steps of the nick translation technique are shown in Figure 5.15. Reverse transcriptase is once again used to synthesise a complementary DNA strand alongside an mRNA template provided with an oligo(dT) primer. Next an RNase (not a DNase as discussed in Chapter 4) is used to nick the RNA in the RNA–DNA hybrid. DNA polymerase 1 is then used to replace the nicked RNA strand with a DNA strand using the RNA fragments as primers.

Whichever technique is used it is clear that cDNA provides an alternative way of cloning. Instead of using restriction endonucleases to break up a genome (Figure 5.11) one can take the **mRNA from a tissue or cell population** and copy it into cDNA.

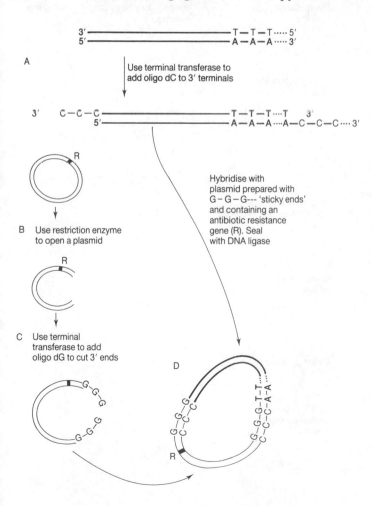

Figure 5.16 Cloning with cDNA. (A) Terminal transferase is used to add an oligo-dC sequence to the 3′ ends of the cDNA. (B) An appropriate plasmid is opened with a restriction enzyme to produce blunt-ended strands. (C) Terminal transferase is used to add an oligo-dG sequence to the the 3′ blunt ends. (D) DNA ligase is used to seal the cDNA into the plasmid. Amplification can now be induced in the usual way

This is obviously of great value if one is looking for **tissue-specific proteins**—as one frequently is in molecular neurobiology. A **terminal transferase** enzyme is then used to add a homopolymer tail of nucleotides to the 3' end of each strand of the cDNA double helix and the result inserted into a suitably prepared vector. This sequence of steps is shown in Figure 5.16.

The cDNA library prepared in this way will (in theory) contain all the genes which are being transcribed at the time in the tissue examined. It will, however, be biased towards the genes which are being most actively transcribed at that time. Nevertheless the library may include genes whose existence, and whose product, was otherwise unknown.

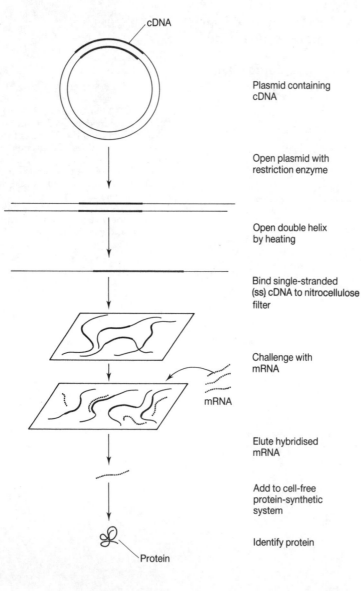

cDNA

Plasmid containing
cDNA

Open plasmid with
restriction enzyme

Open double helix
by heating

Bind single-stranded
(ss) cDNA to nitrocellulose
filter

Challenge with
mRNA

mRNA

Elute hybridised
mRNA

Add to cell-free
protein-synthetic
system

Identify protein

Protein

Figure 5.17   Identification of a gene in a cDNA library by translation of complementary mRNA and identification of the product. This procedure depends on the protein being easily identified by physiological, biochemical or immunological techniques

5.10 FISHING FOR GENES IN A cDNA LIBRARY

There are several procedures for finding the gene of interest in a cDNA library. One much used technique (as we shall see in subsequent chapters) is analogous to that described in Section 5.8. It depends on the amino acid sequence of at least a small section of the gene product being known. If this is the case then an oligonucleotide probe can be prepared—as described in Section 5.8. The cDNA corresponding to the protein can then be 'fished' out by the hybridisation technique described.

Another technique (Figure 5.17) depends on the identification of a gene product by immunological, biochemical or patch-clamping physiological techniques (for the last of these techniques see Chapter 9). In this procedure plasmids containing cDNA are created as described in Section 5.9. It can be arranged that in a colony of bacteria no cell receives more than *one* plasmid. The cells are then separately cloned, lysed, their plasmids extracted, the DNA double helices broken open by heating, the resultant single-stranded DNA bound to nitrocellulose filters, and finally challenged with mixtures of mRNA obtained from the tissue. Only complementary mRNA will be bound. This can later be separated, added to a **cell-free protein-synthetic system** and protein manufactured. **It may then be possible to identify the protein by standard biochemical, immunological or physiological techniques.** Having put aliquots of the cDNA clones on one side during the procedure one can now go back to them and pick out the clone which contains the gene. The cDNA in this clone can then be **amplified** by recloning and its nucleotide sequence determined.

5.11 SEQUENCE ANALYSIS OF CLONED DNA

The most important application of recombinant DNA techniques in molecular neurobiology has (to date) been in the analysis of the primary sequence (and hence structure and function) of neurobiologically important proteins and polypeptides. We shall meet many examples of this as we proceed through this book. Once the gene corresponding to a protein or polypeptide has been isolated by one or other of the techniques described above it can be inserted into a plasmid or phage and amplified by cloning.

This amplification has proved very important. Several powerful techniques have been developed for sequencing DNA. They all depend on the availability of adequate quantities of DNA 'purified' by one or other of the procedures described above. The two best-known sequencing techniques are those developed by Maxam and Gilbert and by Sanger. Gilbert and Sanger shared a Nobel prize (Sanger's second) for this development in 1980. It is now considerably easier to sequence a stretch of DNA than to determine the amino acid sequence of its protein. Indeed workers at Caltech have recently automated the Sanger sequencing technique. Their 'DNA sequenator' is able to read DNA at a rate of up to 8000 bases/day to an accuracy of about 1%: an order of magnitude greater than had previously been possible. It follows that far more proteins are nowadays sequenced by prediction from their DNA codes than have ever been worked out by direct analysis.

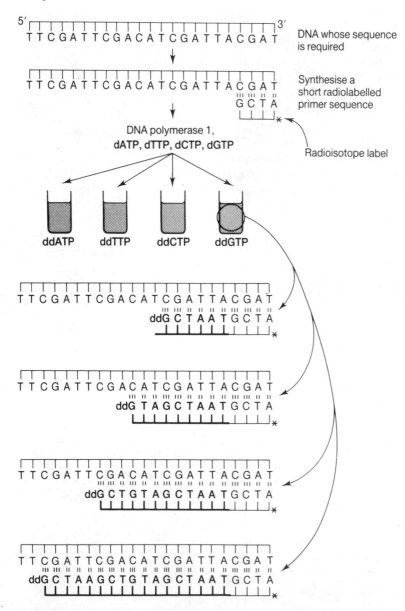

Figure 5.18   Sequence analysis of cloned DNA. The unknown DNA sequence is shown at the top of the figure. A short radioactively labelled primer is synthesised against its 3' end. A reaction mixture of the four deoxribonucleotide triphosphates and DNA polyymerase 1 is prepared in four reaction vessels. A different dideoxynucleotide triphosphate (ddNTP) is introduced into each reaction vessel. The synthesis is allowed to proceed. It is shown that in the right-hand vessel a complementary DNA strand is synthesised alongside the template DNA until a ddG is incorporated. This inhibits any further elongation. As ddG is incorporated randomly a series of fragments of different lengths results. Similar reactions are occurring in the other vessels with the other ddNTPs creating different chain lengths. Finally (*facing page*) the DNA fragments are eluted and separated by electrophoresis. The shortest sequences travel furthest. The sequence of the original DNA can thus be read off the gel. (Modified from Alberts *et al.*, 1987, *Molecular Biology of the Gene*, Menlo Park, California: Academic Press.)

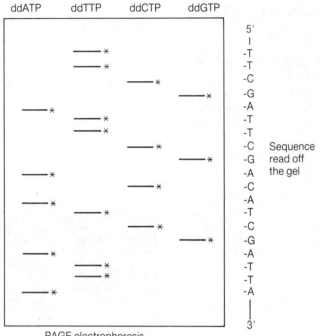

PAGE electrophoresis
Position of fragment detected
by autoradiography

Let us briefly look at **Sanger's technique**. The method is shown diagrammatically in Figure 5.18. It depends on the use of **dideoxynucleotides (ddNTPs)** which, lacking a hydroxyl group at the 3' position, are unable to form phosphodiester bonds with other nucleotides. The DNA strand whose sequence is required is mated with a short primer sequence (radioactively labelled) and incubated with DNA polymerase 1, the four deoxynucleotide triphosphates (dNTPs) and a small amount of one or other of the four dideoxynucleotides. Synthesis occurs, as shown in the figure, **until a ddNTP is incorporated**. This incorporation occurs at random. Hence a random collection of different lengths of DNA are synthesised. These random lengths are then subjected to **polyacrylamide gel electrophoresis (PAGE)**. The latter technique separates DNA fragments **according to their length**. It is able to distinguish between fragments differing in length by just one nucleotide. The position of the fragments on the gel is detected by autoradiography.

As Figure 5.18 shows, four different reactions are run using the four different ddNTPs: ddATP, ddCTP, ddGTP and ddTTP. The reaction products are run alongside each other. By carefully examining the position of the polynucleotide fragments on the gel the nucleotide sequence can be deduced.

5.12 PROKARYOTIC EXPRESSION VECTORS FOR EUKARYOTIC DNA

In some circumstances it is possible to get a bacterial cell to manufacture the protein specified by eukaryotic cDNA. This is of importance in neurobiology where often only very small quantities of a protein or polypeptide are synthesised. It has already been emphasised that the diversity of neuronal proteins exceeds that of other tissues by anything up to five times.

In order to express the information held in the cDNA it is necessary to insert it into an **expression vector**. An example of

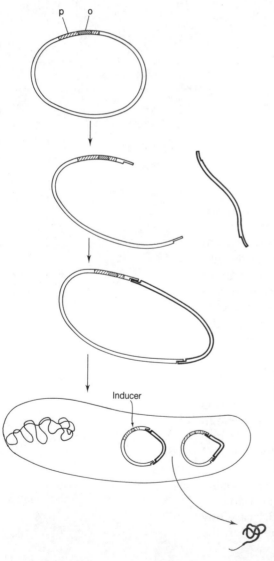

Plasmid with
bacterial promoter (p)
and operator (o) sites

Open plasmid with
restriction
endonuclease

Eukaryotic DNA
prepared with same
restriction enzyme

Seal recombinant
plasmid with
DNA ligase

Insert plasmid into
E. coli and allow
to replicate

Challenge *E. coli*
with appropriate
inducer

Eukaryotic protein
synthesised with
a short
N-terminal bacterial
sequence

Figure 5.19 Expression of a eukaryotic gene by an *E.coli* plasmid. The promoter and operator sequences of *E.coli's lac* operon (see Fig. 3.11) have been inserted into a plasmid. The plasmid is cut with a restriction enzyme and a similarly cleaved fragment of eukaryotic DNA is inserted and ligated. The recombinant plasmid is inserted into *E.coli* and allowed to replicate. In response to the appropriate inducer (in the case of the *lac* operon, lactose) the operon is switched on and the message in the eukaryotic DNA translated into protein. The short length of bacterial polypeptide at the N-terminal end of this protein can usually be removed

such a vector is a plasmid, for instance pBR322, into which has been inserted the **promoter and operator sequences of the** *lac* **operon** from *E.coli*. If a eukaryotic cDNA sequence is inserted next to this region it will sometimes be expressed when the inducer (in this case lactose) is presented. Up to 100 mg of pure eukaryotic protein (for instance proinsulin) have been obtained by this technique. It should be emphasised, however, that it has not proved possible, so far, to express more than a very few eukaryotic genes in bacterial systems. Eukaryotic genes mostly have their own expression signals and also seem to depend on the environment provided by the eukaryotic cell. Indeed attempts to use *E.coli* to manufacture biomedically important proteins on a commercial scale have been fraught with difficulty and disappointment.

5.13 *XENOPUS* OOCYTE AS AN EXPRESSION VECTOR FOR MEMBRANE PROTEINS

One of the best expression vehicles for eukaryotic genes is the large oocyte of *Xenopus*, the clawed toad. This cell may be up to 1 mm in diameter. It is primed, ready to develop into a toad after maturation and fertilisation. It possesses all the appropriate transcriptional and translational machinery in large amounts and 'well-oiled' condition.

mRNA from other cells can be injected into it through a glass micropipette. These mRNAs succeed where endogenous mRNAs—probably due to inhibition by specific binding proteins—fail. The first eukaryotic mRNA to be successfully translated by this system was that coding for rabbit haemoglobin. The oocyte translated this mRNA and manufactured the protein far more efficiently than cell-free systems.

Neurobiologists are particularly interested in membrane proteins—receptors, channels, pumps, etc. The first neuro-biological protein to be expressed by this system was **nAChR**. The mRNA was cloned from the electric organ of the electric ray *Torpedo marmorata* and then injected into *Xenopus* oocyte. It was shown that **functional nAChR channels** appeared in the oocyte membrane. The oocyte translation machinery was thus able to read the *Torpedo* mRNA, synthesise the protein, and perform the post-translational processing required to glycosylate, assemble the subunits, and insert the whole complex in the membrane.

The presence of ACh activated channels in the oocyte membrane could be demonstrated by standard physiological techniques. Their properties seem almost (though possibly not quite) identical to their properties in the nervous system.

Many other chemical- and voltage-activated channels have

subsequently been expressed in *Xenopus* oocyte. These include **GABA-activated channels** from the chick brain; **ACh-activated channels** from cat muscle; **serotonin-, neurotensin-** and **substance P-activated channels** from rat brain; **kainate** and **glycine** receptors from bovine retina; **glycine-, GABA-** and **serotonin-activated channels** from human fetal cerebrum, and **voltage-activated Na⁺** and **K⁺ channels** from rat and human fetal brain and cat muscle.

It is clear that the *Xenopus* oocyte is an extremely valuable system for molecular neurobiology. It enables one to transplant, so to speak, molecular entities from regions (brain, retina, etc.) where they may be exceedingly difficult to study to a robust system where they can be investigated at leisure. Moreover **site-directed mutagenesis** (to be outlined in the next section) allows the neurobiologist to slightly alter the mRNA message and thus cause the synthesis of slightly different channel proteins. This allows the investigation of structure–function relationships: how much, for instance, does the alteration of one amino acid at a known and specific point in the channel affect its physiological properties? Finally the oocyte system can be used in a sense backwards: that is it can be used to express an unknown mRNA. If physiological investigation of the oocyte membrane subsequently shows it to possess a rare channel then the cloning methods described in the preceding sections allow for the amplification of the mRNA and determination of the channel-protein primary sequence.

5.14 SITE-DIRECTED MUTAGENESIS

Recombinant DNA technology also enables us to carry out a sort of 'reverse genetics'. Instead of finding a phenotypic change and *then* looking to see which genes have caused this change and how, we can now proceed in the reverse direction: we can engineer a known change in a gene and then observe the phenotypic result.

One of the most interesting and powerful of these techniques involves the insertion of one or more altered nucleotides into a gene. In this way one can arrange matters so that the gene codes for a protein with one or more unusual amino acids at specific points in its primary sequence.

In order to achieve this result one has first to determine the base sequence of a cloned DNA molecule. It is then possible to synthesise an oligonucleotide of some ten to fifteen bases, complementary to the region of interest, but with **a few mismatches**. This oligonucleotide is then mixed with single-stranded DNA from the cloned gene and provided the hybridisation conditions are correct complementary base pairing will take place. The mismatched base pairs will form a tiny loop in the

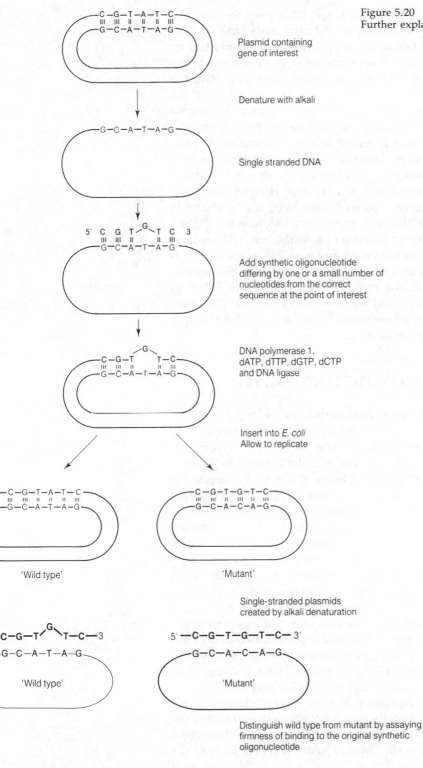

Figure 5.20 Site-directed mutagenesis. Further explanation is given in the text

middle of the oligonucleotide sequence. DNA polymerase 1 will then synthesise a complementary strand to the rest of the plasmid using the **mismatched sequence as a primer**. The plasmid is then inserted into *E.coli*, where it wil replicate in the usual way. The outcome of the replication is two different types of plasmid: a 'wild-type' and a **mutant**.

The final thing which has to be done is to separate the mutant plasmid from the wild-type. This can be done by creating a single-stranded plasmid by alkali denaturation and then using **a radio-labelled oligonucleotide identical to the inserted mutant sequence**. This will find and label the mutant plasmid. But it is likely (especially if only one or a very few base changes have been made) to find the wild-type as well. However, if one begins to raise the temperature the wild-type begins to lose its slightly mismatched probe sooner than the perfectly matched mutant. Thus the mutant can be detected and its DNA retrieved. It is usually sequenced to make quite sure that it contains the desired mutation. If all is well the mutant DNA can be amplified by cloning in the usual way and then introduced into an expression vector if the structure or (more usually) the function of the slightly altered protein is to be examined.

5.15 HYBRIDISATION HISTOCHEMISTRY

So far in this chapter we have been considering some of the ways in which our understanding of molecular biology are enabling us to manipulate nucleic acids and the proteins for which they code. In this penultimate section we shall look briefly at a technique which uses this manipulative ability to investigate the anatomy of the central nervous system. This is the technique which has come to be known as hybridisation histochemistry.

We have already noted that the brain is the most heterogeneous of the body's organs. Neuronanatomists, for instance, recognise more than 50 distinct cell types in a structure as comparatively simple as the retina. We have already noted that the brain itself expresses upwards of 125 000 different mRNAs. These messengers specify the multitude of different molecular structures, the neuropeptides, the transmitter-related enzymes, the receptor molecules, etc., which characterise different regions, and different cells, of the brain. Hybridisation histochemistry aims to detect these different mRNAs *in situ*. The technique thus complements other powerful histological techniques such as histo- and cytochemistry, immunohisto- and immunocytochemistry, etc.

In essence *in situ* hybridisation histochemistry involves the production of RNA or cDNA probes complementary to the mRNA being expressed in the cell. The mRNA strands are isolated by the cloning techniques discussed in the preceding sections of this chapter. Probes complementary to the strands are synthesised and then applied to histological sections (frozen or paraffin wax) of the brain or other parts of the nervous system. If the probes find complementary mRNA in the tissue section they attach by Watson–Crick base-pairing; if no complementary mRNA is present in the tissue they can by washed out of the section.

The probes must, of course, be attached to an entity which can be visualised in the microscope. There are many ways in which this can be done. One of the first but still one of the most popular techniques is that of nick translation (Section 4.1.2). In the majority of cases the entity attached is a radioisotope: ^{35}S, ^{32}P or ^{3}H. The location of the probe, after unbound probe has been washed off, can then be located by autoradiography. Radioisotopes are not, however, the only markers available. Various other means of labelling the probe have been tried, including enzymes, fluorochromes and mercury. Perhaps the most promising non-radioactive marker is biotin. This small molecule can be attached to the probe by nick translation and detected in sections prepared for both the light and the electron microscope. It should be noted, however, that the procedure is complex. Biotin cannot be visualised on its own. The techniques of immunocytochemistry are used to conjugate silver or gold particles to the biotin and it is the latter which is ultimately detected in the section.

This short resumé serves to indicate the latent power of the technique. Needless to say the technique is complicated and time-consuming. But, used with caution and in conjunction with other histo- and cytochemical techniques, *in situ* hybridisation promises the development of a truly functional molecular neuroanatomy.

5.16 CONCLUSION

It will have become apparent from the foregoing pages of this chapter that the techniques emerging from molecular biology are wide-ranging, powerful and advancing with great rapidity. They are revolutionising our understanding of biology, including neurobiology.

We have, of course, only scratched the surface of an enormous subject. The techniques outlined, however, have proved of crucial importance in neurobiology. We shall see in the next few chapters that our understanding of the many membrane pumps, receptors and channels which underly the phenomena of neurophysiology has been revolutionised by their application. Membrane proteins, for instance, are notoriously difficult to isolate and analyse. Were it not for recombinant DNA techniques they would have retained their mystery for far longer than now seems likely. Moreover, as we noted in Section 5.14, molecular biology nowadays promises more than 'passive' analysis and understanding. It also promises action and control. Site-directed mutagenesis holds out the prospect of changing the structure of defined parts of neuro-biological proteins. Expression systems such as the *Xenopus* oocyte provide means of studying the functioning of these subtly altered proteins in isolation. Further into the future one can dimly foresee a time when our knowledge of molecular structure and our control over the reverse transcriptases of retroviruses could allow us to attempt gene therapy: i.e. to replace the defective genes respons-ible for neuropatholgies such as PKU, Tay-Sachs disease, Huntingdon's disease and many others (see Chapter 19). If and when such a time comes it will bring a host of problems: financial, legal, ethical. We are already grappling with the outriders of these coming events. It will be essential to have a thorough grasp of the underlying science if rational judgements are to be made.

Chapter 6
Biomembranes

Fernández-Morán once pointed out that if all the membranes intricately folded within the human brain were to be flattened out they would cover the surface of the entire planet. This is a salutary thought. Any electron micrograph will show that the brain is packed full of membranes. Much of the physiology of the brain consists of fluxes of ions across them. We shall soon see that they are complex and heterogeneous down to the molecular level. Perhaps the brain's computing power becomes more understandable if we think of it as a planet-sized membrane operating at the molecular level, each part within at the most a second's communication time with any other.

Biological membranes are built of three molecular species: always **lipids** and **proteins** and in most cases **carbohydrates** as well. The lipids form a universal matrix whilst the carbohydrates and proteins confer specific biological properties.

6.1 LIPIDS

It has been computed that a small patch of membrane with an area of 1 μm^2 is built of some 5×10^6 lipid molecules. It can be shown that different membranes consist of slightly different lipid mixtures and thus have slightly different properties. The lipids found in biological membranes fall into three major groups: phospholipids, glycolipids and steroids (especially cholesterol). Let us look at each group in turn.

Phospholipids. Figure 6.1 shows the molecular structures of a group of four important membrane phospholipids, the **phospho-glycerides**: phosphatidyl choline (= lecithin), phosphatidy ethanolamine (= cephalin), phosphatidyl serine and phosphatidyl inositol. The figure shows that they all consist of two long **fatty acid** chains attached through **glycerol** and a **phosphate group** to a hydrophilic 'characterising group': **choline**, **ethanolamine**, **serine** or **inositol**.

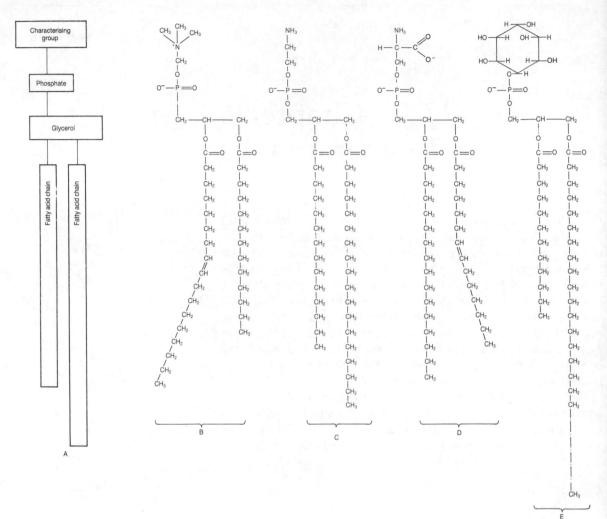

The important feature which all the molecules shown in Figure 6.1. share, so far as membrane structure is concerned, is that they are all **amphipathic** molecules. Moreover they are amphipathic in an interesting way. One end of the molecule, the nitrogen-containing or (in the case of phosphatidyl inositol) the carbohydrate-containing group, is **hydrophilic** whilst the fatty acid chains at the other end of the molecule are **hydrophobic**. This means that phospholipids will line up at an air–water or oil–water interface to form a **monomolecular** layer. The interfaces in cells, however, are always between two aqueous solutions. In such circumstances phospholipids form not monolayers but **bilayers** and in some cases **micelles**.

Phospholipid bilayers are, as may be guessed, extremely fragile structures. The forces holding them together are the same hydro-

Figure 6.1 Phosphogylcerides: (A) schematic diagram; (B) phosphatidyl choline (lecithin); (C) phosphatidyl ethanolamine (cephalin); (D) phosphatidyl serine; (E) phosphatidyl inositol. Note: the fatty acid chains are very variable

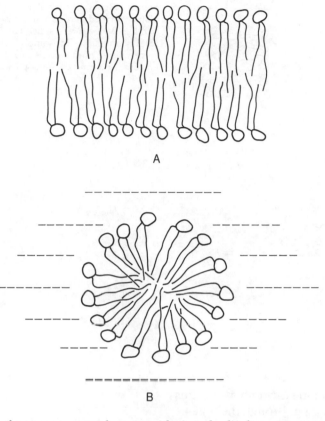

A

B

Figure 6.2 (A) Schematic to show a phospholipid bilayer. (B) Schematic to show a phospholipid micelle

phobic forces we met when considering the higher structures of proteins and nucleic acids. On the other hand if membranes or micelles are disrupted they quickly reseal. This spontaneous sealing is made use of in the formation of **artificial bilayers** and **liposomes**. Both structures have been of considerable use in molecular neurobiology. Artificial bilayers may be constructed across a small pore in a partition separating two aqueous solutions whilst liposomes form spontaneously from phospholipids or mixtures of phospholipids introduced into an aqueous phase of appropriate physico-chemical characteristics. We shall meet with both types of artificial membrane again in future chapters. We shall see that the study of purified channel proteins has been greatly assisted by inserting them into such structures.

The extremely tenuous nature of phospholipid bilayers also means that at room temperatures the individual molecules are in constant motion. Indeed the hydrophobic fatty acid 'tails' of the molecules have, in this respect, been likened to 'a basket of snakes', bending and twisting about in perpetual motion. The interior of the membrane is thus to all intents and purposes an organic fluid. The individual phospholipid molecules, moreover, continually exchange places with each other. They seldom migrate

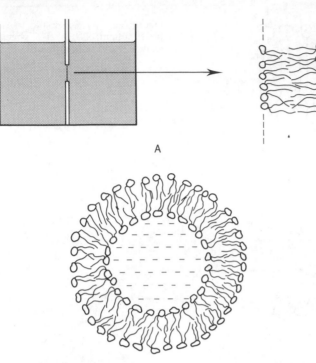

Figure 6.3 (A) Artificial phospholipid bilayer formed across a small hole in a partition between two aqueous solutions. (B) Phospholipd liposome. Note liposomes differ from micelles in that they enclose a volume of aqueous solution

(or 'flip-flop') from one side of the membrane to another—for this would mean their hydrophilic 'heads' passing through the organic phase in the centre of the membrane—but they move laterally within each lipid monolayer with considerable freedom. Indeed their diffusion coefficient is such that it is calculated that they have a lateral velocity (at 37 °C) of about 1 μm/s. This means that the average phospholipid (other things being equal) could travel from one end of an average nerve cell body (diameter, say, 20 μm) to the other in about 20 s. 'Other things', however, as we shall shortly see, are seldom 'equal'!

So far we have distinguished between phospholipids by way of their 'characterising heads': choline, ethanolamine, serine, etc. But phospholipids also differ in the nature of their fatty acid 'tails'. The number of carbon atoms in these tails may vary from 12 to 20. The carbon atoms, moreover, may be linked by **saturated (single)** or **unsaturated (double)** bonds. Both these features have an effect on the nature of the membrane. The shorter the fatty acid tail and the greater the unsaturation the greater the fluidity of the membrane. This is because both features make the tails more difficult to pack compactly within the membrane's core. We shall return to the topic of membrane fluidity when we have considered the nature of some of the other lipids making up the structure of biological membranes.

A

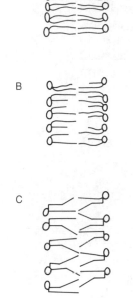

Figure 6.4 Lipid packing and membrane fluidity. (A) The phospholipid fatty acid 'tails' are all fully saturated and of about the same length: they therefore pack compactly. (B) The fatty acid 'tails' differ in length and thus the membrane core is more fluid; (C) the fatty acid 'tails' contain unsaturated bonds and hence, once again, the packing cannot be so tight and the membrane core tends to fluidity

B

C

A second important group of membrane lipids is based not on glycerol but on **sphingosine**. The structure of sphingosine is shown in Figure 6.5.

Figure 6.5 Sphingosine

OH
|
CH₂
|
H—C—NH₂
|
HO—C—H
|
CH
‖
CH
\
CH₂
/
CH₂
\
CH₂
/
CH₂
\
CH₂
/
CH₂
\
CH₂
/
CH₂
\
CH₂
/
CH₂
\
CH₂
/
CH₂
\
CH₃

Sphingosine, like the phosphoglycerides discussed above, is an amphipathic molecule. It possesses a hydrophilic 'head' containing an amino group and a long (13 carbon) saturated fatty acid hydrophobic tail. The 'head' bends round, rather like a hairpin, and forms a point of attachment for other molecules. Thus in cell membranes sphingosine is normally attached to another fatty acid chain to form **ceramide**. Ceramide, in its turn, is often attached through a **phosphate group** to choline to form a quite common membrane constituent: **sphingomyelin**.

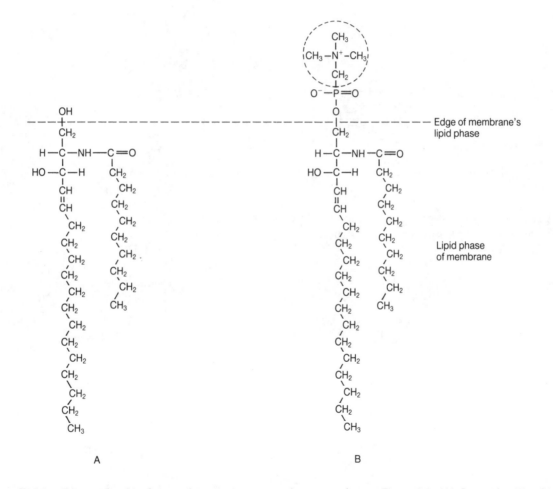

A   B

Glycolipids. Ceramide also forms the starting point for a number of other important constituents of animal cell membranes—the **glycolipids**. These complicated molecules are shown in Figure 6.7. Instead of being attached through a phosphate group to choline we find that ceramide forms a glycosidic linkage to a monosaccharide—**galactose** or **glucose**. **Galactocerebroside**, the simplest of these glycolipids, forms the major glycolipid of the

Figure 6.6 (A) Ceramide; (B) sphingomyelin

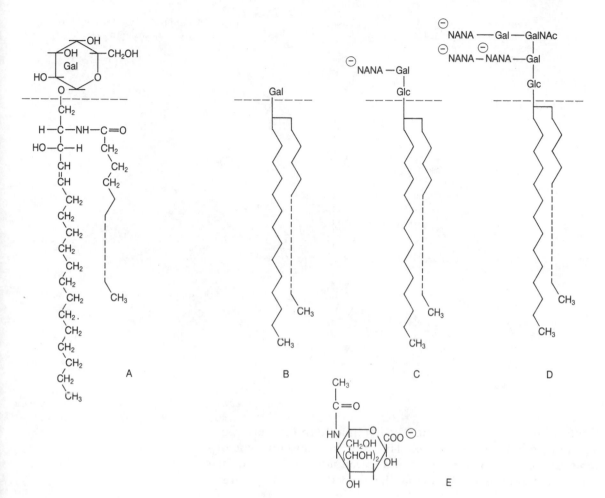

Figure 6.7 Some glycolipids. (A) Galactocerebroside; (B) schematic of galactocerebroside; (C) ganglioside G_{M3}; (D) ganglioside G_{T1}; (E) N-acetylneuraminic acid (NANA). Gangliosides are named according to the number of NANA groups (M = mono, D = di; T = tri, etc.) whilst the number refers to the number of sugar residues subtracted from five. Hence G_{M3} indicates that the ganglioside possesses one NANA and two sugars. Glc = glucose; Gal = galactose; GalNAc = N-acetylgalactosamine; NANA = N-acetylneuraminic acid (= sialic acid)

myelin sheath around axons (up to 40% of the outer monolayer). The other glycolipids, as Figure 6.7 shows, are more complicated molecules containing one or more **sialic acid (n-acetylneuraminic acid)** groups. There are, in fact, at least 30 different varieties. Collectively they are known as **gangliosides**. They are especially plentiful in the membranes of neurons.

Of particular importance in neurobiology is the ganglioside G_{M2}. This is normally transformed into G_{M3} by the enzyme hexosaminidase A. Young children who suffer from the inherited **Tay-Sachs** disease lack this enzyme. Hence G_{M2} accumulates in the nervous system. Cytoplasmic bodies begin to fill the neurons. Patients appear unaffected for the first five or six months of life but they then fail to develop normal mental and motor capacities. Death usually occurs by the third year although, in some cases of late onset, death is delayed until the fifth or sixth years.

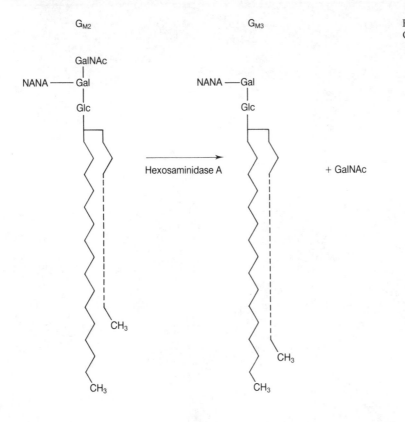

Figure 6.8   Transformation of G_{M2} into G_{M3} by hexosaminidase A

Cholesterol. There is one other type of lipid found in most biological membranes: **cholesterol**. This is a very different type of molecule to the phospholipids and gycolipids we have so far considered. Figure 6.9 shows that the molecule consists of three

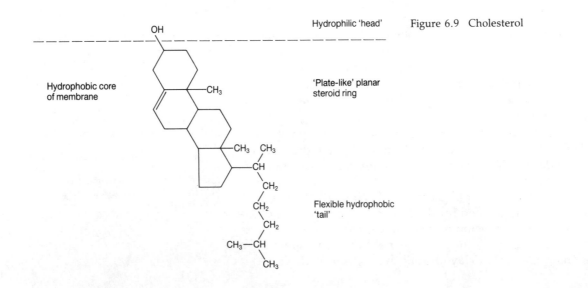

Figure 6.9   Cholesterol

different regions—a hydrophilic 'head' represented by the hydroxyl group, a flat plate-like steroid ring and a flexible hydrophobic 'tail'.

The amount of cholesterol present in biomembranes is very variable (see Table 6.1). Quite large amounts of it are found in some plasma membranes and in myelin, much smaller amounts in intracellular membranes such as ER and mitochondria, and none at all in prokaryotes such as *E.coli*. When it is present it is interpolated between the phospholipid molecules and reduces the fluidity of the membrane.

Table 6.1 Lipid composition of some membranes

Source	Approximate percentages of total extracted lipid								
	CHOL	PC	PE	PS	PI	SP	CE	GA	Oth.
Rat liver[a]									
Plasma memb.	30	18	11	9	4	14	–	–	1
ER (rough)	6	55	16	3	8	3	–	–	–
ER (smooth)	10	55	21	–	7	12	–	–	2
Mitochondria									
inner	3	45	24	1	6	3	–	–	19
outer	5	50	23	2	13	5	–	–	5
Nuclear	10	55	20	3	7	3	–	–	1
Golgi	8	40	15	4	6	10	–	–	–
Lysosomes	14	25	13	–	7	24	–	–	5
Erythrocyte[a]	24	31	15	7	2	9	–	–	
Glial plasma membrane[b]	36	25	7	5	–	5	12	–	8
Axon[c]	32	32	23	7	7	–	–	–	–
Synapse[c]	19	34	28	10	2	3	2	–	–
Myelin[b]	42	10	16	5	–	5	16	–	3
Grey matter[d]	22	26	22	8	3	7	5	7	–
E.coli[a]	0	0	80	–	–	–	–	–	20

CHOL = cholesterol; PC = phosphatidyl choline; PE = phosphatidyl ethanolamine; PS = phosphatidyl serine; PI = phosphatidyl inositol; SP = sphingomyelin; CE = cerebrosides; GA = gangliosides; Oth. = other lipids

Data: [a] Darnell, Lodish and Baltimore, 1986; [b] Bradford, 1985; [c] Cotman and Levy, 1975; [d] Siegel, Albers, Agranoff and Katzman, 1981

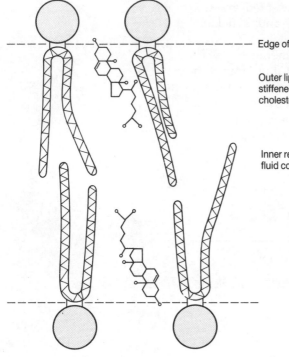

Figure 6.10 Interpolation of cholesterol in a phospholipid bilayer

Edge of lipid phase

Outer lipid layer stiffened by cholesterol

Inner relatively fluid core

6.2 MEMBRANE FLUIDITY

We have already noted that the fluidity of a biomembrane is determined to some extent by the length and saturation of the fatty acid chains forming its core. In artificial bilayers formed of a single phospholipid species there is a sharp **transition temperature**, characteristic of the particular phospholipid, from a gel state to a fluid state. This transition temperature varies in natural membranes, being higher if there is more cholesterol and a greater number of saturated fatty acid chains. As the lipid constitution of a membrane such as that which envelops a neuron must vary from place to place we must suppose that the fluidity also varies from place to place. The neuronal membrane thus can be looked at as if it were a patchwork of different fluidities.

6.3 MEMBRANE ASYMMETRY

Membranes are highly asymmetrical. This can be shown by both biochemical and electron microscopic techniques. The **freeze-fracture** method allows the electron microscopist to cleave the membrane along its plane of greatest weakness—the centre of the lipid bilayer (Figure 6.11). The outer monolayer (= outer 'leaflet') is defined as having an **'exoplasmic' or 'E' face** abutting the extracellular space and an **'exoplasmic fracture' or 'EF' face** which is the fracture plane. The inner monolayer (= inner 'leaflet') is, similarly, defined as having a **'protoplasmic fracture' or 'PF' face** (again the fracture plane) and a **'protoplasmic' or 'P' face** next to the protoplasm.

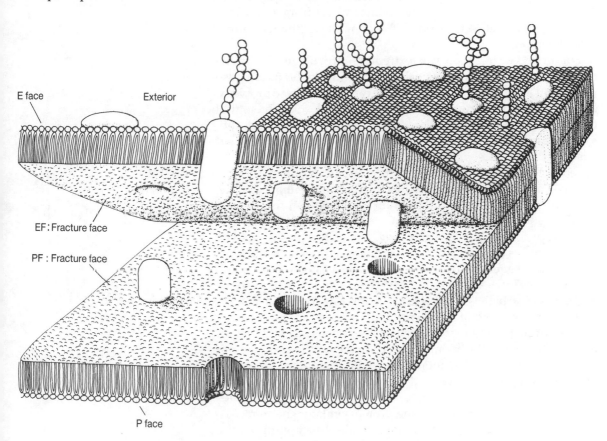

E face

Exterior

EF : Fracture face

PF : Fracture face

P face

One of the most striking asymmetries, so far as the lipids are concerned, involves the glycolipids. These are to be found almost exclusively in the outer monolayer and their oligosaccharide moieties extend from the E face into the extracellular compartment. It has been shown that they have much to do with the processes of cell–cell recognition.

It is also worth noting that significantly more phosphatidyl serine and phosphatidyl inositol are found in the inner monolayer or 'leaflet' than the outer. Reference to Figure 6.1 will show that these phospholipids bear a preponderating negative electrostatic charge. Hence we find that the P face is significantly more negative than the E face.

Figure 6.11 Freeze-fractured membrane showing positions of E, EF, PF and P faces. (Reproduced with permission from B. Satir, 1975, *Scientific American*, **233**(4), 29–37. Copyright © 1975 by Scientific American Inc. All rights reserved.)

6.4 PROTEINS

So far we have been discussing the universal scaffolding of biomembranes. Although the glycolipids are believed to be very
important in intercellular recognition the most important
functional characteristics of most biomembranes is conferred not
by their lipid but by their protein constitution. The quantity of
protein present in biological membranes varies from about 20%
of the mass (myelin) to about 75% of the mass (mitochondrial
inner membrane).

For many years it proved extremely difficult to determine
exactly where proteins were positioned in the membrane and also
the exact nature of the proteins which were there. These problems
have yielded to new biochemical and molecular biological
techniques. **Extraction** by the strong detergent **SDS** and subsequent analysis by **electrophoresis on SDS–polyacrylamide gel**
has been used to separate membrane proteins—more than 50
different types have have been distinguished in one membrane
(that of *E.coli*) alone. **Freeze-fracture etching**, as mentioned in the
previous section, allows the position of proteins in the interior
of the phospholipid bilayer to be examined by electron
microscopy. Last, but far from least, the techniques of genetic
engineering, as described in Chapter 5, are beginning to elucidate
the primary sequence of many membrane proteins.

Figure 6.11 has already indicated the position which proteins
are nowadays believed to occupy in the phospholipid matrix.
They form a mosaic of globular molecules in a flat lipid sea. It
is thus not surprising that this concept has been called the '**fluid-
mosaic**' model of the biomembrane. Some of the proteins are
confined to one or other monolayer, whereas others project all
the way through the bilayer and extend into both the extracellular
and intracellular compartments. We shall meet many examples
of these so-called transmembrane proteins in later chapters. We
shall see that they are fundamental to the functioning of the
nervous system.

In general we can say that transmembrane proteins are so
constructed that they possess a **hydrophobic region or domain**
which is embedded in the lipid core of the membrane and
hydrophilic regions which project into the aqueous extracellular
and intracellular compartments. In comparison with the globular
proteins of the aqueous cytosol the intramembranous domains
of membrane proteins are, in a sense, 'inside-out': their hydrophobic residues project outwards, while their hydrophilic residues
are tucked inside towards their cores. This ensures that they 'stick'
in the lipid bilayer. Membrane proteins, too, whether transmembrane, confined to a single monolayer or merely adhering
to a P or E face, are always asymmetrical. They are constructed

so that one part of their conformation interacts with the lipid bilayer in a specific way. Sometimes they make use of the fact, mentioned above, that the P face is electrically negative compared with the E face. Transmembrane proteins, moreover, never rotate or 'flip-flop' across the membrane—this would entail dragging their hydrophilic ends through the membrane's lipid core and this in normal circumstances is not possible.

Studies which involve the incorporation of enzymatic proteins into artificial lipid bilayers show that the activity of such proteins is conditioned by their lipid environment. Features of the lipid bilayer such as the length of the fatty acid chains, the degree of saturation, the nature of the lipid 'heads', all influence the biological activity of the enzyme. Just as water-soluble enzymes are affected by parameters of the aqueous environment such as pH, so lipid-embedded enzymes are affected by the precise nature of their lipid environment.

We shall meet many examples of transmembrane proteins in the next few chapters—receptors, pumps, ion channels. As an introductory example, however, let us take the very well-known case of **glycophorin**, a protein found in the erythrocyte membrane. Glycophorin, as Figure 6.12 shows, consists of some 131 amino acid residues of which 34 (numbers 62–95) are embedded in the lipid core of the membrane. The great majority of these are hydrophobic residues and one stretch of 23 residues (73–95) consists exclusively of such residues—phe, leu, ile, val,

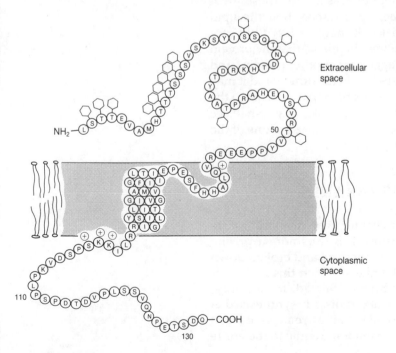

Figure 6.12 Glycophorin in the erythrocyte membrane. The amino acids are symbolised by their single letter codes (see Table 2.1). Oligosaccharide groups are represented by hexagons on the appropriate amino acid residues

try and tyr. It is believed that these residues take the form of an α-helix so that their hydrophobic side chains can project into the lipid phase and the hydrogen-bonding potentialities of their amide groups can be satisfied by the usual α-helical intra-chain linkages. The section of the molecule emerging into the cytosol is composed initially of several positively charged amino acid residues (arg, lys) and these presumably are stabilised by electrostatic attraction to the predominantly negatively charged heads of the phospholipids in the membrane's P face. The amino terminal end of the molecule projects from the E face of the membrane and oligosaccharide groups are attached to many of the ser, thr and asn residues.

6.5 MOBILITY OF MEMBRANE PROTEINS

We have already referred to membrane proteins as floating in a lipid sea. It is not surprising, therefore, to find that they have considerable lateral mobility. Their diffusion coefficients range from about 10^{-9} cm^2 s^{-1} for rhodopsin in retinal rod outer segments (i.e. about 0.1 μm^2 s^{-1}) to about 10^{-11} cm^2 s^{-1} for proteins in other membranes (i.e. about 0.001 μm s^{-1}). In the first case rhodopsin could travel across the diameter of an outer-segment disc in about 10 seconds, whereas at the opposite extreme a protein might require a couple of hours to travel the same distance. There are a number of reasons for these great differences in mobility. It may be, for instance, that the lipid constitution of the membrane makes it more or less fluid (see Section 6.2). Or it may be, as sometimes happens, that the protein is part of a large quasi-crystalline aggregate of other proteins and thus rendered too bulky to move easily. On the other hand it may be stabilised by structures (cell junctions perhaps) external to the membrane (see Section 6.8). Lastly it is possible, as we shall see in Section 6.7, that a membrane protein is anchored to one of the elements of the submembranous cytoskeleton.

6.6 SYNTHESIS OF BIOMEMBRANES

We have noted throughout this chapter that membranes are extremely fragile, tenuous, structures. It is thus not surprising to find that they are continuously synthesised and broken down throughout the life of the cell. The rate at which this is done is often extraordinarily high. It has been calculated, for instance, that the membrane of *Xenopus* retinal rod discs is synthesised at a rate of 3.2 μm^2 min^{-1}. This no doubt is an extreme case but it seems that in many cells an area of membrane equal to the entire surface of the cell is cycled between synthesis and degradation every hour.

The biosynthesis of both membrane proteins and membrane lipids occurs in and on the **rough endoplasmic reticulum (RER)**. We shall discuss the interrelations between ribosomes and endoplasmic reticulum (ER) (which together form the 'rough' endoplasmic reticulum) in Chapter 14. Here we can content ourselves by merely stating that proteins destined for incorporation into membrane (whether plasma membrane or the membranes of intracellular organelles) **never escape into the lumen of the ER but remain trapped in the ER membrane**. This is because the hydrophobic character of the amino acids which follow the signal sequence (see Chapter 14) prevents their squeezing through into the aqueous interior of the ER cisternae. Glycosylation of the proteins begins in the ER and continues as the membrane moves towards the Golgi apparatus. Ultimately small 'transport' vesicles bud off the Golgi body and make their way to the plasma and other membranes where they fuse to form part of the bilayer.

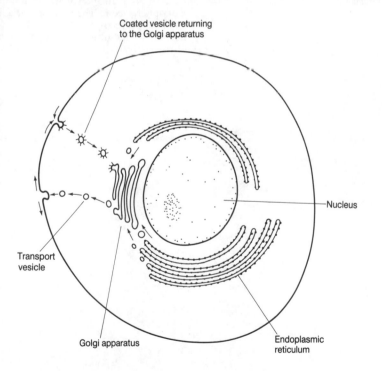

Figure 6.13 Membrane synthesis. The figure shows that not only is fresh membrane being continuously synthesised but also that 'old' membrane is just as continuously resorbed and carried back to the Golgi apparatus

This process is by no means haphazard. Radiolabelling shows that both different lipids and different membrane proteins have quite different turnover rates. Once again the processes of molecular recognition must be at work. In the special case of neurons it is not difficult to show that there is a busy traffic of membrane vesicles in the axon. Some of these vesicles will, of course, contain secretory materials but others will be involved in the membrane turnover process described above. If the flow of vesicles is interrupted by constricting the axon it can be shown that they mount up on both sides of the constriction. In other words there is a flow of fresh membrane material out to the synaptic ending and a counter-flow of old membrane and debris back to the cell body.

We shall discuss the secretory activity of neurons in more detail in Chapter 14.

6.7 MYELIN AND MYELINATION

In the vertebrates (though only rarely in the invertebrates) the axons of both central and peripheral neurons often (not always) become ensheathed in a physiologically very important whorl of

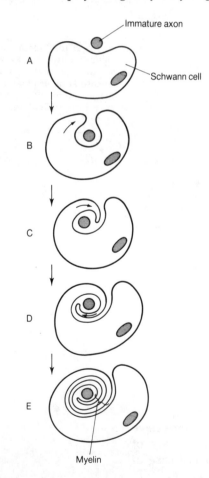

Figure 6.14 Formation of myelin around a peripheral axon. The process starts at (A) and proceeds through to (E) and beyond so that ultimately a tight spiral of perhaps 50 layers of myelin results

membranes: **myelin**. Defect in central myelin leads to the incapacitating condition known as **multiple or disseminated sclerosis (MS)**. The formation and upkeep of myelin is clearly of great importance.

Myelin is formed in both central and peripheral nervous systems by glial cells. In the peripheral nervous system the glial cells responsible are the **Schwann cells**. In the central nervous system **oligodendroglial cells** perform the same task. The myelination process is, however, different in the two cases. Peripheral axons become associated with a sequence of single Schwann cells which form a sort of gutter into which the axon sinks. The opening of this gutter to the extracellular space gradually becomes narrower until its two sides meet to form the **mesaxon**. The mesaxon then begins to grow in length and spirals around the axon, forming first of all a loose spiral of membrane and later a tight whorl. This process is shown diagrammatically in Figure 6.14.

In the central nervous system the process is different. Instead of a single Schwann cell being associated with a single axon it is found that single oligodendroglial cells myelinate many, sometimes up to 50, different axons. This is achieved by the oligodendroglial cells sending out huge extensions of their plasma membranes, sometimes as much as ten times the diameter of their own cell bodies, which wrap around neighbouring axons to form their myelin sheaths. This is perhaps the most remarkable instance of membrane synthesis known. Oligodendroglial cells may synthesise up to three times their own weight of myelin every day.

It can be seen from Table 6.1 that the lipid composition of myelin differs markedly from that of its parent glial cell plasma membrane. It contains significantly more cholesterol and phosphatidyl ethanolamine. Its protein constitution is also very specific. There are two major proteins—**basic protein** and **proteolipid protein**—and a large number of minor constituents of which the most important are the **Wolfgram proteins**.

It is believed that the two major proteins play an important role in maintaining the structure of central myelin. The basic protein (18 000 Da), rich in lysine and arginine residues, is found on the P face of developing myelin. The positive charges of the lysine and arginine residues may attach the protein to this generally negatively charged membrane face, although five N-terminal hydrophobic residues may penetrate the lipid monolayer and also help to hold it in place. The basic protein is also found in peripheral myelin.

The second major protein, the proteolipid protein (30 000 Da), is found only in central myelin, and is a transmembrane protein, extending from one membrane face to the other. This protein

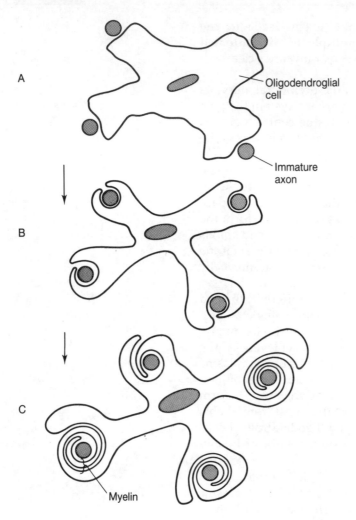

A

Oligodendroglial
cell

Immature
axon

B

C

Myelin

Figure 6.15   Formation of central myelin

projects through the E face of the membrane and, it has been
suggested, penetrates the E face of the adposing membrane
during myelination, thus helping to hold the myelin whorl
together. It also projects through the P face and this projection
is believed to form a hydrophobic surface which may bind with
the hydrophobic surface of a proteolipid in the adposed
membrane or with a hydrophobic surface of an adposed basic
protein. This suggested role of the two proteins in the formation
and stabilisation of central myelin is shown in Figure 6.16.

We have already noted (Section 3.2.2) that well-known
mutations affect the structure of myelin. We saw that the jimpy
mutation in the mouse was due to faulty splicing of the primary
mRNA transcript for proteolipid protein. The genetic programming of both mouse and human basic protein is also becoming
known. It has been shown that in both mouse and humans this

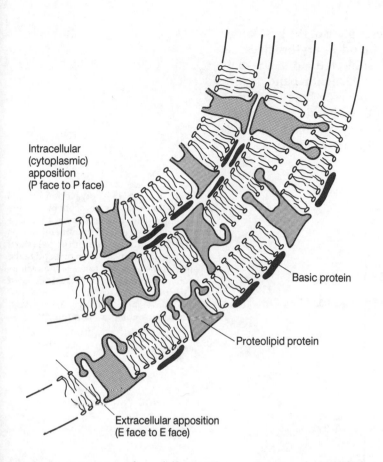

Intracellular
(cytoplasmic)
apposition
(P face to P face)

Basic protein

Proteolipid protein

Extracellular apposition
(E face to E face)

Figure 6.16 Involvement of myelin proteins in the formation and stabilisation of the myelin sheath. For explanation see text. (After Laursen *et al.*, 1984, *Proceedings of the National Academy of Science (USA)*, **81**, 2912–2916.)

protein is present in five different forms, having four different molecular weights: 21.5 kDa, 18.5 kDa, 17 kDa (two varieties) and 14 kDa. Careful genetic analysis shows that the basic protein gene is very lengthy: 30–35 kbp. It can also be shown that the gene consists of seven fairly short exons interrupted by lengthy introns. It turns out that the five different varieties of myelin basic protein are formed by differential splicing of the primary transcript. Thus the 21.5 kDa protein is programmed by all seven exons; the 18.5 kDa type is formed by the omission of exon 2 (coding for 26 amino acids); the two 17 kDa varieties by omitting either exon 6 (coding for 41 amino acids) or exons 2 and 5 (which together code for approximately the same number of amino acids); and, finally, the 14 kDa is programmed by a secondary mRNA which lacks exons 2 and 6 (together coding for 67 amino acids).

6.8 THE SUBMEMBRANOUS CYTOSKELETON

All eukaryotic cells possess some form of **cytoskeleton**. We shall examine the neuron's cytoskeleton again in Chapter 14. Here we will introduce the subject by a brief description of the best-known submembranous cytoskeleton—that found in **erythrocytes**.

If erythrocyte membranes are subjected to SDS–polyacrylamide gel electrophoresis at least **12 major bands** can be detected by staining with the dye Coomassie blue (see Figure 6.17). Some of the most prominent of these bands are caused by proteins involved in the submembranous cytoskeleton, i.e. '**band 3 protein**', '**band 4.1 protein**', **spectrin, actin, ankyrin**.

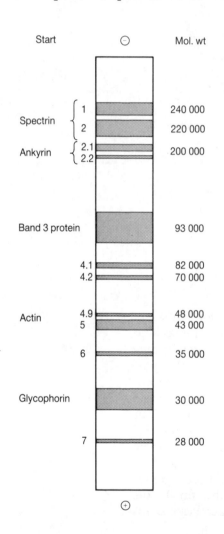

Figure 6.17 SDS–polyacrylamide gel electrophoresis of erythrocyte membrane proteins. The figure shows that if a preparation of erythrocyte membrane is pipetted on to one end of the gel (start) and a voltage applied from one end to the other of the gel ([–] to [+]) the various proteins will migrate at velocities related to their molecular weights. (After Avers, 1986, *Molecular Cell Biology*, Menlo Park, California: Benjamin/Cummings.)

The band 3 protein is the major transmembrane 'anchorage' protein for the submembrane cytoskeleton. It is also believed to function as a channel for small anions. It is both considerably bigger and considerably more complicated than glycophorin. It is a dimer consisting of two identical chains built of no less than

929 amino acid residues each. Figure 6.18 shows that both the N-terminal and the C-terminal end of each dimer are on the cytoplasmic face of the membrane. The C-terminal appears to be bound firmly to the P-face of the membrane. It is this domain of the protein which acts as the anion exchanger. Chloride ions are exchanged for bicarbonate ions—an important aspect of the erythrocyte's job in respiration. The amino acid chain then traverses the membrane, back and forth, probably as an α-helix, ten times. Some of the loops of this great molecule project out beyond the E face and one of these forms a point of attachment for oligosaccharide chains. Finally the N-terminal, as Figure 6.18 shows, projects far into the cytosol and it is this second domain of the molecule which provides firm anchorage for elements of the submembranous cytoskeleton.

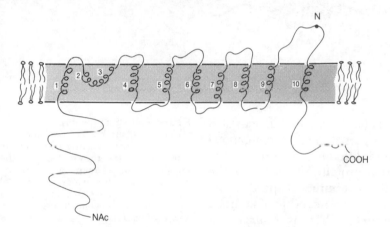

Figure 6.18   Organisation of the band 3 protein in the erythrocyte membrane. The figure shows a spread out 'plan' view. In reality the ten α-helical regions are grouped together (the membrane has, of course, a third dimension) to form a compact unit. This compact structure is believed to be associated with a second similar molecule to form a dimer. NAc = N-acetylated methionine; N = point of attachment of oligosaccahride chain. (After Jay and Cantley, 1986, *Annual Review of Biochemistry*, **55**, 511–538.)

The submembranous cytoskeleton of the erythrocyte consists of at least five proteins: **α- and β-spectrin** (240kD and 220kD, respectively), **band 4.1 protein, actin** and **ankyrin**. Figure 6.19 shows that these proteins form an intricate mesh just beneath the P face of the membrane. They are responsible for maintaining the biconcave shape of the cell. Spectrins are members of a class of submembranous proteins which includes the **fodrins** of epithelial microvilli and neurons. Both spectrins are fibrous proteins and spontaneously assemble to form a two-stranded rope—the $\alpha\beta$ dimer (about 100 nm in length and 5 nm in diameter). Two $\alpha\beta$ dimers join together tail to tail to form an $(\alpha\beta)_2$ tetramer. The spectrin tetramers next form a mesh by interacting with short lengths of actin and these junctions are strengthened by another submembrane protein, the band 4.1 protein. Last, but very far from least, the whole meshwork is anchored to the membrane through the fifth submembrane protein, ankyrin, which joins the free ends of the spectrin tetramers to the band 3 protein.

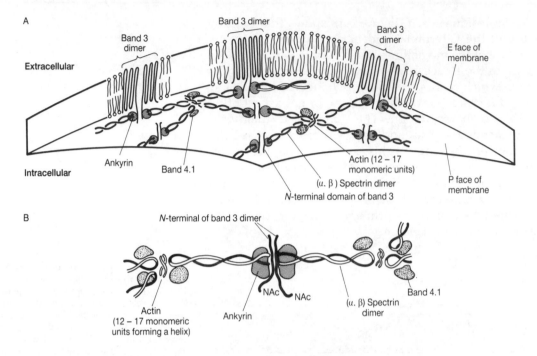

A

Band 3 dimer

Band 3 dimer

Band 3 dimer

Extracellular

E face of membrane

Intracellular

Ankyrin   Band 4.1

Actin (12 – 17 monomeric units)

(α. β) Spectrin dimer

N-terminal domain of band 3

P face of membrane

B

N-terminal of band 3 dimer

NAc   NAc

Actin
(12 – 17 monomeric
units forming a helix)

Ankyrin

(α. β) Spectrin dimer

Band 4.1

Figure 6.19 Submembranous cytoskeleton of an erythrocyte. (A) Schematic diagram to show the disposition of the cytoskeleton on the P face of the membrane. (B) Enlargement to show the organisation of the major cytoskeletal elements. Further explanation is given in the text. (Data from Bennett, 1985, *Annual Review of Biochemistry*, **54**, 273–304.)

A spectrin-like protein, fodrin, is (as mentioned above) also found in neurons. Here again it forms part of the submembranous cytoskeleton. It is both similar to and different from erythrocyte spectrin. It, too, is a tetrameric fibrous protein. Whilst two of the subunits appear to be identical to the α-subunits of spectrin, the other two differ and are named γ-subunits. The fodrin of neurons is thus referred to as an $(\alpha\gamma)_2$ tetramer. There is a surprising amount of fodrin present in neurons, up to 3% of the total protein in some cases. Moreover erythrocyte-type $(\alpha\beta)_2$ spectrin is also found in lesser quantities. It appears that whilst $(\alpha\beta)_2$ spectrin is restricted to the cell body the $(\alpha\gamma)_2$ fodrin is concentrated in the axon.

In addition to the spectrin-like fodrins it appears that homologues of the other characteristic proteins of the erythrocyte cytoskeleton are also found in neurons. **Synapsin**, which is localised in the termini of central and peripheral axons, where it is a component of the walls of synaptic vesicles, is a homologue of band 4.1 protein. A variant of ankyrin is also present in neural membranes. Actin is well represented. It begins to look as if the submembranous cytoskeleton discovered in erythrocytes has a wider significance. Perhaps something rather like it exists in other cells and, in particular, in neurons. Perhaps the fodrin cytoskeleton of neurons anchors ion channel proteins, holding them in position, just as the spectrin cytoskeleton of the erythrocyte holds the anion channel, band 3 protein, in position (see Section 16.5). Indeed fodrin is a major component of **subsynaptic** densities and appears to be concentrated in **synaptic endings** and at **nodes of Ranvier**. This strengthens the belief that it has an anchoring function, for these are domains of a neuron's membrane where channels of one sort or another are particularly densely concentrated it could well be that it is has an anchoring function.

We have emphasised in the preceding account that we are only considering the submembranous cytoskeleton. In the erythrocyte there is little else, but in most cells there is a great deal more. In neurons the cytoskeleton extends deep into the cytosol and is composed of numerous other proteinaceous elements: neuro-tubules, neurofilaments (of various sorts), actin and multifarious binding proteins.

6.9 JUNCTIONS BETWEEN CELLS

There are three major types of junction between cells, each of which serves a different purpose. **Desmosomes** hold neighbour-ing cells in a tissue together, **tight junctions** prevent materials diffusing in the intercellular space between two cells and **gap junctions** allow communication between neighbouring cells. Of these three only the latter two play important roles in the brain.

Tight junctions. Figure 6.20 shows the structure of a typical tight junction. The plasma membranes of the two cells touch each other at intervals, indeed may even fuse, so that all possibility of materials diffusing between them is eliminated. Freeze-fracture electron microscopy shows that the junction consists of globular proteins in both adposed membranes which articulate with each other so that the intercellular gap is completely sealed. Figure 6.20 shows that one such sealing is usually not enough. Two or more seals are usually made and the number appears to vary with the tissue and the diffusional forces which need to be counteracted.

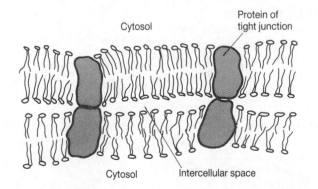

Cytosol

Protein of tight junction

Cytosol   Intercellular space

Figure 6.20 Tight junction. The figure shows two cell membranes joined together by the articulation of large globular proteins

For instance a sequence of six or more tight junctions are made between the epithelial cells which form the wall of the small intestine.

The most important tight junctions in neurobiology are those which are responsible for the 'blood–brain barrier'. It has been known for over a century that small molecules do not escape from the capillaries of the brain as easily as they do from capillaries in other parts of the anatomy. However, the physical basis of this barrier has only fairly recently been elucidated. It appears that it is due to the presence of well-developed tight junctions between the endothelial cells of brain capillaries. The tight junctions between brain endothelial cells are grouped in pairs, thus forming a double seal and effectively preventing the escape of small molecules from the blood. Tight junctions are also developed between the choroid cells lining the ventricles. The brain is thus protected from unwanted chemical influences. The molecules which reach the neurons have to pass through the endothelial (or choroid) cells and possibly are also monitored and filtered by the glial cells, especially astrocytes (see Chapter 1).

Gap junctions. Gap junctions play several important roles in the functioning of the CNS. Indeed they were first discovered in the CNS of the crayfish, where they function as **electrical synapses**. But they have since been found in many non-nervous tissues and have been assigned a great variety of functions ranging from metabolic co-operation between neighbouring cells to the signalling involved in growth and development. Figure 6.21 shows that they are formed once again by proteins developed in both adposed membranes. The proteins are called **connexins** and have a molecular weight of some 25–28 kDa. Six connexins are grouped to form a cylinder surrounding a central hydrophilic canal. This hexagonal structure is called a **connexon** and is adposed to a similar connexon in the adjacent membrane. Thus a hydrophilic pore extends across the intercellular space between one cytosol and the next.

Both human and rat liver connexins have had their amino acid sequences determined by recombinant DNA technology. The technique used was similar to that described in Chapter 5. From a purified preparation of human liver gap junctions a 19 amino acid primary sequence was determined and a matching oligonucleotide probe synthesised. This probe was then used to screen a library of liver cDNA. It hybridised with a cDNA of 1574 bases. The coding sequence of this DNA was found to specify a polypeptide of 283 amino acids. A very similar sequence (differing in only four amino acid residues) was detected by the same technique in rat liver.

One of the most interesting findings to emerge from this

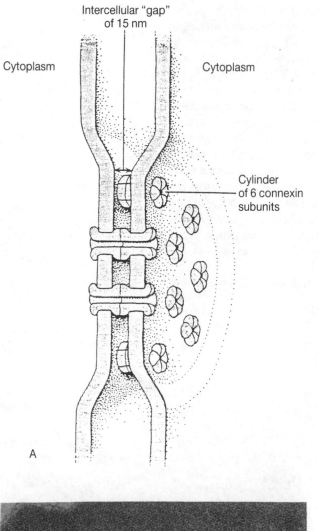

Intercellular "gap"
of 15 nm

Cytoplasm

Cytoplasm

Cylinder
of 6 connexin
subunits

A

B

Figure 6.21 Molecular structure of gap junctions. (A) Diagrammatic representation of gap junction. (B) Electron micrograph of purified suspension of gap junctions. (From *Molecular Cell Biology* by James E. Darnell *et al*. Copyright © 1986 Scientific American Books Inc. Reprinted with permission.)

molecular biology is the marked similarity in the hydropathic profiles of the **connexin protein** and the subunits of the **nicotinic acetylcholine receptor**. These subunits will be considered in Chapter 9. Here, however, it can be said that in each case the primary sequence seems to contain strings of 20 of so hydrophobic amino acids. These hydropathic domains probably form membrane-spanning α-helices (see Chapter 2). It should be noted, however, that whereas the connexon of the gap junction is formed by a group of **six** connexins, the nicotinic acetylcholine receptor consists of only **five** subunits. Thus although the units of which gap junctions and nAChRs are built may be similar and evolutionarily related, they are put together in rather different ways in the two functionally very different structures. We shall outline further the emerging evolutionary relationships between the various proteins of neural membranes in the next four chapters.

Here, however, we should note next that **connexons** are normally arranged in large clusters. In this, again, they resemble the nicotinic acetylcholine receptor. We shall see in Chapter 9 that

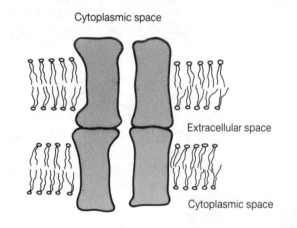

Figure 6.22 Sectional view of a gap junction showing (A) open and (B) closed conformation of connexin subunits in a gap junction.

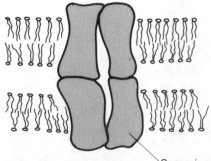

the latter, especially in electric organs, often form huge conglomerations. In the case of connexon clusters the whole structure is believed to provide both a way of transferring metabolites (up to molecular weights of 1.5 kDa) from one cell to another and a pathway of low electrical resistance for electrical signalling. Neighbouring cells are thus both metabolically and electrically coupled. This coupling, moreover, can be controlled. It has been shown that a connexon can exist in various stereochemically different forms—open, partially open and closed—and that these transitions are affected by the concentration of intracellular calcium, by pH and by cAMP.

As with the other membrane proteins we have discussed it seems that the connexons of different tissues are biochemically and presumably functionally somewhat different. Once again we are probably dealing with a family of related proteins having subtly different properties.

In the CNS, gap junctions are perhaps best known amongst glial cells and in the retina. In the nervous systems of leeches and amphibia gap junctions between neighbouring glia cells have been shown to mediate electrical signalling as well as metabolic communication. Although a recent report suggests that glial cells may, after all, be excitable and generate action potentials the conventional wisdom is that any electrical communication is by slow 'local-circuit' currents (see Chapter 11). There have also been observations of gap junctions uniting astrocytes, oligodendroglia and neurons in mammalian central nervous systems. This would, at the least, provide a means of metabolic communication between glia and neurons. This strengthens the case for believing that, in view of the blood–brain barrier, glia provide a vital route for the transport of materials from blood to neuron (see Chapter 1).

Finally the **retina** provides several very interesting cases of gap junctions uniting sensory cells and also neurons together. In all the lower vertebrates so far examined (salamander, toad, fish, turtle) many thousands of **rod cells** are connected by electrically conducting gap junctions. This ensures that stimulation of any one rod cell spreads to a large population. This organisation is not found in mammals; instead it is found that groups of rods connect via gap junctions to **cones**.In all vertebrates, both higher and lower, it is found that gap junctions develop between **horizontal cells** and this once again ensures that excitation is spread laterally through the retina, this time to groups of cones. It is clear that gap junctions, or electrical synapses, play an essential role in the electrophysiology of the vertebrate retina, especially in increasing its sensitivity. No doubt this is part of the underlying organisation which allows a mammalian retina, under optimal conditions, to respond to a single photon in the visible spectrum.

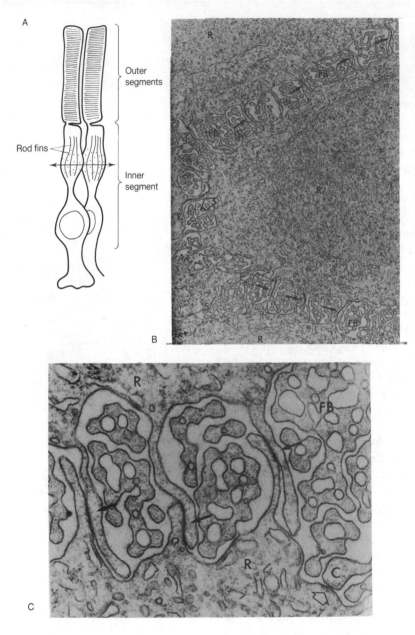

Figure 6.23   Gap junctions in the retina. The figure shows the organisation of the gap junctions which develop between certain types of rod cell in the toad retina. In (A) two rod cells are shown. It is shown that the outer part of the inner segments develop a series of ridges or 'fins'. In (B) a transverse section ($\times 10\,000$) at the level of the arrow in (A), is shown. The fins of adjacent rod (and, indeed, cone) cells interdigitate. Gap junctions are made between the fins of adjacent cells. In this way large groups of rod (and cone) cells are electrically interconnected. Finally (C) shows a higher magnification electron micrograph ($\times 32\,000$) of three of these interdigitations (R = rod cell inner segment; C = cone; FB = fibre basket (glial cell process); the solid arrows point to the gap junctions; open arrow points to a close apposition between a cone fin and a rod fin). (From Gold and Dowling, 1979, *Journal of Neurophysiology*, **42**, 292–310; with permission.)

6.10 CONCLUSION

This chapter has covered a very wide and rapidly advancing topic. The next four chapters build on the fundamental concepts of membrane structure and function developed here, applying them to the specific characteristics of nerve cell membranes. Thus in

Chapter 7 we look at a superfamily of important membrane receptors and note how their action depends on the ability of proteins (so-called G- or N-proteins) to shuttle to and fro in the lipid bilayer of the membrane to influence distant membrane-embedded enzymes. Because the response time of these receptors is comparatively long-lasting (tens of milliseconds) they have been termed '**class 2**' receptors. In the next chapter we consider the very important role which biological membranes, and especially neuronal membranes, play in separating ionic solutions of different concentrations. We shall see that transmembrane proteins act as 'pumps' creating and maintaining these all-important ionic imbalances. In Chapters 9 and 10 we examine the way in which membrane proteins act as gates and thus control the flow of ions across neural membranes. We shall see that there are two cases. First, in Chapter 9, we shall look at gates controlled by chemical ligands. In many instances these gates open and close very rapidly (less than a millisecond), and the effect on the membrane potential is consequently also very rapid. Although, like the receptors discussed in Chapter 7, they respond to chemical agonists the mechanism and rapidity of response are so different that they are distinguished from the former as '**class 1**' receptors. Finally in Chapter 10 we consider voltage-controlled gates. These again are many and various. Normally they act very rapidly and are responsible for the ion flows underlying innumerable electrophysiological phenomena, especially the all-important action potential.

Chapter 7
G-coupled receptors

At the end of Chapter 6 we noted the various types of junction which hold cells together and, in the case of gap junctions, allow communication between a cell and its nearest neighbours. This of course is an absolute condition of multicellularity. Else, as the poet says, ''Tis all in pieces, all coherence gone/ All just supply and all relation.' The nervous system is, of course, the great exemplar of this intercellular signalling and co-ordination. But on a lesser scale the phenomenon is shown by all the cells of a multicellular body.

7.1 MESSENGERS AND RECEPTORS

In this chapter we shall begin a discussion of some of the mechanisms by which one cell can communicate with another. This is usually (not always) accomplished by way of chemical substances. This immediately entails two things: first the production and release of appropriate molecules and second the recognition of these molecules by other cells once released. Details of the synthesis and release of these chemical signals will be considered in Chapters 14 and 15, whilst the biophysical and biochemical response of the **target cell** forms the subject matter of Chapter 16. The initial recognition of the signal or messenger depends, however, on the nature of the **receptors** embedded in the target cell membrane.

Receptors are large protein molecules which usually span the membrane—often many times. They possess sites (comparable to the active sites of enzymes) which are stereochemically designed to fit specific messengers. Neurons are far from being the only cells to possess such molecules in their membranes. Probably most cells in multicellular organisms possess membrane receptors. They are especially well known in cells which respond to circulating hormones.

The messenger or signal molecule (whether it be a hormone or a neurotransmitter) exerts its influence by first binding to the

167

receptor to form a **receptor–ligand complex**. This initial step then sets in train a specific set of responses in the target cell. What these responses are depends on the biochemical nature of the receptor. Thus the same messenger may cause very different results with different receptors.

Until quite recently the study of neural receptors has been the province of neuropharmacologists. Their approach has been to distinguish and differentiate between receptors in terms of the pharmacological agents which switch them on and off. These agents are called **agonists** and **antagonists** (= **blockers**), respectively. A very large number of such agents have been discovered. Not all of them induce maximal responses in the receptor. Thus pharmacologists distinguish between full agonists and partial agonists, and between full antagonists and partial antagonists.

A complex and somewhat confusing nomenclature for receptors has grown up in neuropharmacology. The convention has been to name the receptor after its full agonist. Thus we shall meet NMDA receptors, quisqualate receptors, kainate receptors, benzodiazepine receptors, and many more as we proceed through the pages of this book. This is a valuable way of discriminating between receptors and, especially, between receptor subtypes. There are, however, difficulties with this taxonomy. First, full agonists at one receptor are sometimes partial agonists at another; second, the neuropharmacologist's agonist is frequently not the same molecule as the naturally occurring transmitter for which the receptor is 'designed'. Moves are accordingly afoot to reorganise and clarify the terminology. It is possible that the advent of molecular neurobiology and the consequent understanding of the molecular structure and relatedness of receptors will play a role in this clarification. Meanwhile we shall have to continue with the customary system, always bearing in mind its capacity to confuse.

Let us turn next to the response of the target cell when a receptor–ligand complex is formed. There are two major cases. First, as we shall discuss in the present chapter, the detection of the signal may lead to a complex membrane-bound biochemistry which ultimately leads to biochemical alterations within **the detecting cell or in its plasmalemma**. In other cases, as we shall see in Chapters 9 and 10, the chemical signal may open **ion channels** in the detecting cell's membrane, thus leading to a change in the **electrical voltage** across that membrane.

Finally, in this introductory section, it is important to draw a distinction between **primary messengers** and **secondary messengers**. In the nervous system the primary messenger is the neurotransmitter (or neuromodulator) released from the presynaptic terminal. This crosses the synaptic cleft or gap (or it may diffuse further in the intercellular space) and unites with the receptor in the subsynaptic membrane to form the ligand–receptor complex. This may (certainly not always) lead to the production of a 'second messenger' on the cytoplasmic face of the subsynaptic membrane. This second messenger then diffuses into the cytoplasm, where it may elicit one or more biochemical effects. One such effect, which we shall come across frequently, is the activation of a **protein kinase**. Once activated this multimeric enzyme phosphorylates (with the help of ATP) one or other of the many biologically active proteins present in a cell—an enzyme, a channel protein, a nuclear histone, etc. The phosphorylation, which is of the OH group of the side chain of a **serine, threonine** or **tyrosine** residue (see Table 2.1), either inhibits or activates the protein to which the residue belongs. The protein is dephosphorylated back to its original condition by one of the phosphatases with which the cytosol abounds.

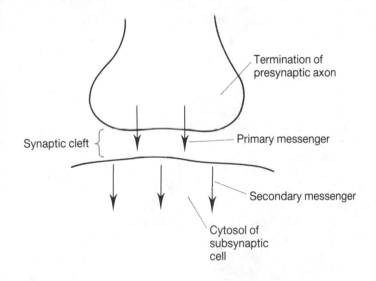

Figure 7.1 Primary and secondary messengers

Neuronal membranes have many different receptors designed to detect many different primary messengers. In this chapter we shall consider four of these receptors in depth: the **β-adrenergic receptor (β-AR)**, the **muscarinic acetylcholine receptor (mAChR)**, the **substance K receptor (SKR)** and the **visual pigment proteins (opsins)** of vertebrate photoreceptor cells. These receptors have been chosen because their molecular structure is now well understood and they also seem to form a superfamily of evolutionarily related proteins. They also share a common intramembranous method of signal amplification and a similar second messenger system. This mechanism, as we shall see, capitalises on the lateral mobility of proteins in biomembranes and on the fact that the lipid bilayer holds such proteins in close proximity to each other: they cannot diffuse away into the cytosol. This device is so effective that it seems that several other types of receptor, e.g. dopamine receptors and adenosine receptors, act through a similar molecular mechanism. They may well all form part of the same molecular superfamily.

7.2. THE β-ADRENERGIC RECEPTOR (β-AR)

The biochemistry and pharmacology of **noradrenaline** (= **norepinephrine**) will be discussed more fully in Chapter 15. Here we shall merely note that it is a member of a class of neuroactive molecules sharing a common six-membered ring structure— **catechol**. As noradrenaline and its congeners (though not adrenaline itself) also possess amine groups this whole family of important neurotransmitters is commonly referred to as the **catecholamines**.

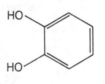

Figure 7.2   Catechol

Four subtypes of membrane receptor have been identified for adrenaline and noradrenaline, and four receptor subtypes have also been identified for the closely related catecholamine— dopamine. These different receptor subtypes have been identified by pharmacological studies using different agonist and antagonist drugs (see Table 15.4). The adrenaline receptors (which also accept noradrenaline) are classified as α_1, α_2, β_1 and β_2. All these types of adrenergic receptor have been found in tissues outside the nervous system. The β_1-receptors, in particular, are known to exist in cardiac muscle membrane. They accept circulating adrenaline from the adrenal medulla and cause the heart to beat more rapidly. Agents such as practolol (the so-called β-blockers), which bind strongly to cardiac β_1-receptors and hence displace adrenaline, are prescribed for angina and other cardiac conditions.

In recent years the **β_2-receptor (β-AR)** has been cloned and its amino acid structure determined. It is therefore this receptor and its action that we shall consider in this section.

The cloning procedure used was similar to that described in Chapter 5. First the β-adrenergic receptor was isolated and purified by biochemical techniques. After having made quite certain by immunology that a small peptide fragment of the purified β-adrenergic receptor (β-AR) was indeed a fragment of the receptor its amino acid sequence was determined and a complementary oligonucleotide probe prepared. The probe was then used to fish out the β-AR gene from a hamster genomic gene library. This gene was then cloned in a plasmid vector and its nucleotide sequence analysed.

The primary structure deduced from the β-AR gene shows that the receptor consists of a protein built of 418 amino acids. Analysis of the sequence for hydrophobic amino acids shows there to be seven hydropathic segments, suggesting that there are seven membrane-spanning helices. In this, as we shall see, the receptor resembles the muscarinic acetylcholine receptor, the substance K receptor and the various opsin molecules found in the outer segments of retinal photoreceptor cells.

Figure 7.3 Conformation of the β_2-adrenergic receptor. The N-terminal end of the molecule projects into the extra-cellular space and two asparagine residues (N) are believed to bear oligosacccharide chains (represented by hexagons). The polypeptide chain then spans the membrane as an α-helix seven times (numbered 1 to 7 in the figure). The molecule ends with a lengthy carboxy-terminal domain which projects into the cytoplasm. (After Dixon *et al.*, 1986, *Nature*, **321**, 75–79.)

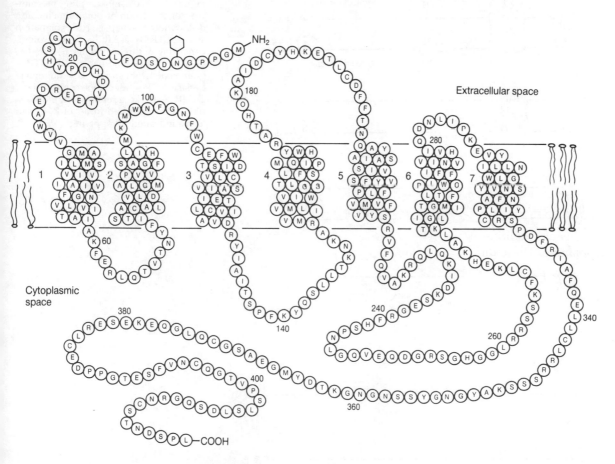

We have already noted that β-ARs are coupled to a compli-cated multimolecule membrane biochemistry. It can be shown that two other membrane molecules are involved—the **G (sometimes called 'N') proteins** and **adenylate cyclase (C)**. These proteins are embedded in the cytoplasmic 'leaflet' of the membrane. Let us examine their interaction.

In Figure 7.4 the interaction of the three membrane proteins is schematised. First of all it should be noted that in the absence of an appropriate signal in the form of noradrenaline all three membrane proteins—β-AR, G and C—are 'floating' free in the membrane. No doubt they are shuffling to and fro and occasionally bumping into each other, but they do not stick together. It should also be noted that the G-protein is composed of **three subunits—α, β and γ**. The G-protein is so-called because it unites with a guanosine phosphate—either **GDP** or **GTP**. The figure shows that in the 'free-floating' condition GDP is attached to the α-subunit of the G-protein.

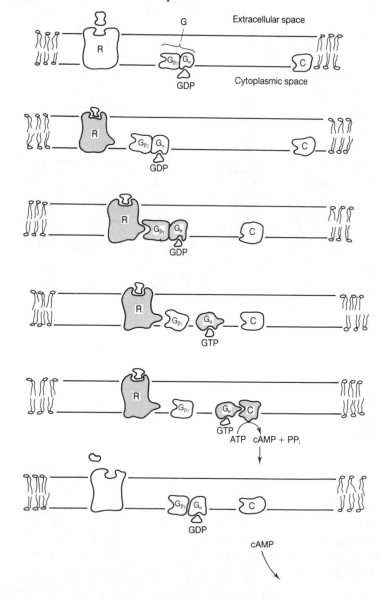

Figure 7.4   Collision-coupling mechanism for the action of noradrenaline at a β₂-adrenergic synapse. For explanation see text. R = β-AR; G = G-protein, consisting of three subunits: α, β and γ; GDP = guanosine diphosphate; GTP = guanosine triphosphate; C = adenylate cyclase; ATP = adenosine triphosphate; cAMP = cyclic adenosine monophosphate. The activated forms of R, G and C are indicated by stippling

When noradrenaline arrives on the outside of the membrane and interacts with the β-AR a whole set of changes occurs. First the presence of noradrenaline changes the **conformation** of the β-AR. It has been suggested that ligands (such as the catecholamines) which affect the β-AR do so by intercalating among the transmembrane helices, thus altering the disposition of the membrane-embedded part of the molecule. We shall see later that something analogous occurs when the opsins are photoactivated.

The altered conformation of the membrane-spanning segment of the β-AR has the effect of rendering it very '**sticky**' to the β and γ subunits of the G-protein. On coming into contact with the β-AR the G-protein not only sticks but undergoes a transformation which causes its α-subunit to come free and to **release its GDP in exchange for GTP**. Not only this but the freed α-subunit itself undergoes a conformational change which allows it to stick to **adenylate cyclase**. This, in turn, activates the adenylate cyclase, which can then catalyse the dephosphorylation of ATP to form **cyclic AMP (cAMP)**. cAMP is perhaps the most important of the cell's internal, or 'second', messengers. It diffuses into the cytosol where it may, as we shall see in later chapters, exert a number of biochemical changes. The α-subunit of the G-protein, meanwhile, dephosphorylates its bound GTP to GDP (i.e. in contact with membrane-bound adenylate cyclase it acts as a GTPase), dissociates from the adenylate cyclase and assumes its original conformation. When it collides with the βγ complex it forms the αβγ complex of the inactive G-protein again—ready for the whole cycle to start once more.

A further complexity is added to this already rather intricate scenario by the finding that the α-subunit of the G-protein exists in two forms: a form (α_i) which inhibits and a form (α_s) which stimulates the cyclase enzyme.

What is the biological significance of this complicated mechanism? It looks as though the system confers several benefits. First, a single noradrenaline molecule may cause the synthesis of several hundred cAMP second messengers. This is because the activation of a single β-AR may lead to the dissociation of tens of G-proteins (remember membranes have a third dimension!). In turn the union of an α_s with a cyclase enzyme may lead to tens of cAMPs being synthesised before the α-subunit dephosphorylates its GTP. The system can thus lead to a considerable amplification of the signal.

Second, the system only works so long as the β-AR is in receipt of a noradrenaline. Once the neurotransmitter is removed the G-protein mechanism is switched off. Thus not only amplification is achieved but also rapid shut-down.

Before leaving the β-AR and its associated G-proteins two further points should be noted. First, that the G-protein system we have met here is also to be found in several other receptor systems, including the muscarinic acetylcholine receptor which we shall consider next, and, somewhat modified, in the opsin systems of the rod outer segment. Second, we should note that the cAMP, which as we have seen, is the end-product of the whole intricate mechanism, can often work back and effect the flux of K^+ and/or Ca^{2+} through their channels (see Chapter 10). In this way comparatively long-lasting effects on membrane potential can be achieved. This may be done directly or, more usually, by cAMP acting on a protein kinase which phosphorylates the hydroxyl group of a serine, threonine or tyrosine residue of a channel protein (Figure 7.5).

Figure 7.5 Modification of channel conductance by cAMP. cAMP, shown approaching from the left-hand side of the diagram, interacts with a large tetrameric enzyme—a protein kinase (PK). PK breaks up into its constituent subunits (regulatory (R) and catalytic (C)). The catalytic subunits catalyse the phosphorylation of the channel protein, using ATP as both an energy and a phosphate source. The channel conductance is altered. The channel protein is ultimately dephosphorylated by a protein phosphatase

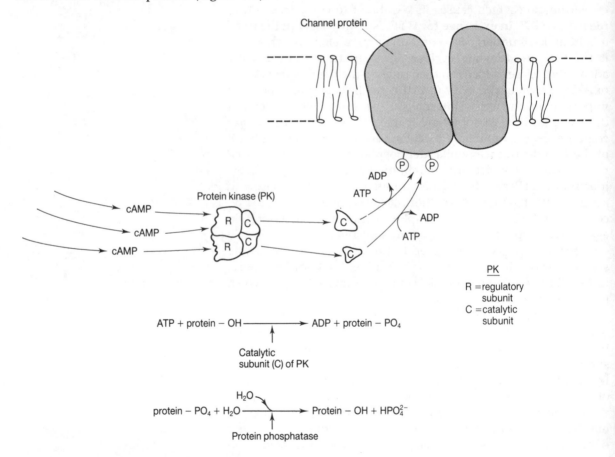

7.3: THE MUSCARINIC ACETYLCHOLINE RECEPTOR (mAChR)

Acetylcholine (**ACh**) was the first neurotransmitter to be discovered, by Loewi in 1922. ACh, or **cholinergic**, synapses are now known to exist in both the peripheral and central nervous systems. In the peripheral nervous system of vertebrates the neuromuscular junction is always cholinergic and it was here that the pharmacology of ACh was first investigated. We shall look further at this pharmacology in Chapter 15.

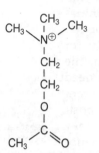

Figure 7.6   Acetylcholine

Before going any further it is important to make a distinction between acetylcholine's **muscarinic** and **nicotinic** action. These two completely different effects are due to the interaction of ACh with different receptors. This is a first and striking example of the importance of receptors in neural membranes. Acetylcholine's nicotinic action is shown at the junction between motor neurons and skeletal muscle, in some central synapses and as we shall see (spectacularly) in the electric organs of electric fish. It is an action which can be mimicked by **nicotine**—hence the nomenclature. Muscarinic synapses, on the other hand, are found on smooth muscle, cardiac muscle and outnumber nicotinic synapses in the brain by a factor of ten to a hundred. Muscarinic synapses are not affected by nicotine but can be activated by **muscarine**.

We shall discuss the well-known molecular neurobiology of the nicotinic acetylcholine receptor in Chapter 9. We shall see that its action is very different from that of the muscarinic receptors we are about to discuss. Instead of the fairly long lasting and biochemically complex response of muscarinic receptors we shall see that the nicotinic receptor responds extremely rapidly and then shuts off. Let us, however, turn our attention to the subject of this section: muscarinic acetylcholine receptors (**mAChRs**).

We have just noted that in the brain muscarinic synapses outnumber nicotinic synapses by a factor of ten to a hundred. It is thus not surprising that the first muscarinic acetylcholine receptor to be cloned was obtained from the brain—the brain of a pig.

Once again the technique involved the use of oligonucleotide hybridisation probes prepared from partial amino acid sequence data. The probes were used to fish for mAChR DNA from a cDNA library prepared from porcine cerebral mRNAs. The cDNA obtained in this way was cloned and injected into the *Xenopus* oocyte. The oocyte expressed the cDNA in the form of receptors in its membrane which showed all the functional and binding characteristics of the M1 subtype of mAChR.

As implied in the previous paragraph there are various **subtypes** of the mAChR: Four subtypes—M1, M2, M3 and M4—are distinguished, principally by their differential affinities for the anti-ulcer drug **pirenzepine** and its analogues. The M1 mAChR can be detected through its very high affinity for pirenzipine. It was this antagonist which was used to define the cDNA expressed in *Xenopus* oocyte and confirm that it was indeed the M1 mAChR. It is not yet known whether the different subtypes are due to differential post-transcriptional or post-translational processing of a single gene product, or whether they are the products of different genes. The balance of evidence favours the latter interpretation.

The protein moiety of the M1 subtype of mAChR has a molecular weight of 51.4 kDa and consists of 460 amino acids. In addition there is a large carbohydrate moiety which makes up about 26% of the mass of the entire molecule.

Figure 7.7 Conformation of M1 muscarinic acetylcholine receptor. For explanation see text. Hexagons represent oligosaccharide chains attached to asparagine (N) residues in the amino-terminal end of the molecule. As was the case in the β_2-adrenergic receptor there are seven transmembrane α-helices. The cytoplasmic loop between transmembrane helices 5 and 6 is, however, very much longer than in the adrenergic receptor. (After Kubo *et al.*, 1986, *FEBS Letters*, **209**, 367–392.)

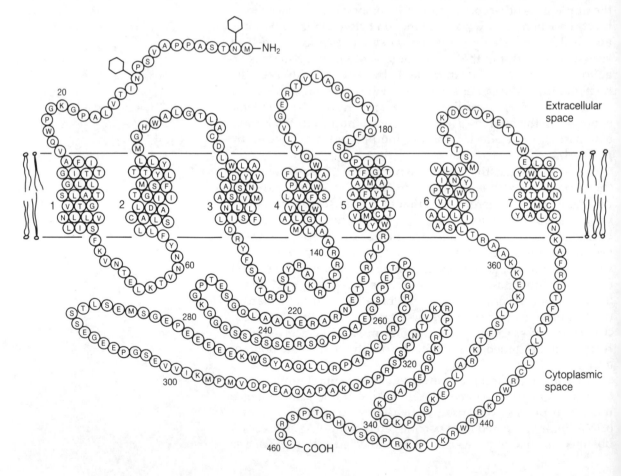

The customary hydropathic analysis indicates that the molecule has seven transmembrane α-helices. This conformation, of course, is analogous to that which is displayed by the β-AR. The amino-terminal end of the molecule lies on the E face of the membrane and carries two potential N-glycosylation sites. The extensive carbohydrate moiety mentioned above is attached at these positions. The carboxy-terminal tail contains a number of serine and threonine residues which may be involved in cytoplasmic phosphorylation.

Muscarinic receptors resemble β-adrenergic receptors in acting through G-protein collision-coupling. It has been shown that porcine M1 mAChR activates an α_i (i.e. inhibitory) G-subunit and hence **switches off** adenylate cyclase. Other subtypes of mAChR may activate α_s (i.e. stimulatory) subunits and thus **stimulate** the cyclase enzyme. These various effects on the cyclase enzyme control the quantity of cAMP in the cell. We have already noted the effects which this 'second messenger' may have when discussing the β-adrenergic receptor above. An end result of a 'cascade' of biochemical interactions may be to modulate (by phosphorylation) the conductance of, for instance, K^+ channels. Indeed it is known that one of the consequences of activating a muscarinic synapse is down-modulation of the **leak channels** which are largely responsible for the resting potential across nerve cell membranes. This has the extremely important consequence, as we shall see in Chapter 11, of depolarising the membrane.

The M2 muscarinic receptor, present in porcine cardiac muscle, has also been cloned and analysed. It is slightly larger than the M1 subtype, consisting of 466 amino acids. But like M1 it possesses seven transmembrane helices and its amino acid sequence is very similar. Indeed there is 82% homology if both conservative substitutions and identical amino acids are counted.

The M2 mAChR also works through a G-protein system. It is believed, however, that the mechanism is rather different from systems we have considered previously. It appears that the M2 mAChR is linked to a G-protein on the P face of the membrane which only binds GTP when ACh binds on the E face (see Figure 7.8). The whole (GTP – G-protein – mAChR – ACh) complex then interacts with a potassium channel (not the leak channel mentioned above, nor the Hodgkin–Huxley 'delayed rectifier' channel which plays so vital a role in the recovery phase of an action potential), ensuring that the latter stays in the open state for longer than normal. Interaction with the K^+ channel, however, leads to the hydrolysis of GTP to GDP and the separation of the mAChR – G-protein complex and the closing of the channel. Whether this mechanism is at work in the brain is not known. In atrial cells the 'up-modulation', leading to a hyperpolarisation, slows the pacemaker.

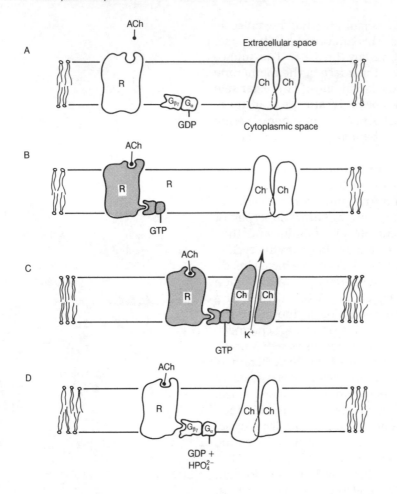

Figure 7.8 Control of a K$^+$ channel by mAChR-coupled G-protein. Ch = channel protein; other symbols as in Fig. 7.4. For explanation see text

The M2 subtype is not confined to cardiac muscle. It is also found in the medulla and pons of the brain. Other subtypes of the muscarinic acetylcholine receptor are also found in the brain. Rapid progress is being made in their analysis. Use is being made of the emerging realisation that the receptors are all members of an evolutionarily related family. All of them show considerable amino acid homology in their transmembrane segments. Consequently oligonucleotide probes prepared against the most conserved of these segments (the second) are likely to stick to all four mAChR cDNAs. This turns out to be the case. When a porcine cerebral cortex cDNA library was screened the probes hybridised with four different cDNA sequences. These presumably correspond to the M1, M2, M3 and M4 mAChR subtypes. Indeed there is evidence for even more subtypes. It looks as though each of these mAChR subtypes responds in a (slightly) different way to acetylcholine.

It is clear that mAChRs which work through a G-protein collision-coupling mechanism can exert very diverse effects. The full range and complexity of these effects have yet to be elucidated. But the possibilites of long-lasting modulation of various channel conductivities and of biasing metabolic activities in the recipient cell are legion. The muscarinic activity of ACh is very different from the discrete, rapid, effects characteristic of its nicotinic action (see Chapter 9). Perhaps it is not surprising that mAChRs are so much more prevalent in the brain than nAChRs.

7.4 THE SUBSTANCE-K RECEPTOR (SKR)

We saw in Chapters 3 and 4 that a group of small peptides, the tachykinins, were synthesised in the brain (and, indeed, elsewhere). These molecules, which include substance K and substance P, are synaptically active (see Chapter 15). Their receptors, however, are only sparsely represented in neural membranes. If it were not for the new techniques of molecular biology it is doubtful if their structure and function could have been determined.

Figure 7.9 Conformation of the substance-K receptor. There are seven transmembrane helices. The N-terminal end of the polypeptide chain is believed to be bonded to myristic acid, which is embedded in the membrane. (Reprinted with permission from Masu *et al.*, 1987, *Nature*, **329**, 836–838. Copyright © 1987, Macmillan Magazines Ltd.)

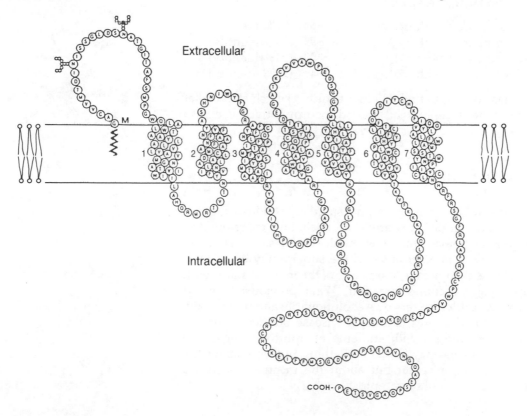

Extracellular

Intracellular

COOH-

In essence the technique adopted was to generate a population of mRNAs from a bovine stomach cDNA library. Substance K, and the other tachykinins, are not, as we noted above, confined to cerebral tissue. Once having obtained a mixture of mRNAs it was necessary to select out the strand coding for substance K. This was done by using the *Xenopus* oocyte system. The appearance of receptors responsive to substance K and to a lesser extent to the other tachykinins (but not to non-tachykinin peptides) in the oocyte membrane indicated that the appropriate mRNA had been injected. After a number of further fractionations and purifications a single SKR clone was obtained from which the nucleic acid sequence for the receptor could be obtained.

The substance-K receptor was shown to have a molecular weight of 43 066 Da and to consist of 384 amino acid residues. The customary hydropathic analysis of the sequence showed that there were seven transmembrane segments. It is thus very obviously a member of the family of receptors we have been considering in this chapter.

Analysis of the amino acid homology between SKR and other members of the superfamily of 'seven-transmembrane segment' receptors confirms their mutual relatedness. If the comparison lumps together identical residues and conservative substitutions then the similarities are as follows:

SKR compared with opsin: 46% (21% identity)
SKR compared with β_2 AR: 39% (24% identity)
SKR compared with M1 mAChR: 38% (24% identity)
SKR compared with M2 mAChR: 34% (22% identity)

It will be fascinating to find whether future research shows that the membrane receptors of related neuropeptides are also members of this molecular superfamily.

7.5 RHODOPSIN

It may seem odd to consider the photopigment rhodopsin alongside the β-adrenergic, muscarinic acetylcholine receptors and substance K receptors. But, as we shall shortly see, it is in fact very obviously a member of the same superfamily of receptor proteins. Here, if anywhere, the power of the molecular approach to neurobiology becomes apparent. What previously seemed poles apart is suddenly seen to be evolutionarily and functionally closely related. Students of cardiac disease suddenly share a common deep interest with students of ophthalmology. The action of β-blockers may tell us something not only about the cardiac adrenergic receptor but about the means by which a photon stimulates a photoreceptor!

In this section we shall only consider rhodopsin and its associated G-protein (often called **transducin (T)**). The organisation of rhodopsin into rod cell outer segments and the further biochemistry of photoreception will be considered in Chapter 12.

Rhodopsin is a ubiquitous photopigment. Not only is it found in the retinal rod cells of all vertebrates but is also widespread as a photopigment in invertebrates. A relative, **bacteriorhodopsin**, is found in the 'purple membrane' of *Halobacterium halobium*, where it acts as a 'proton pump' across the membrane. In all cases rhodopsin consists of a membrane-embedded protein, **opsin**, and a light-sensitive pigment group, **retinal**.

Retinal absorbs light in the visible range (λ = 400–600 nm). Its structure is shown in Figure 7.10. The figure shows that it can exist in two forms—an '**11-*cis*'** form and a lower energy '**all-*trans*'** form. The primary event in photoreception is the absorption of a photon of visible light by 11-*cis*-retinal. This provides the activation energy necessary for the transition between the 11-*cis* and all-*trans* form.

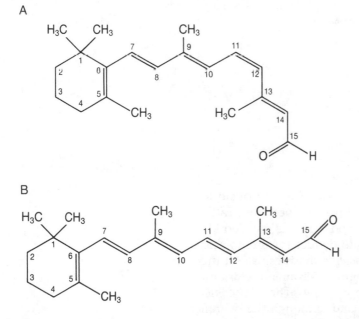

Figure 7.10 (A) 11-*cis* and (B) all-*trans*-retinal

It is the 11-*cis* form of retinal which is attached to opsin in the rhodopsin molecule. The attachment is by way of a **Schiff base** linkage to a lysine residue in the opsin. Transformation into the all-*trans* form breaks this linkage and leads to the dissociation of retinal from opsin. This initiates a cascade of biochemical, biophysical and physiological events which ultimately leads to a visual sensation.

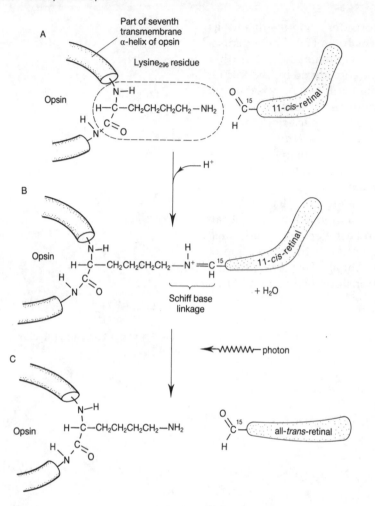

Figure 7.11 Linkage of 11-*cis*-retinal to lysine$_{296}$ of opsin. The linkage, as shown, takes the form of a Schiff base. This linkage is disrupted by a photon of appropriate energy. 11-*cis*-retinal is transformed to all-*trans*-retinal and diffuses out of the opsin molecule

Let us turn now to the structure of opsin. The first opsin to have its amino acid sequence analysed was derived from cattle eyes. Subsequently the usual methods of oligonucleotide hybridisation have enabled biologists to deduce the amino acid sequences of human, sheep and *Drosophila* rhodopsins. All the vertebrate rhodopsins have a chain length of 348 amino acids and show a high degree of sequence homology. The *Drosophila* rhodpsin consists of 373 amino acids and, although the overall sequence homology with bovine rhodopsin is only 37%, portions of it are sufficiently similar to be picked out by a bovine oligonucleotide probe. The overall conformation of *Drosophila* rhodopsin and its disposition in the membrane is remarkably similar to that of the mammalian photopigment.

Hydropathic analysis suggests that once again there are seven transmembrane segments—numbered from one to seven from the amino-terminal end. The carboxy-terminal projects from the

P-face of the membrane into the cytoplasmic space and the amino-terminal projects into the lumenal space within the rod discs (see Chapter 12). The transmembrane helices of both *Drosophila* and bovine rhodopsin and all the loops except that between helix five and six have exactly the same number of residues. The extra amino acid residues in *Drosophila* occur at the amino- and carboxy-terminal ends and in the five/six loop.

Figure 7.12 Bovine rhodopsin. The structural similarity to both the β_2-adrenergic and the mACh receptor molecules is clear. Once again the amino-terminal end bears oligosaccharide groups and there are seven trans-membrane α-helices. The black lysine residue (K) is that to which retinal is attached (see Fig. 7.11). The stippled residues in the carboxy-terminal end of the molecule are those which are phos-phorylated by rhodopsin kinase (see Fig. 7.14 and text). For orientation of the molecule in the outersegment disc see Figs 12.9 and 12.11. (After Lefkowitz *et al.*, 1986, *Trends in Pharmacological Sciences*, **7**, 444–448.)

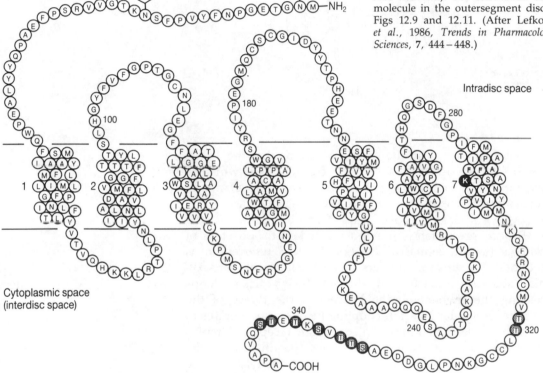

Figure 7.12 shows the seven opsin helices spread out in the usual plan form. It is believed that within the membrane they are grouped to form a somewhat 'dented' cylinder (Figure 7.13). The retinal pigment group is located deep down in the centre of this cylinder. The lysine residue to which it is attached through the Schiff base linkage is residue 296 in bovine opsin and is tentatively residue 319 in *Drosophila*.

The precise chemical environment surrounding retinal, i.e. the exact nature of the adjacent amino acid side chains from all seven helices, determines the wavelength to which the retinal will be maximally responsive. On receipt of an appropriate photon 11-*cis*-retinal will unbend into the all-*trans* form and this causes a

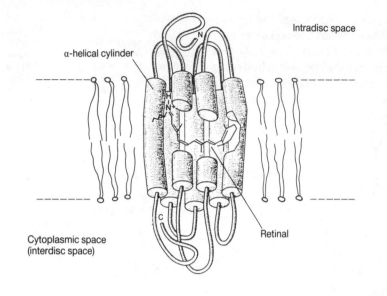

α-helical cylinder

Intradisc space

Cytoplasmic space
(interdisc space)

Retinal

Figure 7.13   Three-dimensional diagram of rhodopsin molecule in the rod disc membrane

conformational change in the opsin. It may be that the 11-*cis*-retinal holds the opsin in a strained configuration which is released once the Schiff base linkage is broken. The change in conformation, however, has far-reaching consequences.

For, as we indicated above, rhodopsin (like the β-AR, the mAChR and, presumably, the SKR) is linked to a system of G-proteins (in the retina, as we noted, often referred to as T-proteins). The linkage appears to be through the carboxy-terminal sequence and especially through the cytoplasmic loops connecting the transmembrane helices on the P-face of the membrane. A similar collision-coupling mechanism operates to that which we described for the β-adrenergic receptor. There is a difference however. Figure 7.14 shows that instead of the α-subunit of the G-protein (G_α or T_α) acting on adenylate cyclase to produce cAMP, the α-subunit in rod disc membranes acts on **cGMP phosphodiesterase (PDE)**.

Figure 7.14 shows that when the large trimeric PDE enzyme is activated it opens the cyclic GMP ring to form 5'-GMP. cGMP, as we shall see in Chapter 12, is believed to keep the rod cell in a depolarised state. As we noted when discussing collision-coupling in the β-AR system the mechanism allows considerable amplification of the signal to occur. Receipt of one photon may result in several hundred cGMPs being affected. Transformation of a number of cGMPs into their straight-chain forms consequently leads to a hyperpolarisation of the membrane and this in turn to a sequence of neurophysiological events ending in the activation of one or other parts of the visual system in the brain.

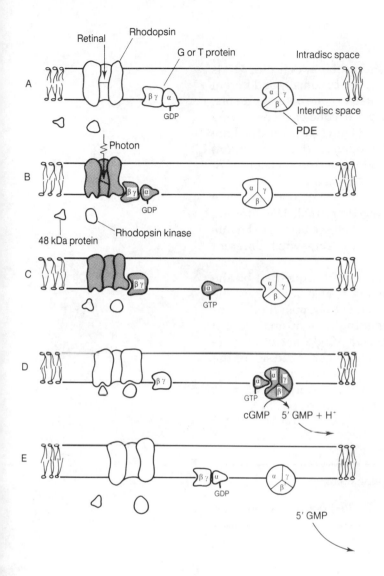

Figure 7.14. Collision-coupling in rod disc membrane. For explanation see text. PDE = cGMP phosphodiesterase. The figure shows that PDE is activated by the α-subunit of the G (or T) protein. Once activated PDE is able to open the ring structure of cGMP. The consequences of this change are discussed in Chapter 12. The photoactivation of rhodopsin is switched off by rhodopsin kinase and the 48 kDa protein

The conformational change undergone by opsin when retinal's Schiff base linkage is broken has further consequences. The changed contour of the cytoplasmic domain allows another two proteins to attach—**rhodopsin kinase** and the so-called 48 kDa protein. Rhodopsin kinase uses phosphate groups from ATP to phosphorylate as many as nine serine and threonine residues in opsin's carboxy-terminal tail (see Figure 7.12). It seems likely that this alters the conformation of the cytoplasmic domain in such a way that the interaction with the G-protein is prevented. Thus the photoactivation of the phosphodiesterase is switched off. The rod-cell returns to its resting state.

7.6 CONE OPSINS

Colour vision is widespread in the animal kingdom. It depends on the presence of pigments which absorb maximally at different wavelengths. These pigments are located in **cone outer segments**. In the human retina there are three types of cone pigment, having absorption maxima at 420 nm (blue), 530 nm (green) and 560 nm (red). The absorption maximum of rhodopsin (for comparison) is at 495 nm. Differential stimulation of the three categories of cone pigments is the first step in colour vision.

The cone pigments, like rhodopsin, consist of a protein (**cone opsin**) attached by a Schiff base linkage to **retinal**. The differing absorption maxima are believed (as we shall see below) to be due to the three different opsins providing somewhat different chemical environments for retinal.

The three human cone opsins have been sequenced by the customary techniques of gene cloning. Table 7.1 shows the sequence similarity with each other and with human rhodopsin. It can be deduced from this table that the cone opsins and rod opsin form a family. It appears that a single ancestral gene duplicated twice at least 500 Ma ago to give genes coding for the rod opsin and the red and blue cone opsins; a much more recent duplication of the red opsin gene, perhaps only 40 Ma ago, resulted in a gene coding for the green cone opsin.

Table 7.1 Homologies of rod and cone opsins

	Percentage sequence homology			
	Rod opsin	Blue opsin	Red opsin	Green opsin
Rod opsin	100	75	73	73
Blue opsin	42	100	79	79
Red opsin	40	43	100	99
Green opsin	41	44	96	100

Data from Nathans (1986). Values below the 100% diagonal are percentage identical residues; values above the diagonal are percentage identical plus conservative substitutions

The usual hydropathic analysis indicates that the cone opsins have retained the seven membrane-spanning helices of rhodopsin. All the cone opsins have a lysine corresponding in intramembranous position to the all-important lysine in rhodopsin which forms the Schiff base linkage with retinal. There is also considerable amino acid homology in the cytoplasmic loops between the transmembrane helices. We saw in the preceding section that these loops may well be involved in the vital interaction with the G-protein. Finally the carboxy-terminal tail, though not strongly homologous to rhodopsin, nevertheless contains a number of threonine and serine residues which, it will be remembered, are phosphorylated in rhodopsin to switch off its photoactivation.

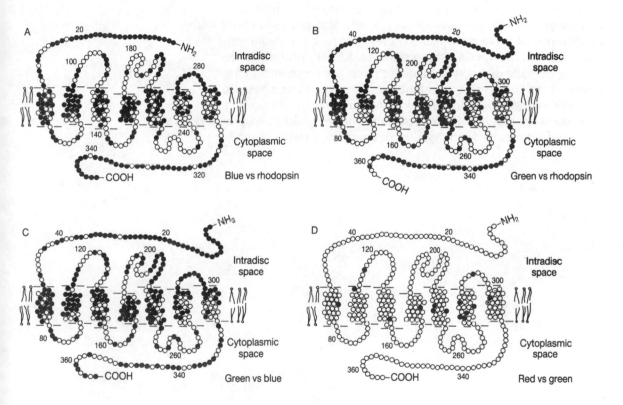

Although each of the cone opsins has, as already indicated, a lysine corresponding to rhodopsin's lysine 296 the distribution of charged amino acid side chains in its vicinity, and the overall charge in its environment, vary. The net intramembranous charge for the blue pigment (λ_{max} = 420 nm) is +1, whilst that for the green and red pigments (λ_{max} = 530 and 560 nm) is −1, and that for rhodopsin (λ_{max} = 495 nm) is 0. It may well be that these differences and other subtle biochemical and electrical variations are at root responsible for the different absorption maxima of the different pigments in our retinae, and thus for our appreciation of colour.

Figure 7.15 Comparison of the human visual pigments. The black residues indicate altered amino acid residues. It can be seen that blue and green cone opsins differ radically from rhodopsin and from each other (see Table 7.1). In contrast the red pigment differs only slightly from the green. The lysine residue to which retinal is attached is marked by a central dot in each drawing. For further explanation see text. (After Nathans *et al.*, 1986, *Science*, **232**, 193–202.)

It can be seen from this brief account that the molecular analysis of the visual pigments is providing not only a synthesis of biochemistry and neurophysiology, but also beginning to establish a comparative molecular anatomy with all the evolutionary implications which that entails.

7.7 CONCLUSION

In this chapter we have reviewed some of the intricate bio-chemistry which the fluid-mosaic structure of biological membranes allows. We have also achieved a first glimpse of how the determination of molecular structure has revealed evolution-ary relationships among receptors which had formerly been considered quite distinct. In the next chapter we begin on another vastly important aspect of membrane biology: their ability to separate solutions of different ionic concentration. It does not take very much knowledge of neurophysiology to recognise that upon this ability depends the whole working of the brain.

Chapter 8
Pumps

So far in this book we have been considering the biochemistry and molecular biology of neurons and neuronal systems. Now it is time to broach a second major theme in molecular neurobiology: **the part which membranes play in separating ionic solutions** and all that follows from this. Ionic fluxes, as we remarked at the end of Chapter 7, underlie the functioning of the nervous system. In the nineteenth century the great physicist James Clark Maxwell imagined a demon controlling a trapdoor between one compartment and another of a thermodynamic system. Such a demon, he suggested, could by judicious opening of the door allow only atoms above a certain energy to pass from one compartment to the other and hence cause the never yet experienced phenomenon of one part of an isolated system warming up whilst the other part cooled. It was later pointed out that for such a thought-experiment to be realised Maxwell's demon would need to be informed about the energy of the atoms in his two compartments—and information (as the twentieth century has discovered) has a thermodynamic cost. This is not the place to discuss the interrelations between thermodynamics and information theory: Maxwell's demon has only been introduced to emphasise the importance of gates and gate-keepers in membranes.

We shall consider in some detail the gates and channels in neural membranes in Chapters 9 and 10. In this chapter we shall look at some of the pumps which produce the inequality in ionic concentration across membranes in the first place. If such concentration differences did not obtain, membrane gates and channels, no matter what their sophistication, would be of no value; neurophysiology (as we know it) could never have come to be. Table 8.1 shows the concentrations of some important ions inside and outside nerve and muscle cells.

8.1 ENERGETICS

First of all let us look briefly at the energetics of creating and maintaining transmembrane concentration differences. How

Table 8.1 Ionic concentrations inside and outside some relevant cells

Ion	Intracellular concentration	Extracellular concentration
1. Squid giant axon		
	mM/kg H_2O	mM/kg H_2O
K^+	400	20
Na^+	50	440
Ca^{2+}	0.4	10
Mg^{2+}	10	54
Cl^-	100	560
Organic anions	385	–
2. Mammalian muscle cell		
	(mM)	(mM)
K^+	155	4
Na^+	12	145
Mg^{2+}	30	1–2
Ca^{2+}	1–2	2.5–5
	(Only about 10^{-4} is free)	
Cl^-	4	120
Organic anions	approx. 150	
3. Cat motor neuron		
	(mM)	(mM)
K^+	150	5.5
Na^+	15	150
Cl^-	9	125

much energy does it need to pump an ion across a membrane to establish a concentration gradient and to hold that concentration gradient in place? If we neglect the transmembrane voltage the appropriate equation is quite easy to derive.

First of all we need to define an important parameter: the **chemical potential**. In essence the notion of a chemical potential is analogous to the better-known electrical and gravitational potentials. It is a familiar idea that electrons will flow from a region of high electrical potential to one of low potential; similarly objects placed in regions of high gravitational potential will fall towards regions of lower potential. The same idea obtains in the world of chemistry. Molecules and/or ions will move from states of high chemical potential to states of low potential.

The chemical potential of a substance, A, in phase α, is symbolised as $\mu_A{}^\alpha$. Its value is given by the following expression:

$$\mu_A{}^\alpha = \mu_A{}^O + RT \ln x_A{}^\alpha \qquad 8.1$$

where $\mu_A{}^O$ is chemical potential of A in a pure phase of A and $x_A{}^\alpha$ is the mole fraction of A in phase α (NB: in a pure phase of A, $x_A{}^\alpha = 1$) and 'ln' is $\log_e$, the 'natural' logarithm.

Now for all biological calculations $x_A{}^\alpha$ may be taken as $C_A{}^\alpha$—the **concentration** of A in phase α.

Having defined a chemical potential let us see how it can be used to determine the amount of energy required either to pump materials across membranes against their concentration gradients or, vice versa, the amount of energy which could (theoretically) be tapped when materials flow 'downhill' along their concentration gradients. The situation under consideration is shown in Figure 8.1.

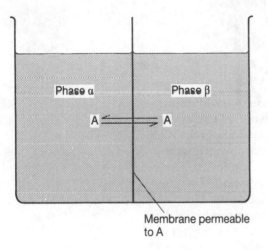

Phase α   Phase β

A ⇌ A

Membrane permeable
to A

Figure 8.1 A permeable membrane separates two solutions of substance A. When $\mu_A{}^\alpha \neq \mu_A{}^\beta$ there will be an overall movement of A across the membrane until equality of chemical potential is achieved

By definition $\mu_A{}^\alpha \neq \mu_A{}^\beta$. Let us suppose that $\mu_A{}^\alpha < \mu_A{}^\beta$, then:

$$\Delta\mu_A = \mu_A{}^\beta - \mu_A{}^a \qquad 8.2$$

$$= (\mu_A{}^o - \mu_A{}^o) + RT \ln \frac{C_A{}^\beta}{C_A{}^\alpha}$$

i.e. $\Delta\mu_A = RT \ln \dfrac{C_A{}^\beta}{C_A{}^\alpha} \qquad 8.3$

This expression gives the 'free energy' (symbolised as ΔG) which is available to do work when the chemical substance passes from its high potential to its low potential state. Let us now simplify the symbolism a little. Let us remove the signs indicating the two phases, α and β, in which our solute is supposed to be present and merely refer to the concentration of the solute on either side of the partition as C_1 and C_2. We can then write:

$$\Delta G = RT \ln \frac{C_1}{C_2} \qquad\qquad 8.4$$

If we now insert the usual values for R and T, i.e. R (the gas constant) $= 8.31$ J K^{-1} mol^{-1} and T (temperature in Kelvins) $= 310$ K (i.e. 37 °C), then:

$$\Delta G = - [(8.31 \text{ J K}^{-1} \text{ mol}^{-1}) \times 310 \text{ K}] \ln \frac{C_1}{C_2}$$

$$= - 2576 \ln \frac{C_1}{C_2} \text{ J mol}^{-1} \qquad\qquad 8.5$$

Let us make use of eq. 8.5 to determine the quantity of energy required to pump a sodium ion from inside to outside a neuron. In this calculation it is important to note that we do not take into account any electrical forces which may be (probably are) acting on the ion. We shall consider these in detail in Chapter 10. There we shall see that the gradient up which an ion is pumped is given by the Nernst equation, which takes into account the electrical as well as the concentration differences of ions on the two sides of a membrane. Here, however, let us introduce the subject by substituting in eq. 8.5 the values given in Table 8.1 (cat motor neuron) for Na$^+$ outside ($[\text{Na}^+]_O$), i.e. 150 mM, and Na$^+$ inside ($[\text{Na}^+]_i$), i.e. 15 mM, the neuron. The energy required to pump a mole of sodium ions from the inside to the outside against this concentration gradient at 37 °C is given by:

$$\Delta G = 2576 \ln \frac{150}{15} \text{ J mol}^{-1}$$

$$= 5932 \text{ J mol}^{-1}$$

Now a mole of Na$^+$ consists of 6×10^{23} ions (i.e. Avogadro's number of ions). It follows that 5932 J are required to pump this quantity against the prevailing concentration gradient—and unless the pumping mechanism is 100% efficient (which it isn't) considerably more.

To determine the minimum amount of energy required to pump a single ion out of the neuron is a simple matter:

$$\frac{5932}{6 \times 10^{23}} \sim 1 \times 10^{-20} \text{ J}$$

Now the majority of biochemical activities are driven by energy derived from energy-rich phosphate bonds, principally those of ATP. We shall shortly see that membrane pumps are no exception to this rule: the energy required to pump ions against their concentration gradients is also derived from the energy-rich phosphate bonds of ATP. We have just worked out how much energy is required to pump a sodium ion out of a neuron against its concentration gradient. Let us see how many 'energy-rich' phosphate bonds have to be hydrolysed to provide this energy.

The ΔG for the dephosphorylation of ATP to ADP + P_i varies somewhat according to the concentration of ATP. Let us take -12 kcal mol^{-1} as a reasonable value for the situation we are considering. Remembering that **1 cal = 4.18 J** it follows that one energy-rich bond is equivalent to about **50 160 J mol^{-1}**.

Hence the dephosphorylation of a *single* ATP to ADP would yield approximately

$$\frac{5 \times 10^4}{6 \times 10^{23}} \sim 8 \times 10^{-20} \text{ J}$$

It follows that the hydrolysis of one energy-rich phospate bond will yield sufficient energy to transfer approximately **eight sodium ions**.

These calculations have, as we have already noted, assumed that the pump is 100% efficient and, as we emphasised at the outset, have totally neglected the contribution of electrical forces. They have also totally omitted any consideration of the complex biochemical mechanisms underlying the operation of the pump. It is thus somewhat surprising that they yield an answer so close to the experimentally determined value. It has been shown (as we shall shortly see) that three sodium ions are pumped out in exchange for two potassium ions pumped in for the expenditure of one energy-rich phosphate bond.

This short excursion into the energetics of pumping will, it is hoped, have given the reader some feel for the quantities of energy and the numbers of molecules and ions involved.

8.2 THE SODIUM/POTASSIUM PUMP

The sodium/potassium pump is ubiquitous. It is found in the plasma membranes of practically all animal cells. It pumps Na$^+$ ions out of a cell and at the same time pumps K$^+$ ions in the opposite direction. It is thus an example of an 'antiport' mechanism. **Three sodium ions** are pumped **out** whilst **two potassium ions** are pumped **in** during one cycle of operation. The pump is energised by the dephosphorylation of ATP, as mentioned above, and one complete cycle is fuelled by the hydrolysis of one molecule of ATP to ADP. The ATPase which catalyses this dephosphorylation is dependent on the presence of both Na$^+$ and K$^+$ ions. The Na$^+$ ions have to be within the cell, the K$^+$ ions outside. The pump is inhibited by cardiac glycosides such as **digitalis** and **ouabain**, which affect the K$^+$ site on the external surface. The Na$^+$ + K$^+$-ATPase is clearly of fundamental importance in maintaining the ionic concentrations upon which, as indicated above, the entire functioning of a nervous system depends.

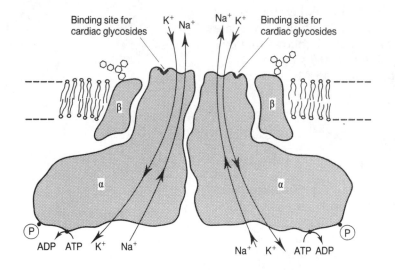

Figure 8.2 Conceptual diagram of the Na$^+$ + K$^+$ pump. The schematic diagram shows that the Na$^+$ + K$^+$ pump is a dimer, each unit of which consists of two subunits—a large catalytic or α-subunit and a smaller glycoprotein β-subunit. The major part of the catalytic subunit lies in the cytoplasmic space. This cytosolic domain has a site for dephosphorylating ATP and another site for the attachment of ATP's γ-phosphate. The extracellular surface of the α-subunit possesses a site for cardiac glycosides such as ouabain and digitalis. The β-subunit is much smaller and bears a short oligosaccharide chain on its external face. It is also believed to be sensitive to cardiac glycosides

The sodium/potassium pump can be isolated from the membranes of several types of cell including mammalian kidney cells and the electric organs of eels and rays, where it is highly concentrated. As Figure 8.2 shows it appears to consist of two identical units, each of which, in turn, consists of two subunits. The larger of the two subunits, the α-subunit, has a molecular weight of about 100 kDa, and consists of 1016 amino acids (sheep kidney) or 1022 amino acids (*Torpedo*, the electric ray). The smaller β-subunit, a glycoprotein, has a molecular weight of 55 kDa. The α-polypeptide is the catalytic subunit. The smaller β-polypeptide is almost 20% carbohydrate by mass. Its exact function is not clear. Its close union to the α-subunit is, however, necessary if the α-subunit is to function as an ATPase.

cDNA libraries prepared from sheep kidney and *Torpedo* electroplax have been probed by radiolabelled oligonucleotides prepared from known amino acid fragments of the α-polypeptide. This technique (which was described in outline in Chapter 5) yields DNA clones from which complete amino acid sequences of the α-polypeptide can be deduced. It turns out that there is 85% amino acid homology between the α-polypeptides derived from these two species. This shows remarkable conservatism when it recalled that a common ancestor of sheep and electric ray can have lived no later than 400 Ma ago.

Examination of the polypeptide for hydropathic domains suggests that the amino acid chain spans the membrane no less than eight times whilst the central part of the molecule forms a large cytosolic domain (see Figure 8.3). The cytosolic domain contains the ATP binding and hydrolysis sites. The ouabain binding site, on the other hand, is to be found on the outside of the membrane, possibly between the third and fourth trans-membrane helices. It is not yet completely clear where the ion pore(s) is (are) although the evidence suggests that it (they) runs through the α-subunit between the fourth and fifth helices. A schematic diagram showing the disposition of the polypeptide in the membrane is shown in Figure 8.3.

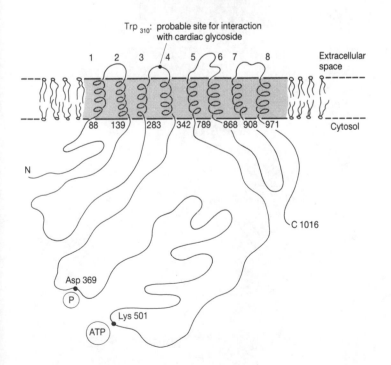

Figure 8.3 $Na^+ + K^+$-ATPase catalytic subunit. The major part of the α-subunit is located in the cytosol. It is attached to the membrane by eight transmembrane helices. The largest cytosolic domain (residues 342–789) provides the phosphate binding site (Asp_{369}) and the ATP hydrolysis site (Lys_{501}). A tryptophan residue (Trp_{310}) on the outer face of the membrane between transmembrane helices 3 and 4 is believed to be the site with which cardiac glycosides interact. The figure represents only a two-dimensional plan of the molecule: in reality both the cytosolic and the transmembrane domains would be folded in upon themselves. (Data from Schull, Schwartz and Lingrel, 1985, *Nature*, **316**, 691–695.)

196 *Pumps*

It is believed that the binding of an Mg^{2+}-ATP to the catalytic subunit at lysine 501 leads to a dephosphorylation with the transference of the cleaved phosphate (i.e. the **γ-phosphate**) to aspartate 369 (see Figure 8.3). The energy released in the dephosphorylation brings about an extensive conformational change in the molecule involving at least 80 amino acid residues.

Figure 8.4 Schematic to show the operation of the $Na^+ + K^+$ ATPase. (A) Na^+ ions and ATP approach the pump's cytosolic domain; K^+ ions approach from the extracellular compartment. (B) Na^+ ions find their binding sites on the α-subunit and ATP is hydrolysed to ADP. (C) The γ-phosphate from ATP is transferred to the phosphate binding site and the α-subunit undergoes a conformational change so that three Na^+ ions are discharged to the exterior. (D) K^+ ions bind to the extracellular surface and a continuation of the conformational change impels two K^+ ions into the cell and releases the phosphate group. The catalytic subunit returns to its original state

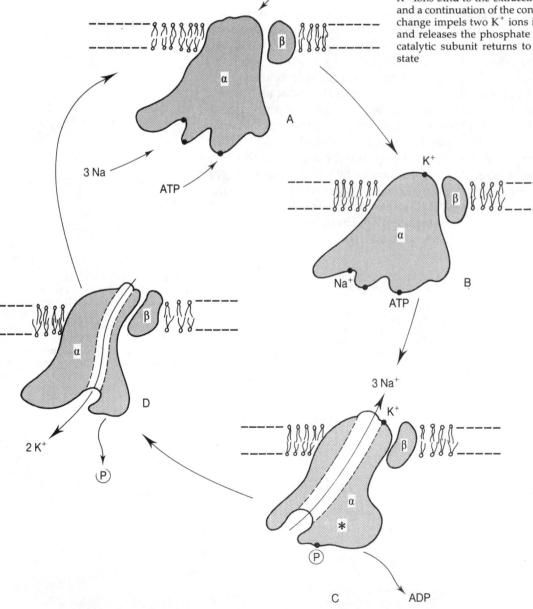

It is suggested that this conformational change consists in a transition from an α-helical to a β-sheet structure. The conformational change impels three sodium ions out of the cell. The new conformation also allows two potassium ions to bind to the extracellular side of the subunit. This leads, in its turn, to a reverse conformational change which both frees the γ-phosphate from aspartate and impels the two K^+ ions into the cell. Thus at the end of this sequence of events one ATP has been hydrolysed to ADP, three sodium ions have been extruded, two potassium ions pumped into the cell, and the catalytic subunit has resumed its original conformation.

We shall shortly see that the structure of the $Na^+ + K^+$ catalytic subunit is similar to the Ca^{2+}-ATPase of muscle sarcoplasmic reticulum (and indeed also similar to the K^+-pump of bacteria). It seems that pumps form yet another group of evolutionarily related proteins.

8.3 THE CALCIUM PUMP

In Chapter 10 we shall note the great importance of the Ca^{2+} ions in neurons, especially at synapses. We shall return to this in more detail in Chapter 14. We can note here, however, that there is very steep concentration gradient of (free) calcium ions between the inside and the outside of neurons (see Table 8.1). There is thus just as great a need for a pump to extrude the Ca^{2+} ions, which as we shall see flow in during a membrane depolarisation, as there is for a pump to move K^+ and Na^+ into and out of an axon after an action potential.

A calcium pump is present in the membranes of most cells. Judged by its immunological reactivity it takes slightly different forms in different cells. Immunologically distinct forms of the calcium pump have been detected in fast twitch and slow twitch skeletal muscles, cardiac muscle, erythrocyte membranes, etc. The pump has, however, been most intensively studied in the system of internal membranes found in striped muscle fibres—the **sarcoplasmic reticulum (SR)**. The SR constitutes a reservoir of Ca^{2+} ions. The contraction of striped muscles is dependent on triggering by Ca^{2+} ions and hence the concentration of calcium ions in the vicinity of the contractile elements (actin, myosin, etc.) is very critical. It is for this reason that the sarcoplasmic reticulum provides such a rich source for the calcium pump. Indeed it appears that the pump forms up to 80% of the SR membrane.

It comes as no surprise therefore that the first gene coding for a calcium pump was isolated from the SR of rabbit skeletal muscle. Essentially the same technique of oligonucleotide hybridisation cloning was used as was employed to isolate the gene coding for the $Na^+ + K^+$-ATPase. From the nucleotide base sequence obtained in this way the amino acid sequence of the pump was deduced. Again it turned out to be a huge protein consisting of 997 amino acids.

By examining the polypeptide chain for hydropathic domains the position of the molecule in the membrane can as usual be deduced. It is believed that there are no less than ten transmembrane segments which may be in either the β-sheet or α-helical conformation. In addition to the membrane-spanning segments the molecule also possesses a large and intricate tripartite cytosolic domain. Five 'stalks' project into the cytoplasm connecting the transmembrane segments of the protein with these three large cytosolic domains. Each domain is believed to have a different function. The first is concerned with Ca^{2+} binding and transportation; the second, the phosphorylation domain, with acceptance of the γ-phosphate from ATP; and the third, the nucleotide domain, is concerned with ATP attachment. These three cytosolic domains are believed to be folded together so that they can work interactively as a unit. Evidence from electron microscopy and optical diffractometry support this interesting structure.

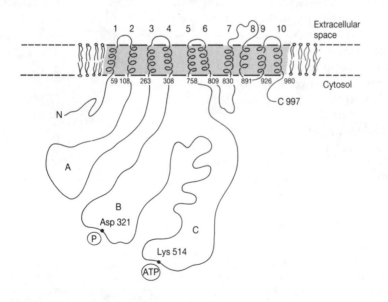

Figure 8.5 Structure of the rabbit SR Mg^{2+} dependent Ca^{2+}-ATPase. It can be seen that the molecule bears a striking resemblence to the $Na^+ + K^+$ ATPase catalytic subunit (Fig. 8.3). The large cytosolic region can be divided into three major domains. The first domain, A (residues 132–238), is believed to be concerned with the transport of Ca^{2+} out of the cytosol; the second, B (residues 330–505), is involved in phosphorylation; the third, C (residues 505–680), has to do with ATP hydrolysis. Asp_{321} is at the centre of the phosphate binding process and Lys_{514} is essential for the ATPase activity. The molecule is believed to be attached to the membrane by ten transmembrane helices. It should be borne in mind that the diagram represents only a two-dimensional plan: in reality both the cytoplasmic and the transmembrane domains would be folded in upon themselves. (Data from MacLennan *et al*, 1985, *Nature*, **316**, 696–700.)

For every two Ca^{2+} ions transported by the pump one ATP molecule is dephosphorylated. The pump also depends on the presence of Mg^{2+} ions; indeed there may be a counter-transport of one Mg^{2+} ion inwards for every two Ca^{2+} ions pumped out. Because free calcium ions are in such very low concentration within a cell the calcium pump is very specific, and has a very high affinity for the ion. The pump is, moreover, controlled by the quantity of Ca^{2+} in the cytosol. If the concentration rises beyond about 10^{-4} mM the pump increases its rate of working. In the erythrocyte membrane this has been shown to be due to the presence of an important regulatory protein, **calmodulin**, as part of the pump. This binds excess cytosolic Ca^{2+}, undergoes a conformational change, and causes the work rate of the Ca^{2+} pump to increase.

Finally, as mentioned in the preceding section, it is possible to find remarkable similarities between the Mg^{2+}-dependent Ca^{2+}-ATPase and the catalytic subunit of the $Na^+ + K^+$ ATPase. Analysis of the hydropathic segments of the molecules indicates striking homologies The phosphorylation and ATP-binding sites are in the same position and except for three regions where segments of $\geqslant 20$ amino acids have been inserted or deleted from one or other of the proteins homologous structural features are obvious. There is no doubt that the calcium and sodium/potassium pumps have evolved from a common ancestor.

Figure 8.6 Comparison between the Mg^{2+}-dependent Ca^{2+}-ATPase and the $Na^+ + K^+$-ATPase. (A) The amino acid homology between sheep kidney $Na^+ + K^+$-ATPase (NKA) and rabbit cardiac Ca^{2+}-ATPase (CA) is shown (amino acids represented by letter symbols, see Table 2.1). Only sequences with greater than 30% homology are compared and gaps have been added to maximise the homology; homologous residues are indicated by a dot.(B) Hydropathic plots for the two pumps. Hydrophobic regions are drawn above the horizontal axis and hydrophilic regions below it. The parallelograms represent the homologous regions shown in (A) and their positions along the polypeptide chain. The numbers along the NKA plot indicate the position of the major hydrophobic regions (transmembrane helices). P = the phosphate binding site; A = the ATP binding site. (Reprinted by permission from Shull, Schwartz and Lingrel, 1985, *Nature*, **316**, 691–695. Copyright © 1985, Macmillan Magazines Ltd.)

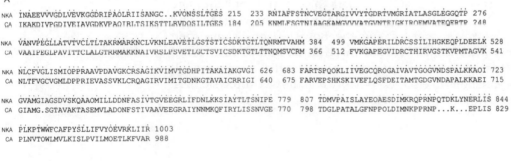

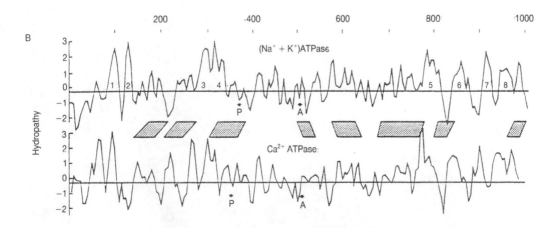

8.4 OTHER PUMPS AND TRANSPORT MECHANISMS

Plasma membranes possess many other metabolically driven pumps. Some of these are linked to the pumping of Na^+ ions across the membrane. Others are connected to the movement of H^+ ions. One pump which is of considerable importance in neurobiology is that which extrudes chloride ions from the neuron. Rather little is known about this pump. Chloride ions are not in electrochemical equilibrium across the membranes of most neurons (see Chapter 11). This indicates that a pump ultimately depending on metabolic energy must exist. In some cases it is believed the energy is derived from the ATP–ADP system; in other cases the energy may be derived from the distribution of other ions (for instance H^+ ions) across the membrane.

The several metabolically driven pumps we have considered in this chapter are very effective in establishing concentration differences of ions across neuronal and glial cell membranes. In the next chapters of this book we shall examine the ways in which neuronal membranes are able to control the fluxes of ions back down their electrochemical gradients. Neurons are, of course, not the only types of cell able to exert this control, but they are certainly the most accomplished. We shall see how ligand- and voltage-controlled gates shape the flows of ions along their gradients and we shall see how these flows, in their turn, affect the electrical polarity of neuronal and neuroglial membranes. It is these variations in electrical polarity that the electrophysiologist picks up with his probing electrode.

Chapter 9
Ligand-gated channels

In Chapter 6 we met a first example of a gate controlling a transmembrane channel in the variable open/shut states of the **gap junction connexon**. In this chapter and the next we shall consider some of the many other gates and channels which have been developed in neural cells. Until the advent of genetic engineering and patch-clamping their structure and function were extremely difficult to study. They are sometimes present as only a few molecules per cell and, moreover, are hidden from conventional biochemical techniques by insertion in the lipid biomembrane. Nonetheless, as we shall see in the next few chapters, a great deal of neurophysiology ultimately depends on the their presence and operation.

Membrane 'gates' or 'channels' may be divided into two categories: those which are controlled by **chemical molecules (ligands)** and those which are controlled by transmembrane **voltage**. In fact this division is not absolutely clear cut. Ligands have an affect on some voltage-dependent gates and, vice versa, transmembrane voltage is now known to influence at least some ligand-controlled gates. Nevertheless, for the purposes of exposition, we shall consider each in turn.

Both ligand-controlled and voltage-controlled gates depend for their physiological effect on there being a concentration and/or an electrochemical gradient across the membrane. Opening and shutting of these gates allows ions to flow across the membrane in the direction in which the gradient is inclined. This, in turn, results in the various electrical phenomena which the neurophysiologist picks up when investigating the nervous system: action potentials, postsynaptic potentials, electrotonic potentials, receptor potentials, generator potentials, etc. These concentration differences, ultimately due to the membrane pumps which we considered in the previous chapter, are shown in Table 8.1.

In this chapter we shall consider ligand-gated channels and in the next we shall turn our attention to voltage-controlled gates.

We shall proceed as follows. We shall begin by describing the best-known of all the ligand-gated channels—the **nicotinic acetylcholine receptor (nAChR)**. We shall then go on to discuss two other ligand-controlled gates, the **GABA$_A$** receptor and the **glycine** receptor. We shall see that the molecular structure of these latter two receptors is sufficiently similar to that of the nAChR to indicate that they, too, are all members of an evolutionarily related superfamily. Finally we shall look at another well-known group of ligand-gated channels: those which respond to excitatory amino acids.

9.1 THE NICOTINIC ACETYLCHOLINE RECEPTOR

As mentioned above the type example of a ligand-controlled gate is the nicotinic acetylcholine receptor (nAChR). We have already met this entity several times in previous chapters. Its structure is nowadays very well known.

We noted in Chapter 7 that cholinergic receptors can be divided into two major classes: nicotinic and muscarinic. In that chapter we looked at the muscarinic receptor in some depth. We saw that it was coupled to a complex membrane molecular biology involving G-proteins and cyclase enzymes. The response of the nAChR is, as we shall shortly see, simpler and much more rapid. Although the nAChR is mostly known from peripheral sites it is also to be found in the central nervous system. Recent reports have localised it in the hippocampus, ventro-lateral geniculate nucleus, amygdala and hypothalamus.

Finally, in this introductory section, it should be noted that it is a little misleading to refer to *the* nicotinic acetylcholine receptor. For, like most of the other receptors we have considered and shall consider, nAChRs vary from one organism to another and from one part of a given organism to another. Brain nAChRs, for instance, differ from peripheral nAChRs in their constitution and pharmacology. Peripheral nAChRs themselves differ: those on 'fast' muscles have different response times to those on 'slow' muscles. Nicotinic acetylcholine receptors form yet another closely knit evolutionary family.

9.1.1 Structure

The most concentrated source of nicotinic acetylcholine receptors is to be found in the **electric organ (electroplax)** of electric fish—the elasmobranch electric ray *Torpedo* and the teleost electric eel *Electrophorus* (= *Gymnotus*). Electroplaxes develop from muscle somites and their innervation is via cholinergic neuromuscular junctions. These are far larger and far more numerous than in normal skeletal muscle. The whole organ is very rich in ACh, nAChRs and the associated enzymes of cholinergic synapses. Indeed electron micrographs of electroplax postsynaptic membranes show extremely dense populations of nAChRs. Discharge of the electric organ can generate as much as 600 V. Finally it is worth noting that cartilaginous and bony fish diverged at least 400 Ma ago. Their electric organs, apart from some differences in detailed physiology, are thus remarkable instances of convergent evolution. In spite of the great period of independent evolution their nAChR's are also, as we shall see, very similar.

Figure 9.1 Freeze-fracture electron micrograph of the E-face of the post-synaptic membrane of *Torpedo* electric organ. The acetylcholine receptors are arranged in rows, probably on the crests of the junctional folds of the postsynaptic membrane (see Chapter 14). Each AChR can be seen in this surface view˙ to resemble a tiny doughnut. The scale bar represents 0.1 μm. (From Hirokawa, 1983, *Structure and Function of Excitable Cells*, New York: Plenum Press, pp. 113–141; with permission.)

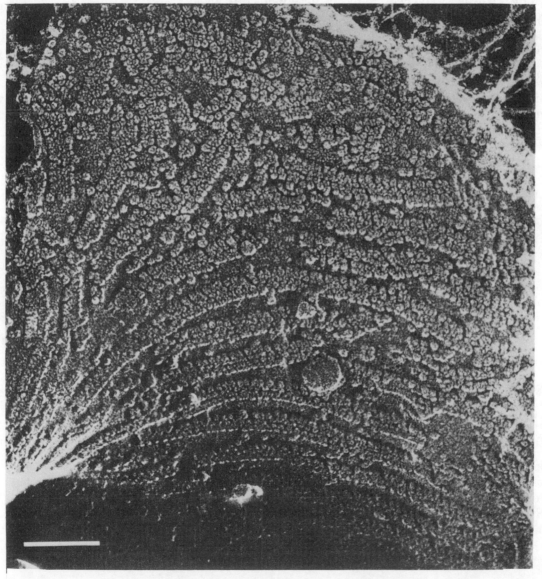

The first molecular-biological studies of the nAChR thus used the very rich source provided by electric organs. Many sophisticated techniques have been employed. It is, for instance, possible to obtain purified samples of the nAChR by making use of some snake neurotoxic peptides, the favourites being **Najatoxin (NajaTX)** from the cobra *Naja naja siamensis* (sometimes called just **cobratoxin**) and **α-bungarotoxin (α-BuTX)** from the snake *Bungarus multicinctus*. These neurotoxins bind specifically to the nicotinic acetylcholine receptor. Thus if α-BuTX is bound to a solid chromatography substrate and a solubilised preparation of electroplax membrane run through the substrate nAChR will be caught by the α-BuTX and held. In fact α-BuTX binds nAChR so firmly that it is almost impossible to wash it off the column. CobraTX binds less firmly and hence provides a better substrate.

After purification of electroplax nAChR by snake venom chromatography it is eluted, denatured with SDS (see Section 6.4) and subjected to SDS–polyacrylamide electrophoresis. Staining with Coomassie blue reveals four bands of material (Figure 9.2). These correspond to four subunits—α, β, γ and δ— in order of increasing molecular weight.

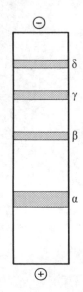

Figure 9.2 SDS-polyacrilamide gel electrophoresis of the nicotinic acetylcholine receptor. Electrophoresis separates the four subunits by molecular weight. The α-subunit travels furthest (mol. wt $\simeq$ 40 000 Da), the β is next (mol. wt $\simeq$ 49 000 Da), then comes the γ-subunit (mol. wt $\simeq$ 57 000 Da) and heaviest of all is the δ-subunit (mol. wt $\simeq$ 65 000 Da). The electrophoresis also shows that there are two copies of the α-subunit for each copy of the β,δ and γ subunits

Although the *Torpedo* electroplax is sufficiently rich in nAChR to yield milligrams of the purified receptor the method of choice for determining primary structure is nowadays via the recombinant DNA techniques described in Chapter 5. Small amino acid sequences can be determined from subunit material eluted from the electrophoresis bands. These can be used, as described in Chapter 5, to construct short oligonucleotide probes. The probes, in turn, are used to screen a cDNA library prepared from electroplax mRNA. The cDNA corresponding to the probe can then be cloned.

It is next necessary to ensure that the cDNA isolated by this technique does in fact code for the nAChR. This can be done by transcribing it into mRNA and introducing this into an expression system. Clearly the mRNA for all four subunits must be injected. As indicated in Chapter 5 the expression system is normally *Xenopus* oocyte. To ascertain that the protein expressed in the oocyte is indeed nAChR can be achieved in two ways. First, one can examine the oocyte membrane by electrophysiological techniques to establish that it now possesses channels responsive to ACh. Second, one can subject the oocyte membrane to SDS–polyacrylamide gel analysis alongside α-toxin-purified nAChR from *Torpedo* electroplax and establish that the same protein is present.

Finally, having satisfied oneself that the isolated cDNA is indeed the nAChR gene, one can then use one or other of the standard techniques described in Chapter 5 to obtain its base sequence. Having the base sequence it is then possible, knowing the genetic code, to predict the primary structure of the nAChR.

The outcome of this sophisticated molecular biology has been to show that *Torpedo* nAChR is multimeric protein with a total molecular weight of some 268 kDa. It consists of five subunits: two α-subunits (each consisting of 461 amino acids), one β-subunit (493 amino acids), one γ-subunit (506 amino acids) and one δ-

Figure 9.3 Primary sequences of the *Torpedo*, calf and human nAChR α-subunits. The amino acid sequences have been aligned to achieve maximum homology. Amino acids are represented by single letter code (see Table 2.1). The positive numbering commences at the N-terminal of the mature peptide; negative numbers refer to the signal sequences. Large letters indicate identical residues, dotted lines enclose conservative substitutions. Vertical arrows represent intron splice junctions. S——S shows the disulphide linkage between two cysteine residues in the vicinity of the ACh binding site. M1, M2, M3 and M4 indicate transmembrane helices. (Reprinted by permission from Noda *et al.*, 1983, *Nature*, **302**, 528–532. Copyright © 1983, Macmillan Magazines Ltd.)

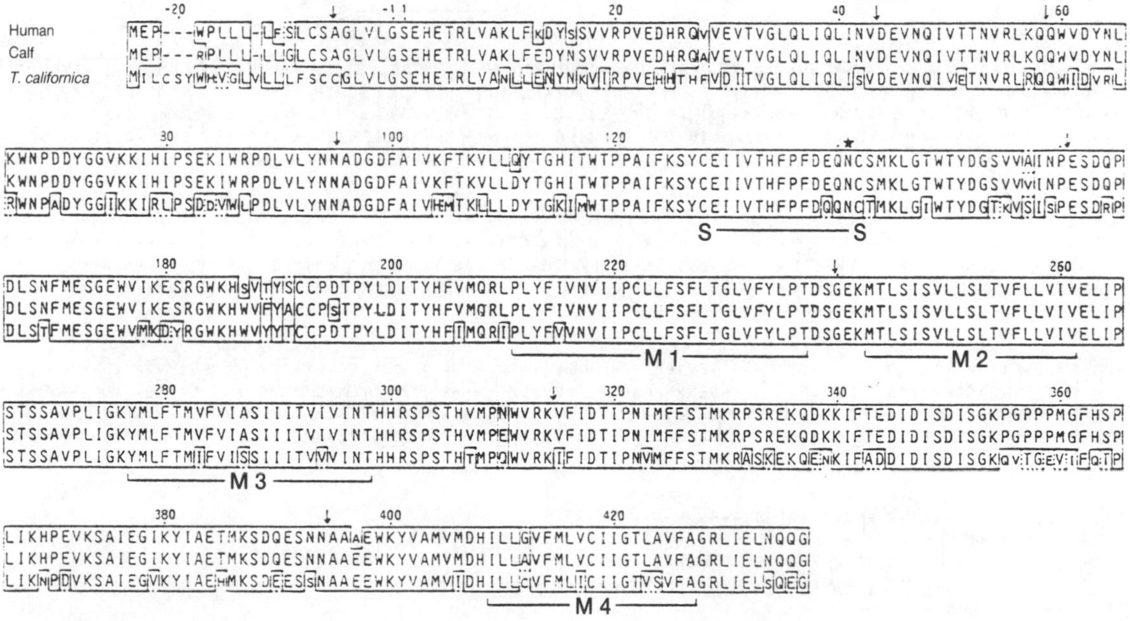

subunit (522 amino acids). A pentameric structure has been shown to exist in all the vertebrates so far examined. The subunits making up the pentamer may, however, differ. There is some evidence, for example, that rat brain nAChR consists of three α- and two β-subunits ($\alpha_3\beta_2$). The amino acid sequences of human, calf and *Torpedo californica* α-subunits are shown in Figure 9.3.

Inspection of the figure shows that there is very considerable amino acid homology between these three evolutionarily widely separated AChR subunits. Figure 9.3 also indicates the hydrophobic stretches of the α-subunit. The position of these hydrophobic stretches in the primary sequences of the other three subunits, as Figure 9.4A shows, is very similar. This suggests that all subunits derived by three successive duplications of an original ancestral gene. Indeed, as we noted in Chapter 4, the nAChR present in the nervous systems of some insects appears to be a homopentamer ($\psi\alpha_5$) and hence perhaps similar to the ancestral vertebrate complex.

A

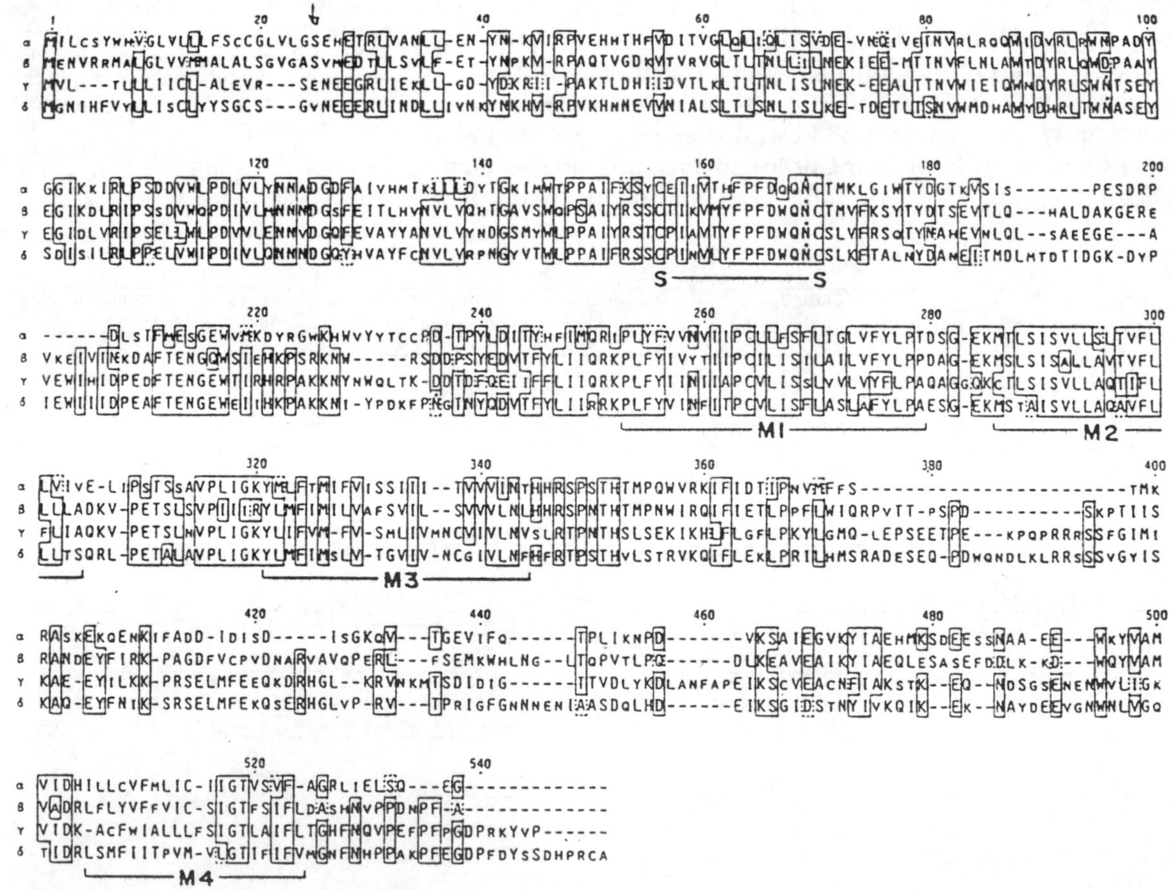

(Figure 9.4A: multiple amino acid sequence alignment of four nAChR subunits (α, β, γ, δ), residue positions numbered 1–540+, with disulphide bond (S—S) and hydrophobic membrane-spanning regions M1, M2, M3 and M4 indicated.)

B

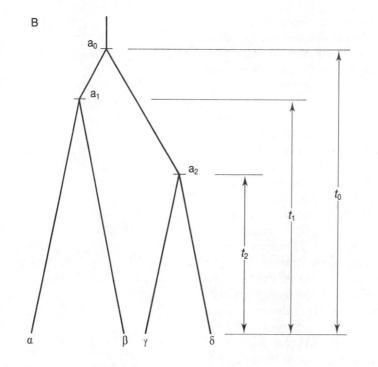

Figure 9.4 Primary sequences of the α-, β-,γ- and δ-subunits of *Torpedo* nAChR and possible evolution of the nAChR gene. (A) *(facing page)* Note that the numbering of these sequences commences from the N-terminal methionine residue of the signal peptide. To compare the residue numbers with those in Fig. 9.2 it is necessary to count from residue ser_{25} (arrowed). The four sequences in the figure have been aligned to achieve maximum homology. Gaps ($-$) have been inserted to achieve this maximum. Identical residues are enclosed by continuous lines. Dashed lines enclose conservative substitutions. Otherwise as for Fig. 9.3. (B) Examination of the similarities in the amino acid sequences of the α-, β-, γ- and δ-subunits suggests that they all evolved from a common ancestor by three gene duplications, a_0, a_1 and a_2. Making certain assumptions about the rate of change it is estimated that $t_1 = 0.82t_0$ and $t_2 = 0.65t_0$. (From Numa *et al.*, 1983, *Cold Harbour Symposia on Quantitative Biology*, **XLVIII**, 57–69; with permission.)

The hydrophobic amino acid stretches indicate which parts of the various subunits are embedded in the membrane. The amino-terminal end of the molecule extends into the extracellular space and the amino acid chain then loops through the membrane five

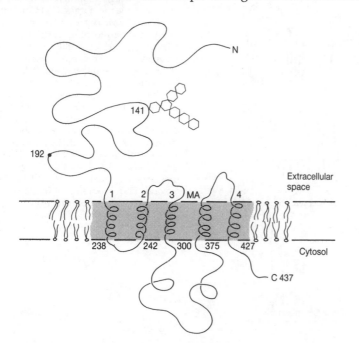

Figure 9.5 Disposition of human α-subunit in a membrane. The first 210 residues of the subunit are located in the extracellular space. Glycosylation occurs at residue 141 (asn). The binding site for acetylcholine is believed to be close to residue 192 and 193 (both cys). Five helices span the membrane. Helices 1,2,3 and 4 are hydrophobic; helix MA is amphipathic.

times so that all its hydrophobic segments assuming an α-helical formation are embedded in the lipid bilayer. The carboxy-terminal end emerges ultimately into the intracellular compartment. As all five subunits have similarly placed hydrophobic sequences they are all believed to take up a similar disposition across the membrane.

Lastly, how are the five subunits of the pentamer arranged with respect to each other? If sufficient electon microscope images of a symmetrical structure can be obtained the fuzzy individual images can be superimposed and the 'noise' averaged out to give a much clearer representation. This has been done with samples of electroplax membrane to give a clear image showing that viewed from the surface the nAChR has fivefold symmetry. Indeed this image strongly suggests that the five subunits are grouped around a central pore (Figure 9.6B). This structure is supported by the observation that one of the transmembrane segments (MA) of each subunit is amphipathic rather than strictly hydrophobic. In other words it apppears that one face of the MA α-helix is hydrophobic and the other polar. It is the latter face which faces inward toward the pore. The outcome of all this sophisticated work is the structure shown in Figure 9.6(C).

Each nAChR pentamer has a diameter of about 9 nm and a central pore of 2 nm. The pentamer projects 7 nm into the synaptic

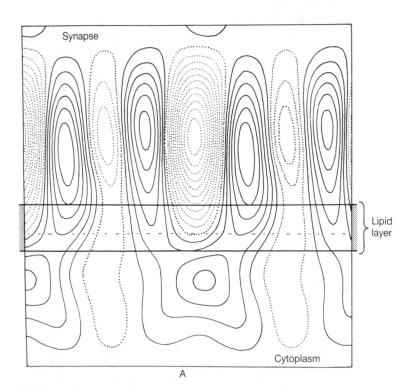

A

Figure 9.6 Pentameric structure of the nicotinic acetylcholine receptor in the postsynaptic membrane. (A) Computer-analysed EM representation of the acetylcholine receptor: vertical section. (B) (*facing page*) Computer-analysed EM of acetylcholine receptors seen end-on. Note five-fold symmetry. (C) (*facing page*) Drawing of acetylcholine receptor. The fivefold structure is shown; the position of the ligand and/or neurotoxin binding sites are shown on the α-subunits; the internal cup-shaped channel is shown by dotted lines. ((A) and (B) reprinted by permission from Brisson and Unwin, 1985, *Nature*, **315**, 474–477; Copyright © 1985, Macmillan Magazines Ltd. (C) from Stroud, 1981, *Proceedings of Second SUNYA Conversation in the Discipline of Biomolecular Stereodynamics*, ed. R.H. Sarma, vol. 2, New York: Adenine Press, with permission.)

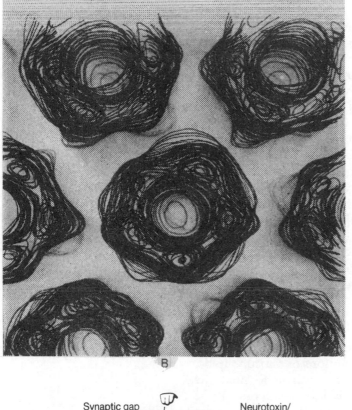

B

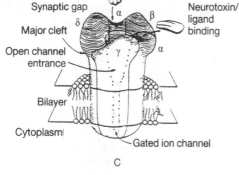

C

cleft. This ensures that it stands proud of any extracellular
basement membrane which may be present (see Figure 14.16).
It will be recalled from Chapter 2 that the collagen-like 'tail' of
the important cholinergic enzyme, acetylcholinesterase, is also
believed to be inserted into this membrane at neuromuscular
junctions. On the other side of the cell membrane the nicotinic
acetylcholine receptor protrudes some 3 nm into the cytoplasm.
Studies with small cations suggests that the maximum diameter
of the channel is no more than 0.80 nm (= 8 Å).

9.1.2 Function

In recent years a number of sophisticated techniques have been developed which enable detailed examination of membrane channels to be undertaken. Many of these have been used to investigate the properties of the nicotinic acetylcholine receptor. Purified nAChR derived from snake venom affinity chromatography can be inserted into **liposomes and/or lipid bilayers** and its physiological properties examined in isolation. Alternatively **patch-clamping** techniques allow the investigation of individual nAChRs expressed in oocyte membranes. **Biochemical** and **electron microscopical** techniques may be used to find the sites on the subunits which bind α-bungarotoxin, thus indicating where ACh normally attaches. Finally the techniques of **site-directed mutagenesis**, outlined in Chapter 5, can be used to alter the primary structure of one or more of nAChR's subunits and the effect on function examined by one of the above techniques. Results from all these approaches enable us to home in on the biophysics of the channel. As these are all techniques of general applicability let us look briefly at each in turn.

Liposomes. In Chapter 6 (Figure 6.3) we noted that because of the amphipathic nature of phospholipds it is not difficult to form liposomes from either pure or mixed solutions of phospholipids. Simple single-layered liposomes are too fragile to hold the comparatively huge nicotinic acetylcholine receptors. It is, however, possible to manufacture large multilayered liposomes by subjecting phospholipid suspensions to repeated cycles of freezing and thawing.

If such multilayered liposomes are created from a suspension of phospholipids and purified nAChR it is found that the latter

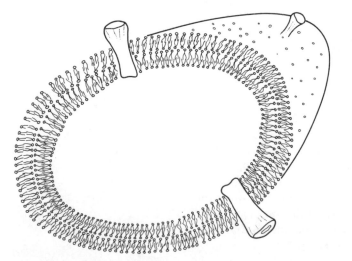

Figure 9.7 Incorporation of nAChRs into a liposome. Three nicotinic acetylcholine receptors have become incorporated into a liposome. Liposomes large enough to hold large multimeric structures such as nicotinic acetylcholine receptors are multilamellar structures formed by a cycle of freeze – thaw steps from suspensions of small liposomes

become incorporated into the structure. In most cases the nAChRs are incorporated in such a way that their α-bugarotoxin binding sites face outwards. It can be arranged that the liposomes form around radioactive Na⁺ and/or K⁺ ions. It can then be shown that these ions are released when ACh is added to the liposome suspension. Furthermore tubocurarine, an antagonist of ACh, prevents the ACh-activated release of these ions. Finally, the liposomal channels can be examined by the patch-clamp technique, described below.

Bilayers. There are several techniques for constructing artificial bilayers. One technique, as shown in Figure 6.3, is to form a bilayer across a small aperture (0.2–1 mm diameter) made in a partition separating two aqueous compartments. A defined phospholipid suspension is then introduced into one compartment and into the other a suspension of liposomes containing nAChR. A bilayer containing the nicotinic receptor forms across the aperture.

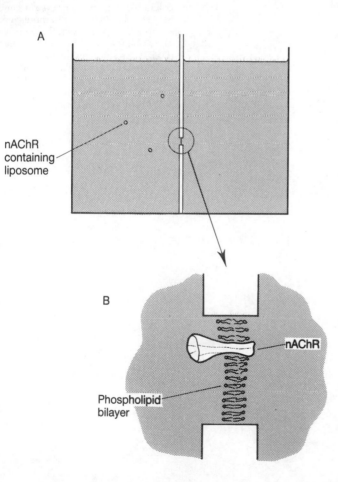

A

nAChR
containing
liposome

B

nAChR

Phospholipid
bilayer

Figure 9.8 Incorporation of nAChRs into an artificial bilayer. (A) An approximately 200 μm hole is made in a teflon partition separating two aqueous buffer solutions. A defined phospholipid bilayer is formed across the aperture. Liposomes incorporating nAChRs are added to one compartment. (B) Enlarged view. A liposome has fused with the artificial bilayer and its nAChR is now incorporated in the phospholipid bilayer

An alternative technique for constructing bilayers is to make use of the spontaneous formation of a monolayer by phospholipids at an air/water interface. It is then possible to allow liposomes containing nAChR to diffuse into the monolayer, thus creating an nAChR containing bilayer. There are several other techniques for forming artificial bilayers and the interested reader should consult the volume of the *Biophysical Journal* mentioned in the bibliography and/or the book edited by Miller.

Patch-clamping. The **patch-clamping** technique was introduced to neurophysiology in 1976 by Erwin Neher and Bert Sakmann. It has revolutionised the investigation of the physiological

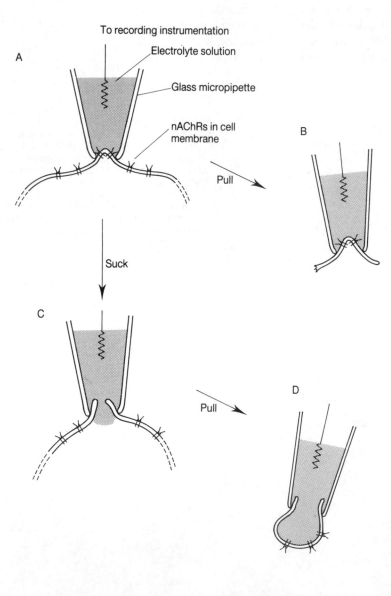

Figure 9.9 Various types of patch-clamping. (A) The recording micropipette is attached to the cell by gentle suction. (B) A sharp pull detaches the cell membrane. The result is an 'inside-out' patch. (C) Alternatively the preparation in (A) can be subjected to a more vigorous suction. This tears open the membrane. The result is a 'whole-cell voltage clamp'. (D) If (C) is subjected to a sharp pull the membrane is removed from the cell but spontaneously seals to provide an 'outside-out' patch

properties of ion channels. It enables the physiologist to examine the fluxes of ions through *single* channels. The essence of the technique is to place a glass micropipette (tip diameter about 0.5 μm) on to the membrane of interest. A very high resistance (10 GΩ) seal is made between the pipette tip and the membrane. This is essential if currents in the sub-picoamp range are to be detected. The micropipette is filled with an electrolyte and hooked up to electronics so that the flow of current across the membrane can be measured. The micropipette can also be used to 'clamp' the membrane patch at a predetermined voltage. Further details of 'voltage clamping' are given in Section 13.1 and in Figure 13.2. The membrane may be left *in situ* or by the application of gentle suction it may be detached from the cell and examined in isolation. The major varieties of this crucial technique are shown in Figure 9.9.

Figure 9.9 shows the various types of preparation which can be obtained: cell-attached patch, whole-cell voltage clamp, inside-out patch, outside-out patch. It is worth noting, especially in the detached patches, that the membrane is sucked into the pipette mouth in an 'omega' form. This means that the area of membrane from which the measurements are made is considerably larger than the area of the pipette tip. This observation is important when calculations of the number of channels per membrane area are made.

Membranes may be obtained from nerve, muscle or other cells, genetically engineered oocytes, liposomes or artificial bilayers. The currents detected by the technique are, of course, minute—to be measured in picoamps (pA). But they are quite sharp. They are due to the opening and shutting of *single* ion channels. If and when a second channel opens in the patch the current doubles in magnitude.

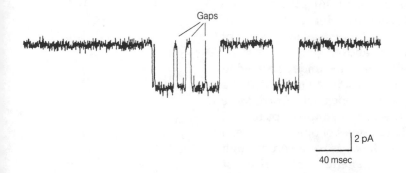

Gaps

2 pA

40 msec

Figure 9.10 Patch-clamp recording of a single nAChR channel. Recording from a rat muscle cell in culture in the presence of 5 μM ACh and the membrane potential at -70 mV. A 'classical' open/shut single-channel event is shown on the right. On the left the trace shows several rapid closings of the gate. (From Barrantes, 1983, *International Review of Neurobiology*, **24**, 259–341; with permission.)

In Figure 9.10 it can be seen that in a rat cultured muscle cell one channel opens for about 30 ms. When the membrane is held at -70 mV a flow of 5 pA of current occurs during that time. The current flow is governed by Ohm's law:

$$I = gV$$

where I is the current, V is the applied voltage and g is the conductance. The magnitude of the current will therefore vary according to the applied voltage and the conductivity of the channel. In the case of the nAChR channel it can be shown that the frequency of opening depends on the quantity of ACh applied.

It is easy to calculate how many ions flow through the channel in the opening event shown on the right hand side of Figure 9.10. It will be recalled that 1 A $= 1$ C s^{-1} and that one mole of univalent ions carries a faraday ($= 96\ 500$ C) of electricity. It will also be recalled that a mole is Avogadro's number (N_A) i.e. 6×10^{23}, of particles. It follows that:

$$\frac{[5 \times 10^{-12}\ C\ s^{-1}] \times [30 \times 10^{-3}\ s] \times [6 \times 10^{23}\ ions\ (g\ ion)^{-1}]}{96\ 500\ C\ (g\ ion)^{-1}}$$

$$= \frac{9 \times 10^{10}\ ions}{9.6 \times 10^4}$$

$$= approx.\ 1 \times 10^6\ univalent\ ions$$

This is a considerably larger flow than normally occurs through single nAChR-controlled channels in the subsynaptic membranes of cholinergic neuromuscular junctions. It can be shown that in this position the gates open on average for only about 3 ms instead of the 30 ms of the cultured muscle cell in the example. Furthermore the flow of ions is dependent (as we have just seen) on the driving voltage. For any given ion this is the difference between the membrane potential (V_m) and the Nernst potential of the ion (V_I) (for further analysis see Chapter 16). This difference diminishes as the membrane discharges. Hence the flow of univalent ions in physiological conditions is several orders of magnitude less than that worked out above.

The initial studies with the patch-clamp technique seemed to show that, as indicated on the right-hand side of Figure 9.10, the nAChR channel existed in just two states—open and closed. More recently it has been shown that this is too simple a picture: it seems that there are in fact two different types of open and several different types of closed state. We shall see as we go on through this book that this complexity is a general characteristic of membrane channels. Furthermore it can be shown that prolonged binding of agonist molecules to the nAChR leads to **desensitisation**. It is found, in other words, that if the agonist is allowed to remain on the receptor for a period of seconds to minutes the channel begins to close. This time period is three to four orders of magnitude greater than that required for opening the nAChR gate (microseconds to milliseconds). It may be that separate binding sites are responsible for activation and desensitisation. It is clear that the patch-clamp technique is beginning to show us something of the molecular complexity which underlies the operation of ligand-gated channels.

Biochemical and electron microscopic techniques. Biochemical and electron microscopic techniques provide a means of determining where the ACh site is located on the receptor. The most usual technique for locating this site is to make use, once again, of the snake-bite venom, α-bungarotoxin. It can be shown that synthetic sequences of amino acids 173–204, and more precisely 185–196, in the α-subunits bind this ACh antagonist. It is consequently believed that it is this part of the pentamer, projecting from the E face of the postsynaptic membrane (see Figure 9.5) which acts as the ACh site. More particularly the cysteine residues at positions 192 and 193 have been implicated.

Electron microscopy provides an alternative approach to the localisation of the ACh site. In essence what is done is to take electron micrographs of nAChRs in the postsynaptic membrane with and without the addition of α-bungarotoxin. By computerised subtraction of the second image from the first the position of toxin can be located. Knowing that the toxin occupies the ACh site on the α-subunits the position of these subunits in the EM image can be deduced.

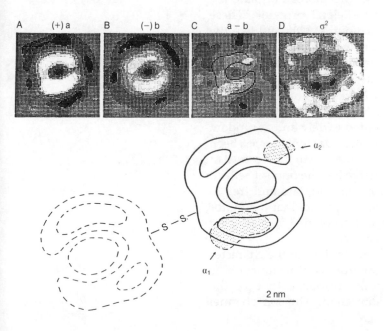

Figure 9.11 Localisation of α-BuTX on the two α-subunits of the nAChR pentamer. (A) Averaged EM image of a negatively stained acetylcholine receptor to which α-BuTX has been bound. (B) The image without the toxin. (C) The image obtained when the computer subtracts (B) from (A). (D) Plot of the standard error of the difference between (A) and (B): the lowest error occurs where there is no toxin. The technique thus allows the localisation of the toxin on the receptor. It is concluded (lower part of figure) that the toxin is located over two parts of the receptor (seen end-on) and these consequently are deduced to be the α-subunits. S—S represents a disulphide bond which is known to link the δ-subunits of adjacent receptor molecules. (From Barrantes, 1983, *International Review of Neurobiology*, **24**, 259–341, with permission, after Zingsheim *et al.*, 1982, *Nature*, **299**, 81–84.)

Finally in this section on function, it can be shown that the nAChR chanel only opens when **two** ACh molecules are attached. When the first ACh binds to its site on the α-subunit it causes a change in the conformation of the nAChR proteins which leads to the probability of another ACh binding to the second α-subunit being enhanced. When both ACh molecules are attached the nAChR pentamer once again changes its conformation, leading to a brief opening of the channel through which ions can flow down their concentration gradients. We shall return to the pharmacology of the nicotinic acetylcholine channel in Chapter 15.

9.1.3 Development

Figure 9.12 shows the major steps in the synthesis and assembly of the nAChR complex in muscle fibres. The synthesis occurs in the rough endoplasmic reticulum (RER) as described in Section 6.6. The assembly of the five subunits into the mature pentamer occurs in the Golgi apparatus and the receptor moves from that position, incorporated in a transport vesicle, to its final home in the folds of the motor endplate. It would seem reasonable to suppose that a similar sequence of events obtains in neurons. In this case the transport vesicles budding off the Golgi apparatus would have to be moved along the dendrites to the appropriate postsynaptic membrane. Alternatively if, as seems likely, many brain nAChRs are presynaptic (i.e. modulating transmitter release) then the transport vesicles would be carried from the perikaryon to the bouton in the axoplasmic flow (see Chapter 14).

Figure 9.12 shows that nAChRs in the motor endplate are associated with submembranous cytoskeletal proteins. These proteins have a molecular weight of about 43 kDa and like the submembranous cytoskeletal elements we discussed in Section 6.7 presumably hold the nAChR pentamers in position. They are probably attached to the submembranous stretch of the subunit polypeptide chain between M3 and M4 (see Figure 9.5).

During embryology it is found that before the motor neurons reach the muscle nAChRs are distributed widely and at random in the sarcolemma. Only when a neuromuscular junction has been established are the nAChRs concentrated beneath it. Removal of the junction by sectioning the motor nerve has the opposite effect: the nAChRs are released from the motor endplate and free to diffuse in the sarcolemma once again. It appears that the motor neuron is able to exert a concentrating effect on nAChRs, floating like icebergs in the muscle-fibre membrane.

Yet more interestingly it is found that in the calf the character of the nAChR changes when a neuromuscular junction is established. It can be shown that the response time of the acetylcholine receptor to ACh is shortened. The ion channel

Figure 9.12 Synthesis and assembly of nAChRs in muscle fibre. (A) Co-translational insertion of nAChR subunit polypeptide into cisternal space of ER. (B) N-glycosylation. (C) Termination of translation. Ribosome and mRNA separate. Subunit polypeptide is inserted in its characteristic position across the membrane. Signal peptide cleaved from subunit polypeptide. (D) Assembly of the receptor from two copies of α-, and one copy of the β-,γ-, δ-subunits. This occurs in the Golgi body. (E) Transport in transport vesicle to sarcolemma. (F) Transport vesicle recognises appropriate place in sarcolemma and the two membranes fuse. (G) The five nAChR subunits cluster to form the mature nACh receptor. Their C-terminals become associated with the submembranous cytoskeleton. Their N-terminals project up beyond the thick basement membrane of the neuromuscular junction. For further discussion of the synthetic process see Chapter 14. (After Merlie *et al.*, 1983, *Cold Spring Harbor Symposia on Quantitative Biology*, **XLVIII**, 135–146.)

→

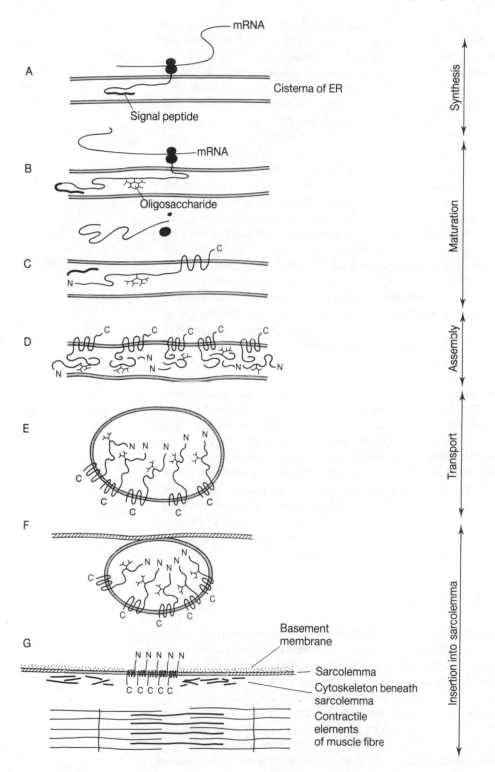

remains open for only about a quarter of the duration that it stayed open in fetal muscle. The response time of the whole muscle fibre consequently becomes three or four times more rapid.

It has been shown that this change in response time is due to the replacement of the γ-subunit in the nAChR pentamer by a different polypeptide—the ϵ-subunit. The ϵ-subunit differs from the γ-subunit in about 50% of its residues. Its hydropathic profile, however, is homologous to that of the γ-subunit and hence its disposition in the membrane is believed to be similar.

It seems, therefore, that when a neuromuscular junction is formed on **mammalian** muscle an ϵ-gene is switched on and the γ-gene switched off. Immediately after innervation both types of subunit are present. Later only the ϵ-subunit can be detected. The acetylcholine receptor at the adult mammalian neuromuscular junction is thus an $\alpha_2\beta\epsilon\delta$ pentamer. This alteration in subunit constitution is very reminiscent of the similar situation in the haemoglobin tetramer which we discussed in Section 4.3. It will be recalled that there, too, fetal forms (ϵ- and γ-) of one of the subunits (the β-subunit) are found. The $\alpha_2\beta\epsilon\delta$ pentamer is confined to the subsynaptic membrane of the mammalian neuromuscular junction; non-innervated sarcolemma retains the familiar $\alpha_2\beta\gamma\delta$ complex.

Myasthenia gravis. Myasthenia gravis is one of the autoimmune diseases. For some as yet unknown reason antibodies are synthesised against the body's own nAChR complexes. The nAChRs are, in consequence, progressively destroyed. This results in increasing muscular weakness. Normally neuro-muscular junctions possess a superabundance of nAChRs. ACh released by motor neuron terminals on to the motor endplate is easily taken up by the nAChRs. But as more and more nAChRs are inactivated ACh becomes less and less able to initiate muscle contraction. Sustained muscular activity becomes progressively more difficult and ultimately impossible.

9.2 The GABA$_A$ RECEPTOR

Two important inhibitory transmitters (**γ-aminobutyric acid (GABA)** and **glycine**) are found in vertebrate central nervous systems (see Chapter 15). GABA is found in the brain and glycine is found in the spinal cord and brain stem. In both cases they exert their effect by controlling a channel specific to small anions. When they open chloride ions course through and, as we shall see in Chapter 16, lead to a hyperpolarisation of the membrane. In this section we shall consider the GABA receptor.

We shall see in Chapter 15 that there are at least two distinct subtypes of GABA receptor. The **GABA$_A$** receptor subtype is believed to be situated in subsynaptic membranes and the **GABA$_B$** subtype in presynaptic membranes. Whereas the GABA$_A$ receptor directly controls a chloride channel the GABA$_B$ receptor acts through a collision-coupling mechanism involving G-proteins. The action of GABA is thus, like acetylcholine, mediated through two very different types of subsynaptic receptor. In this section only the **GABA$_A$** receptor will be considered.

The pharmacology of the GABA$_A$ receptor subtype has been intensively studied. It appears to have binding sites for at least four types of drug. These include GABA itself, the benzodiazepines, picrotoxin and the barbiturates. Just as it is possible to purify the nAChR on an α-toxin column so it is possible to make use of the GABA$_A$ receptor's affinity for benzodiazepine to purify it on a benzodiazepine column. Accordingly it is this subtype of GABA receptor which has been subjected to detailed molecular analysis.

After purification the GABA$_A$ receptor turned out to consist of two α- (48 800 Da) and two β-subunits (51 400 Da): $\alpha_2\beta_2$. The two subunits were then used to prepare oligonucleotide probes and these in turn used to screen calf and/or adult bovine cerebral cortex cDNA libraries. Full-length cDNAs were ultimately fished out which, on decoding, yielded amino acid sequences for the two subunits. The α-subunit was shown to consist of 429 amino acids and the β-subunit of 449. Comparison of the amino acid sequences of the two subunits showed that 57% of the residues were either identical or conservative substitutions.

To ensure that the entire GABA$_A$ receptor had been obtained the mRNAs for the two subunits were expressed in the *Xenopus* oocyte system. The oocyte does not normally possess GABA receptors in its membrane. After injection of the putative GABA$_A$ mRNA large conductances of chloride across the membrane in response to the external application of GABA could, however, be detected. This proved beyond doubt that the entire channel protein had been synthesised by the oocyte and consequently that the entire gene for GABA$_A$ had been cloned.

The usual analysis of the amino acid sequence for hydrophobic stretches showed there to be four regions of sufficient length (i.e. about 20 residues) to form α-helical spans of the membrane. This was the case in both subunits. These transmembrane helices are designated M1, M2, M3 and M4, analogously to the similarly named four hydrophobic transmembrane stretches of the nicotinic acetylcholine receptor. There is, however, no evidence in the GABA$_A$ receptor for an amphipathic segment such as is found in the nAChR (MA).

A proposed structure for the GABA$_A$ receptor is shown in Figure 9.13. As the receptor consists of two α- and two β-subunits there are 16 membrane-spanning helices. It is known that the channel diameter can be no more than 5.6 Å at its narrowest point. It is not geometrically possible to pack all 16 α-helices so that each faces the channel's lumen. Some other, as yet unknown, organisation must be adopted. It is known that five α-helices can be arranged to enclose a channel of pore diameter 5.8 Å. Perhaps one helix from each of the four subunits forms the major part of the channel wall, with some small contribution from each of the other three. Future research will, no doubt, solve this interesting problem in molecular anatomy.

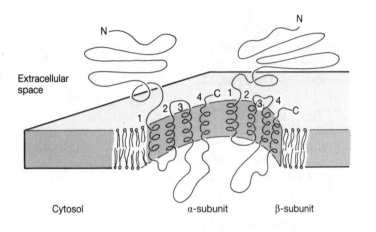

Figure 9.13 Schematic of the GABA$_A$ receptor. The α- and β-subunits are shown schematically in a cut-away part of the membrane. Bear in mind that the schematic shows only a plan view of the helices. The true three-dimensional disposition is undoubtely more complex (see text). The four transmembrane helices in each subunit are numbered. An additional α- and β-subunit make up the complete receptor. (Modified from Schofield *et al.*, 1987, *Nature*, **328**, 221–227.)

9.3. THE GLYCINE RECEPTOR

Next let us look at the **glycine-activated channel**. These channels are found on postsynaptic membranes in the brain stem and spinal cord of mammals. Similar channels are found throughout the vertebrates and in many invertebrates. They are extremely narrow (<5.2 Å) and, like the GABA-activated channels, very selective for anions. Of the ions present on either side of neural membranes they thus allow only Cl$^-$ to pass.

The study of the glycine receptor (GlyR) has been greatly helped by its affinity for **strychnine**. Strychnine thus plays something of the same role for the GlyR that the α-toxins played for the nACh receptor, and bezodiazepine for the GABA$_A$ receptor. The GlyR may, for instance, be purified by chromatography through a column of agarose beads to which has been attached a derivative of strychnine—2-aminostrychnine. The GlyR so purified appears to consist of three polypeptides of 48 kDa, 58 kDa and 93 kDa.

The position of these subunits in the membrane has been clarified by immunoelectron microscopy. Monoclonal antibodies

Figure 9.14 Localisation of the 93 kDa polypeptide of the glycine receptor. (A) The 93 kDa GlyR subunit is labelled by an immunogold technique and examined in the electron microscope. The arrow points to one of the labels. The 93 kDa subunit is clearly on the intracellular side of the subsynaptic membrane. The preparation is of rat spinal cord. (× 100 000). (B) The arrows again point to the immunogold-labelled 93 kDa subunit in the intracellular space. The bars indicate the position of an active zone in the presynaptic terminal (see Chapter 14). Most of the GlyRs lie beneath this active zone although some (arrowed) lie outside it (× 100 000). (From Triller *et al.*, 1985, *Journal of Cell Biology*, **101**, 638–688, with permission.) ⟶

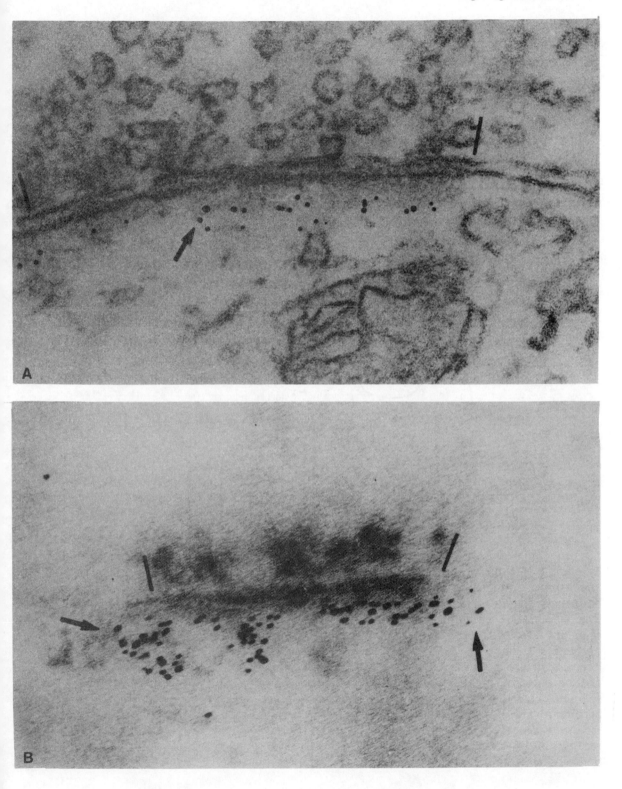

can be prepared against the chromatographically purified GlyR polypeptides. These can then be conjugated to gold and reacted with central synapses. Figure 9.14 shows that the antibody against the 93 kDa polypeptide is located on the cytoplasmic side of the subsynaptic membrane.

The tentative model of the glycine receptor which is beginning to emerge is shown in Figure 9.15. It is thought that the glycine-binding part of the receptor consists of two or three copies of the 48 kDa and one or two copies of the 58 kDa polypeptide. It is likely that the 48 kDa polypeptide forms the ion channel. The 93 kDa polypeptide is associated with this transmembrane complex, but is located on the P face of the membrane where it may possibly interact with the cytoskeleton of the subsynaptic density.

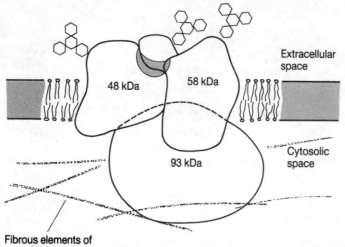

Fibrous elements of
submembranous cytoskeleton

Figure 9.15 Schematic structure of the glycine receptor. The schematic figure shows the putative disposition of the 93 kDa, the 58 kDa and two copies of the 48 kDa subunits. A second 48 kDa subunit is shown behind the first. Glycosylation of the 48 kDa and 58 kDa subunits is shown. The stippled area covering part of the 58 kDa and 48 kDa subunits represents the strychnine binding region

The strychnine-binding subunit of the rat spinal cord glycine receptor (the 48 kDa subunit) has been successfully cloned and its amino acid sequence determined. It consists of 421 amino acids and a precise molecular weight of 48 383 Da. The customary hydropathic analysis reveals that the sequence possesses three transmembrane segments designated M1, M2 and M3. A sequence near the C-terminal is similar to the M4 transmembrane sequences of both the GABA$_A$-receptor and the nAChR and, hence, may also cross the membrane. Unlike the nicotinic acetylcholine receptor the GlyR does not possess an amphipathic sequence (MA). In spite of these differences we once again become aware of a common theme underlying channel architecture. It seems that the various types of nAChR, the GABA$_A$ receptor and the glycine receptor are all members of an evolutionarily related superfamily. This relatedness is borne out by a comparison of the amino acid sequences in the nAChR α-subunit, the GABA$_A$ receptor α- and β-subunits and the 48 kDa glycine receptor. These homologies are shown in Table 9.1.

Table 9.1   Percentage amino acid homologies in the nAChR, GlyR and GABA-R$_A$ receptor subunits

	GABA-R$_{A\alpha}$	GABA-R$_{A\beta}$	GlyR
nAChR$_\alpha$	19 (38)	15 (32)	15 (37)
GABA-R$_{A\alpha}$	100	35 (57)	34 (56)
GABA-R$_{A\beta}$	35 (57)	100	39 (59)

The sequences compared are those of bovine GABA$_A$ receptor (α- and β-subunits), rat 48 kDa glycine receptor and bovine muscle nAChR α-subunit. The first figure in each case represents percent identical residues, the figure in parentheses the percent identical plus conservative substitutions. Data from Bernard, Darlison and Seeburg (1987)

There are many suggestive similarities between the three receptor subunits. The regions of greatest homology are, for instance, to be found in the transmembrane helices. The M2 helix, in particular, is remarkably similar in the GABA$_A$ receptor and the glycine receptor. Although the amino acid homology does not extend to nAChR there is good evidence that the M2 helix in that receptor plays a major role in lining the channel wall. It

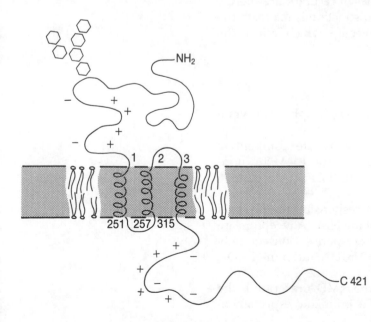

Figure 9.16 48 kDa subunit of the glycine receptor. The schematic figure shows the disposition of the 48 kDa subunit in the membrane. There are believed to be three transmembrane helices, although a fourth towards the C-terminal end may also be present. (After Greeningloh *et al.*, 1987, *Nature*, **328**, 215–220.)

may be, therefore, that the invariance of the M2 helix in the GlyR and the GABA$_A$ receptor indicates that it plays the same role here also. There are many other fascinating aspects of molecular comparative anatomy which our increasing knowledge of this family of ligand-gated ion channels is bringing to light. The interested reader can pursue them in the references given in the bibliography.

9.4 RECEPTORS FOR EXCITATORY AMINO ACIDS (EAAs)

Mammalian brains possess two important excitatory amino acids (EAAs): glutamate and aspartate. They are widely distributed throughout the brain and spinal cord. The EAAs are believed to have two major types of action. In the first case they are known to induce rapid (c. 1 ms) membrane depolarisations. In this respect their action resembles that of the nicotinic acetylcholine receptor. In the second, and perhaps more interesting, case they once again cause a membrane depolarisation but this time of a much longer duration (10–15 ms), often accompanied by other, more complex, events.

Now although the membrane responses to EAAs may be classified into these two major classes there appear to be at least four different types of receptor. It is indeed probable that future research will show up subtle differences in the responses which follow interaction of EAAs with each of these different receptors. At present, however, the different types of receptor are merely distinguished pharmacologically. The distinction is made on the types of agonist and antagonist molecule which affect the receptor:

1. K receptors (agonist: Kainate).
2. Q receptors (agonist: Quisqualate).
3. L-AP4 receptors (antagonist: L-2-amino-4-phosphonobutyrate (L-AP4)).
4. NMDA receptors (agonist: N-methyl-*d*-aspartate; competitive antagonist: D-2-amino-5-phosphonovalerate (D-AP5); non-competitive antagonist: phenylcyclidine (PCP)).

It is found that the K and Q receptors are responsible for the rapid depolarisations mentioned above whilst the NMDA receptors are responsible for the slower, more complex response. Consequently EAA receptors are often classified into NMDA and non-NMDA receptors.

Of the two classes of EAA receptor the NMDA receptor is the better known. It is found throughout the brain and especially in telencephalic structures. Of the latter it is interesting to note that it is particularly heavily represented in the hippocampus. This is especially noteworthy because, as we shall see, the NMDA receptor is suspected of being involved in synaptic plasticity and short-term memory. We shall see in Chapter 18 that the hippocampus is believed to be deeply implicated in these processes.

Let us therefore consider the NMDA receptor in a little more detail. Although it has not yet been isolated and characterised in molecular detail it has been subjected to exhaustive pharmacological analysis. It has also been investigated by patch-clamp analysis of cultured cells, especially cerebellar neurons (probably Purkinje cells) and hippocampal pyramidal cells where, as we noted, the transmitter is known to be present in large quantities.

In contrast to the nACh, $GABA_A$ and Gly receptors, the NMDA receptor appears to be sensitive to the voltage across the membrane in which it is embedded. This, too, makes it appropriate to end the present chapter with a discussion of its characteristics. For, in the next chapter, we shall proceed to a discussion of some very well-known voltage-sensitive channels. The NMDA receptor thus serves as an example of 'hybrid' channel: it is ligand operated, yet sensitive to voltage.

It can be shown that the voltage-dependent opening of the NMDA channel is affected by the presence of Mg^{2+} ions. When these ions are present (and they usually are in physiological conditions) the channel is blocked and small membrane depolarisations have little or no effect. However, when the membrane is depolarised by some 30 mV from its resting state the Mg^{2+} blockade is overcome and the NMDA channel begins to open. As the depolarisation is increased the channel opens wider still. In this respect, as we shall see in Chapter 10, the NMDA channel resembles the Na^+ channel: there is positive feedback between membrane depolarisation and opening of the ion channel.

But which ions pass through the channel? Experiments have demonstrated that Ca^{2+} is the most important ion to flux through, although Na^+ and K^+ ions also pass. In contrast to the NMDA channels the K and Q channels do not appear to open wide enough to allow the passage of Ca^{2+}. They only allow Na^+ and K^+ ions to pass. The fact that the NMDA channels are designed to allow Ca^{2+} ions to flow through into the cytosol from the outside is of great physiological and biochemical significance. We shall see in later chapters how important Ca^{2+} ions are in synaptic transmission and as intracellular 'second mesengers'.

Once the voltage across the NMDA membrane has been reduced sufficiently to overcome the Mg^{2+} blockade the positive feedback effect mentioned above tends to keep the NMDA

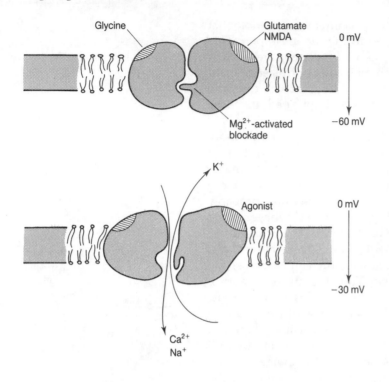

Figure 9.17 Physiological responses of the NMDA-activated channel. (A) The NMDA-controlled ion channel is closed. The figure shows a site for agonist molecules (glutamate, NMDA) and for antagonists (glycine). Agonist molecules will not open the channel at normal membrane resting potentials if Mg^{2+} ions are present. (B) When the membrane is depolarised the Mg^{2+} blockade is removed and agonist molecules can open the channel. Ca^{2+} and Na^+ flow inwards down their electrochemical gradients and K^+ flows out. These ion currents tend to keep the membrane depolarised and hence the channel open

channels open. This accounts for the comparatively long-lasting response which, as we noted at the outset, is characteristic of NMDA receptors. The situation is, however, by no means clear cut. It seems likely that the channel can exist in a number of different sub-states: some more long lasting (10–50 ms) than others (1–3 ms), in some cases fully open, in others in various states of 'partial' opening.

The Mg^{2+}-mediated voltage dependency of NMDA channels could have very important consequences for synaptic physiology. It may, for instance, provide a biochemical basis for an 'AND' gate, and thus for associative learning. The NMDA receptor can only be actuated by an EAA when the membrane in which it is situated is to some extent depolarised. One can suppose therefore that to fire a subsynaptic cell it is necessary for two presynaptic terminals to be active at once: one releasing an excitatory transmitter on to a non-NMDA receptor and the other releasing an EAA on to a nearby NMDA receptor. Perhaps this is why NMDA receptors are so well represented in the hippocampus. We shall return to NMDA receptors in Chapter 18. We shall see that they have been implicated in 'long term potentiation (LTP)', which is much discussed as a biophysical basis for associative learning and short-term memory. We shall also see (Chapter 17) that NMDA receptors may be implicated in the synaptic plasticity of the developing brain.

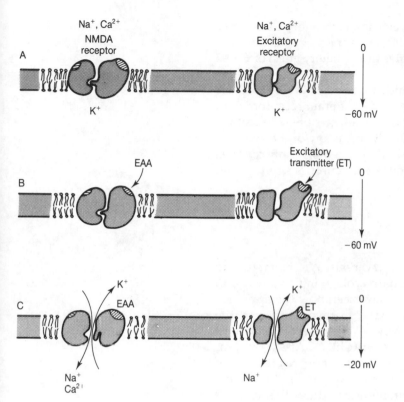

Figure 9.18 The NMDA receptor as a logic gate in a subsynaptic membrane. (A) An NMDA receptor and an excitatory receptor (activated by an EAA or some other excitatory transmitter) are shown in the same subsynaptic membrane. (B) An EAA and (another) excitatory transmitter (ET) is liberated by the presynaptic terminal. (C) The ET opens its ion channel and the membrane depolarises. This removes the Mg^{2+} blockade from the NMDA receptor whose ion channel consequently opens to allow the flow of Na^+, Ca^{2+} and K^+

Finally, it is worth noting that that NMDA receptors may also be involved in pacemaker variations of membrane polarity. We shall see in Chapter 10 that calcium-dependent potassium gates are present in some neural membranes. It is easy to see that if NMDA receptors are activated by an EAA the inflowing Ca^{2+} ions could open nearby gates of this type. The outflow of K^+ ions would tend to repolarise the membrane. This repolarisation would bring into play the Mg^{2+} blockade of the NMDA receptor. The inflow of Ca^{2+} would be cut off. Any cytosolic Ca^{2+} would be quickly bound. The outward flow of K^+ through the Ca^{2+}-dependent channels would cease. The membrane would then be ready for another cycle of depolarisation and repolarisation: perhaps by release of fresh EAAs on to K, Q and NMDA receptors.

The NMDA channel provides a good example of the developing understanding that membrane channels are not the simple 'open'/'shut' mechanisms that they were once thought to be. Indeed the NMDA receptor shows even more subtlety than we have yet discussed. It is known, for instance, to be **potentiated** by external glycine down to a concentration of 10 μM. This tends to pile yet more complexity upon what is already a complex story.

For we saw in Section 9.3 that glycine is an inhibitory transmitter in the brain stem and spinal cord. It now appears that in addition to its inhibitory activity it potentiates the excitatory effect of EAAs at the NMDA receptor.

It is not unreasonable to conclude that in the NMDA receptor we have a better model of the generality of brain receptors than is provided by the better known, but mostly peripheral, nicotinic acetylcholine receptor. It seems likely that many of the synaptic receptors in the brain are, like the NMDA receptor, richly complex in their responses to numerous different neurotransmitters and ions.

9.5 CONCLUSION

Ligand-gated channels are many and various. We shall return to a further consideration of their pharmacology in Chapter 15. In the present chapter, however, we have seen how the approach through molecular biology has begun to reveal order in the otherwise overwhelming complexity. We have seen that at least three major ligand-gated channels—nAChR, $GABA_A$ receptor and GlyR—are members of a single evolutionarily related super-family. It is becoming clear that these receptors, and all their many subtypes, are variations on a single architectural theme. This theme, in its essence, consists of units built of four membrane-spanning α-helical segments (M1, M2, M3 and M4) joined by stretches of hydrophilic amino acids. The peripheral nicotinic acetylcholine receptor is constructed from five of these units, $\alpha_2\beta\gamma\delta$ and $\alpha_2\beta\epsilon\delta$, and there is evidence that central (rat brain) nAChRs are assembled as $\alpha_3\beta_2$ pentamers; the $GABA_A$ receptor consists of two units; the glycine receptor, so far as is presently known, consists of two or three such units. Whether other ligand-gated channels also belong to this family only future research will show.

In the last section of the chapter we briefly discussed the NMDA receptor for the excitatory amino acids glutamate and aspartate. We noted the great complexity of response which this single receptor system displayed. It will be a fascinating topic of future research to determine its molecular structure and relate this structure to the receptor's multifarious function.

Chapter 10
Voltage-gated channels

Excitable cells, as we shall see more fully in Chapter 13, depend on the existence of voltage-controlled gates in their membranes. These gates, once again, are many and various. The most important are those which open to allow the passage of ions such as Na^+, K^+ and Ca^{2+}. It appears that there are at least three types of Na^+ channel, five types of K^+ channel, and three types of Ca^{2+} channel. These channels are responsible for the electrical excitability of nerve and muscle cells and for the sensitivity of sensory cells.

All of these gates respond to voltage changes across the membrane. As we shall see more fully in Chapter 11 the resting potential across most cell membranes is about 50 or 60 mV (inside negative to outside). This may not seem very much. It must be remembered, however, that membranes are very thin—no more than 6 or 7 nm. Hence the voltage drop is in fact very steep. A potential gradient of 60 mV in 6 nm works out as 10^5 V cm^{-1}. We must assume that voltage-sensitive proteins are very delicately poised in this intense electric field. Any change in the potential gradient will affect their conformation—and the open or shutness of any ion channel they may contain.

10.1 THE SODIUM CHANNEL

Just as the acetylcholine receptor was the best known of all the ligand-controlled gates so the Na^+ gate is by far the best known of the voltage-controlled gates. This again is due to its ubiquity and to the existence of very specific marker molecules which can be used to detect it. The Na^+ channel is, as might be expected, highly concentrated in mammalian brain tissue, and it is also found in high concentration in fish electric organs. The probe molecule—**tetrodotoxin (TTX)**—is not this time derived from snake-bite venom but from fish belonging to the family Tetro-

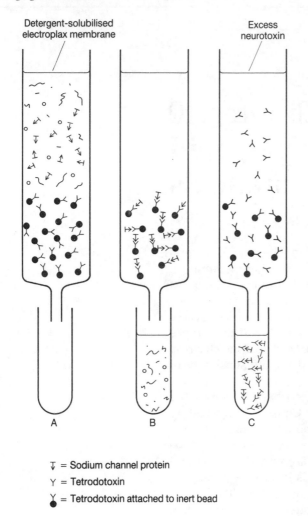

Detergent-solubilised
electroplax membrane

Excess
neurotoxin

A   B   C

$\bar{\text{I}}$ = Sodium channel protein

Y = Tetrodotoxin

Y = Tetrodotoxin attached to inert bead

Figure 10.1 Purification of the sodium channel on an immobilised neurotoxin chromatography column. (A) Detergent-solubilised electroplax membrane preparation is added to the top of the chromatography column. The column consists of inert beads to which have been attached a neurotoxin such as tetrodotoxin. (B) The electroplax preparation flows through the column and only the sodium channel protein is held by the beads. All the other proteins, polypeptides and membrane fragments flow through unimpeded. (C) A suspension of excess neurotoxin is now passed through the column to elute the sodium channel from the beads

Figure 10.2 Doman structure and amino acid sequences of the four regions of internal homology of the sodium-channel protein. (A) The 1820 amino acid sequence contains four homologous domains, I, II, III and IV. The first domain stretches from residue 111 to residue 419, the second from residue 555 to residue 807, the third from residue 989 to residue 1281 and the fourth from residue 1311 to residue 1587. Each homologous domain consists of six transmembrane segments, S1, S2, S3, S4, S5 and S6. (B) Amino acid sequence of the four homologous domains. The six transmembrane segments in each domain are labelled; S4 can be seen to contain a number of positively charged residues (R = arginine, L = lysine) and has been proposed as the voltage sensor. The number of residues in each line of the figure are given on the right; gaps (–) have been inserted to achieve maximum homology; the non-homologous regions of I, III and IV are shown by lines and the number of residues in each indicated in parenthesis; identical residues and conservative substitutions in all four domains are boxed. ((B) Reprinted by permission from Noda *et al.*, 1984, *Nature*, **312**, 121–127. Copyright © 1984, Macmillan Magazines Ltd.) ⟶

dontidae, the best-known example being the Japanese puffer fish. Tetrodotoxin binds very specifically to the Na$^+$ channel, in a one to one fashion. A similar toxin—**saxitoxin**—is synthesised by a dinoflagellate. Once again it binds in a one to one fashion with the sodium channel. Both these molecules inactivate the sodium channel and are hence extremely poisonous.

10.1.1 Structure

Because of the highly specific binding of these neurotoxins the sodium channel can be isolated from detergent-solubilised electroplax membrane fragments by affinity chromatography through a column of bead-immobilised tetrodotoxin or saxitoxin.

The technique shown in Figure 10.1 isolates a 260 kDa glycosylated protein from eel electroplax. When a similar technique is applied to mammalian brain two other smaller polypeptides (39 kDa and 37 kDa) are often found associated with the sodium channels. A different pair of associated polypeptides (45 kDa and 38 kDa) appear to be associated with the sodium channels isolated from mammalian skeletal muscle. It has been suggested that these smaller polypeptides have a regulatory function.

The Japanese group led by Numa have applied recombinant DNA techniques to clone and sequence the sodium channel just

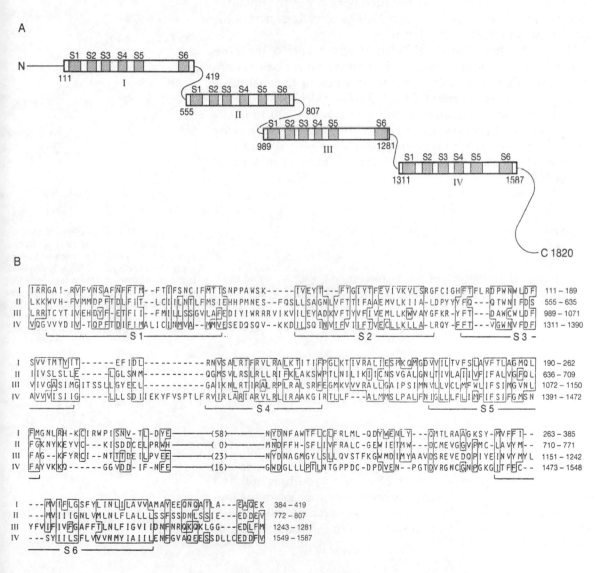

as they had done earlier for the acetylcholine receptor. They were able to show that the major channel protein consists of a single run of 1820 amino acids and consists of four homologous domains of approximately 300 amino acids each. Unlike the acetylcholine receptor the sodium channel protein thus does not consist of distinct subnunits. The homology of the four domains does, however, suggest that they all arose by internal duplication of a single ancestral gene.

Hydropathy analysis indicates that within each 300 residue domain there are six membrane-spanning helices termed S1, S2, S3, S4, S5 and S6. S4 is found to contain a number of positively charged residues (especially arginine and lysine) in addition to hydrophobic residues. It is consequently believed to constitute the 'voltage sensor' which detects change of voltage across the membrane and opens the channel.

Figure 10.3 shows the proposed architecture. Each of the intra-membranous segments of each of the four domains helps to form the wall of the channel. The narrowest region of the channel is believed to be a rectangular 0.31×0.51 nm orifice and the entire channel protein has a diameter of approximately 10 nm. The sodium channel protein thus appears to do with one lengthy amino acid chain what the ligand-gated channels of Chapter 9 and the gap junction of Chapter 6 required multiple subunits to accomplish.

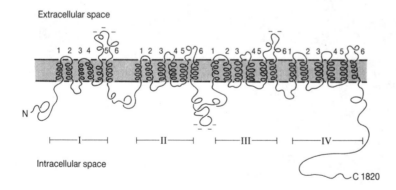

Figure 10.3 Plan of the disposition of the sodium channel in a membrane. In this schematic diagram the transmembrane segments are displayed linearly disposed in the membrane. In reality it is likely that they are clustered together, making use of the third dimension and surrounding the sodium channel. Aggregations of negatively charged residues are indicated by (-) signs

The next phase in the analysis of the sodium channel is to determine the nature of the gating mechanism. We have already noted that the sequence of positively charged residues in the S4 segment is suspected. Presumably the S4 helix of each of the four homologous domains forms part of the channel wall. Further research should allow us to understand in molecular detail its mechanism of action.

0.1.2 Function

The physiology of the sodium channel has been studied by several of the methods by which the AChR was studied (see Section .1.2). In particular the patch-clamp and bilayer techniques have proved important. If a small patch of neural or muscle fibre membrane is clamped some 10 mV positive to its resting potential sodium channels open and current can be recorded as shown in Figure 10.4.

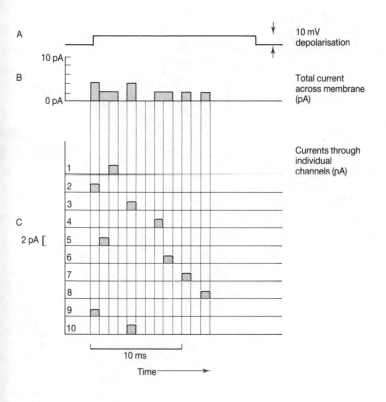

A

B

10 pA

0 pA

C

2 pA [

1
2
3
4
5
6
7
8
9
10

10 ms

Time

10 mV
depolarisation

Total current
across membrane
(pA)

Currents through
individual
channels (pA)

Figure 10.4   Schematic to show current flow through a patch of excitable membrane when clamped 10 mV positive to resting potential. (A) The membrane patch is clamped 10 mV positive to resting potential. (B) The current through the membrane measured in picoamps. (C) The current in (B) is due to the random opening and closing of ten individual sodium channels in the membrane

Figure 10.4 shows that the channels open for about 1 ms and allow about 2 pA of current to pass. A single channel thus has a conductance of about 10^{-11} S i.e. 10 pS. When two channels open at the same time twice the amount of current is recorded. Once a channel has opened it is inactivated and will not open again whilst the membrane remains depolarised. The channel thus exists in three major conformations: closed, open and inactivated. This cycle is shown diagrammatically in Figure 10.5.

A classical recording from a patch-clamped fragment of myotube membrane is shown in Figure 10.6. The membrane patch which possessed only two or three active sodium channels) is

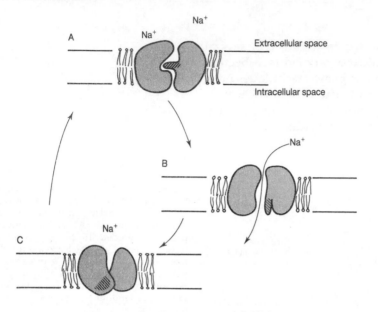

Figure 10.5 Conformational cycle of a sodium channel. (A) In the 'resting' membrane the sodium channel is closed. (B) When the membrane is depolarised the voltage drop is sensed by a 'voltage sensor' and the channel opens. Sodium ions flow through down their electrochemical gradient. (C) After about 1 ms in the open conformation the channel closes. When the membrane returns to its resting voltage the channel assumes its original conformation

held at a voltage some 30 mV below its resting potential to ensure that the Na⁺ gate is closed. It is then depolarised from this holding potential to some 10 mV above its resting potential. This causes Na⁺ channels to open. Each channel remains open on average for 0.7 ms and then closes again. During the open phase 1.6 pA of current flow.

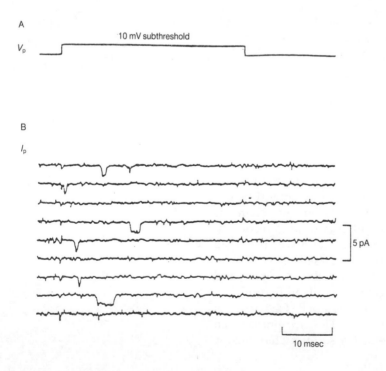

Figure 10.6 Current flux across a patch-clamped fragment of sarcolemma. (A) The membrane patch was hyperpolarised by 30 mV to ensure that all sodium gates were closed. Depolarising pulses of 40 mV were given, ensuring that the membrane was depolarised 10 mV above its resting potential and clamped at that value (trace at (A)). (B) Nine successive records from this patch-clamped membrane. The large downward deflections indicate channel openings. The mean channel current was 1.6 pA and mean lifetime was 0.7 ms. The patch probably contained two or three active channels. In some cases channel openings overlap. The small wiggles represent noise in the recording equipment. (Modified from Sigworth and Neher, 1980, *Nature*, **287**, 447–449; with permission.)

The number of sodium ions which flux through a single sodium channel in the above experiment during its transient open configuration can be calculated in the same way as for the nAChR channel (see Section 9.1.2):

$$\frac{[1.6 \times 10^{-12} \text{ C s}^{-1}] \times [0.7 \times 10^{-3} \text{ s}] \times [6 \times 10^{23} \text{ ions mol}^{-1}]}{96\ 500 \text{ C mol}^{-1}}$$

= approx. 7000 sodium ions (about 10 000 ions ms^{-1})

This is, in fact, a small number compared with the number of sodium ions present. Because tetrodotoxin marks the sodium channel so precisely it is possible to radiolabel the toxin and determine the number of channels present in an area of membrane. We can thus estimate the number of sodium ions cascading in during an action potential if all the channels should happen to open. In rabbit unmyelinated vagus nerve fibres the concentration of channels turns out to be about 100 channels μm^{-2} of membrane whilst in the nodes of Ranvier of myelinated fibres there may be be up to 3000 μm^{-2}. Let us consider an unmyelinated axon with a radius of 6 μm. We need to calculate the quantity of sodium ions beneath a square micrometre of neurilemma. We proceed as follows: the surface area of a cylinder is given by

$$A = 2\pi r l$$

i.e $l = A/2\pi r$

The volume of a cylinder is given by

$$V = \pi r^2 l$$

Hence $V = \dfrac{\pi r^2 A}{2\pi r}$

$$= rA/2$$

But $A = 1$ μm^2, and therefore

$$V = 6/2 = 3 \ \mu\text{m}^3$$

We now have to calculate how many sodium ions there are in a volume of 3 μm^3.

The concentration of Na$^+$ ion in a mammalian motor neuron has been found to be 15 mM (Table 8.1), i.e. 15×10^{-3} M litre^{-1}.

Now

$$1 \ \mu m^3 = 1 \times 10^{-12} \ ml \ or \ 10^{-15} \ litre$$

Therefore 1 μm^3 contains

$$(15 \times 10^{-3}) \times (1 \times 10^{-15}) \ mol \ of \ Na^+.$$

But 1 mol of Na^+ ions consists of 6×10^{23} ions (Avogadro's number). Therefore 1 μm^3 of mammalian axoplasm contains

$$(15 \times 10^{-18}) \times (6 \times 10^{23}) = 90 \times 10^5 \ sodium \ ions.$$

Hence 3 μm^3 of axoplasm will hold 2.7 $\times$ 10^7 sodium ions.

If all 100 channels in the square micrometre of rabbit vagus fibre membrane were to open during the passage of an action potential then $7000 \times 100 = 700 \ 000$ ions will flow into the axoplasm. It can be seen that this constitutes about 3% of the sodium ions inside. It is, of course, unlikely that all the sodium channels will open during any single action potential. It is also obvious that the calculation makes some very unphysiological assumptions. Most importantly it overlooks the fact that during an impulse the potential across the membrane rapidly diminishes and indeed reverses. Hence the driving force behind the sodium ions (remember $I = gV$) rapidly diminishes to zero. Nevertheless it is clear that an axon cannot continue conducting impulses for long without the $Na^+ + K^+$ pump described in Chapter 8 working to re-establish the proper internal and external ionic concentrations.

Finally it should be emphasised that the sodium channel, like the other channels we have considered, is more complex than this first analysis suggests. It appears to be capable of existing in more than just the three states—open, inactivated and shut— which we outlined above. Careful analyses of the patch-clamp records suggests that there are at least three substates of the open condition. This untidy complexity turns out to be characteristic of all the channels which have so far been carefully examined. It shows that we are dealing with complex macromolecular structures—not simple mechanical or electronic valves.

10.2 POTASSIUM CHANNELS

Unlike the nAChR channel and the Na^+ channel no marker toxins have as yet been discovered which are specific for potassium channels. It follows that until the very recent development of genetic engineering techniques there has been no good way of isolating these channels for detailed molecular study. Yet potassium channels are physiologically just as important as the AChR and the sodium channel. In recent years, as we shall see, important progress has been made towards an understanding at the molecular level of one of the potassium channels by application of the methods of molecular genetics in *Drosophila*.

Biophysical studies have shown there to be a number of different potassium channels. In molluscan neurons at least four different types have been identified. All of these channels are voltage-gated but their temporal characteristics and sensitivity to neurotransmitters and 'second messengers' such as Ca^{2+}, cAMP, etc., varies. They have in consequence been termed the **delayed K^+ channel**, the **early K^+ channel, or A-channel**, the **serotonin-dependent K^+ channel** and the **Ca^{2+}-dependent K^+ channel**. The K^+ currents which course through them when they open are termed I_K, I_{KA}, I_{KS} and I_{KCa} currents. In other organisms yet other types of K^+ channels have been detected. Finally it has been found that the major types of K^+ channel can be further classified into subtypes according to their kinetics and single-channel conductances. As the outflow of potassium ions determines the shape and duration of an action potential (Chapter 13) the characteristics of these channels are very important. The mix of channels in its membrane confers personality on an individual neuron.

Furthermore, the duration and magnitude of depolarisation of a synaptic terminal governs, as we shall see, the inflow of calcium ions and this, in its turn, controls the quantity of neurotransmitter released (see Chapter 14). The distribution and mix of potassium channels on synaptic terminals is thus likely to be of considerable importance in the large-scale functioning of the nervous system.

Finally it should be mentioned that *voltage-independent* K^+ channel proteins also exist in cell membranes: these, the so-called 'leak channels', are responsible for the 'passive' diffusion of K^+ ions into a cell and thus for the 'resting potential' (Chapter 11) across the plasma membrane.

10.2.1 Delayed potassium channels (Hodgkin–Huxley channels)

The pioneering work of Hodgkin and Huxley in the 1950s showed that the recovery phase of an action potential, the phase in which the axonal membrane reverts to its normal polarity (see Chapter 13), is due to the efflux of potassium ions. This efflux is through potassium channels which open about 2 μs **after** the membrane has been depolarised. They are voltage-dependent, but not as quick to respond to a change in transmembrane voltage as the sodium channels. They also differ from the sodium channels in remaining open as long as the membrane is depolarised. In other words there is no snapping open and shut but a sustained open state until the membrane regains or surpasses its original polarity. These, then, are the 'classical' delayed K$^+$ channels upon which so much basic neurophysiology turns. The delayed potassium channel may be inactivated by tetraethyl ammonium chloride [(CH$_3$CH$_2$)$_4$N$^+$Cl$^-$] or TEA.

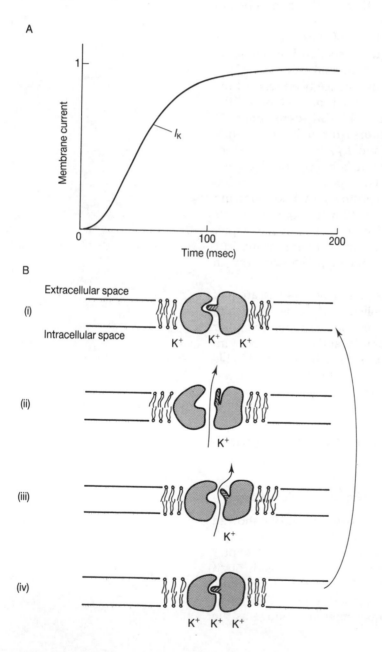

A

B

Figure 10.7 The 'classical' delayed potassium channel.(A) The membrane is depolarised at time zero. The outward potassium current, I_K, commences about 2 μs after time zero. It rises to its full height in about 150 ms. If the membrane is held in a depolarised condition the potassium gates remain open and I_K continues indefinitely. (B) Schematic to show the functioning of the gates responsible for I_K. (i) When the membrane is at its resting potential the I_K gate is closed. (ii) On depolarisation a voltage sensor causes the gate to open. Potassium ions flow down their electrochemical gradient from the intracellular to the extracellular space. (iii) As the membrane recovers its original polarity the gate begins to close and shut off I_K. (iv) On achieving the Nernst potassium potential (i.e. $V_M \simeq V_K$) the gate closes and remains closed until the next depolarisation

10.2.2 Fast potassium channel

Although the delayed K^+ channel is fundamental to the bio-physics of the action potential it may not have been the earliest K^+ channel to develop in evolution. There is evidence for the existence of the fast K^+ current, the A current, in Metazoa from coelenterates, such as *Obelia* and the 'sea-pansy', *Renilla*, through the molluscs, arthropods, to all classes of vertebrates. Indeed the squid giant axon (used by Hodgkin and Huxley in their original work) seems to be very much an exception to the rule in that it does not exhibit this current. Unlike the delayed K^+ current of classical Hodgkin–Huxley biophysics, the fast K^+ current occurs immediately on depolarisation and switches off within 10–100 ms whether the membrane has been repolarised or not. Thus this current and (presumably) the responsible channel resemble the Na^+ current and channel far more than they resemble the slow K^+ current and channel. Two other features distinguish I_{KA} from the classical I_K. First, the I_{KA} channel opens when the membrane is more hyperpolarised (i.e. less depolarised) than is required for the opening of the I_K channel; second, the I_{KA} channel is not inactivated by TEA but by another blocker which has no effect on I_K—**4-aminopyridine (4-AP)**.

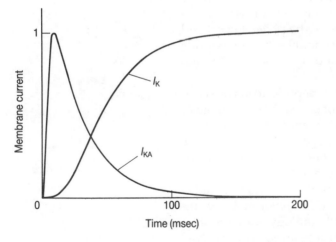

Figure 10.8 I_K and I_{KA}. The membrane is depolarised at time zero. The figure shows the relationship of the fast I_{KA} and delayed I_K potassium currents

The function of I_{KA} in excitable cells has been the subject of a great deal of discussion. Several roles have been proposed. **First** and foremost the channel is probably important in ensuring that a neuron does not fire when a small 'subthreshold' stimulus is applied. This is due to the fact that the very rapid opening of the fast channel allows a quick outflow of K^+ ions which repolarise the membrane. We shall see the significance of this when we come to consider the generation of action potentials in Chapter 13.

Second, it has been suggested that as the channel is active when the membrane is hyperpolarised it may act to increase the duration of the afterhypolarisation (AHP) following a spike (see Chapter 13). **Third**, it has been shown that the fast potassium current is affected by a number of modulating agents: Ca^{2+}, serotonin, α-adrenergic agonists and other agents all seem to be able to reduce the flow of potassium ions through this channel. This implies that these agents have some control over the shape and duration of an action potential.

A valuable approach towards an understanding of the fast channel have recently become possible by way of **Drosophila genetics**. **Shaker** mutants show leg-tremor under ether anaesthesia. Voltage-clamp techniques show that the condition is due to a defect in the I_{KA} channel which results in an abnormally broadened spike. This defect shows itself not only in the leg muscles but also in all the other muscles of *Drosophila*'s anatomy. It seems that the mutation affects a gene coding for a fast channel protein(s). As *Drosophila* genetics is very well known this at once opens the possibility of a genetic attack on the structure of the fast channel.

The challenge has been accepted. cDNA clones have been isolated from the shaker region of the *Drosophila* genome. There is good evidence that this cDNA specifies the polypeptide structure of the fast channel. Indeed it can be expressed in the *Xenopus* oocyte system, where it shows all the physiological and pharmacological properties of the I_{KA} channel. The polypeptide has a molecular weight of 70 200 Da and consists of 616 amino acids.

Hydropathic analysis shows the polypeptide to have six or seven transmembrane segments. This, of course, at once suggests an analogy with one of the four homologous domains of the sodium channel protein. Even more suggestive is the outcome of a comparison of the two amino acid sequences. It can be shown that a stretch of 120 amino acids in the putative potassium fast channel protein (304–435) is 27% identical (47% if conservative substitutions are added) to a stretch (1360–1496) in *Gymnotus* sodium channel protein. The centre of homology is an arginine-rich region in the sodium channel which is believed to be involved in voltage-gating. Indeed the general design of this region with alternating hydrophobic and hydrophilic residues is remarkably similar to the S4 segment of the homologous domains of the sodium channel and, as we shall see below, the calcium channel. It is beginning to look as though the *Drosophila* fast channel protein is evolutionarily related to both the sodium and calcium channel proteins. We noted above that the fast potassium channel is of great antiquity. It may be, therefore, that it represents the ancestral channel protein from which the sodium and calcium

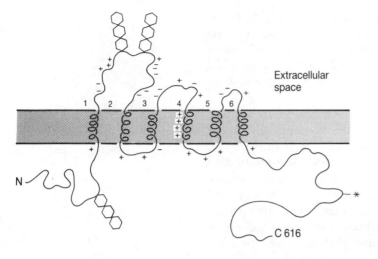

Extracellular space

N

Intracellular space

Figure 10.9 Structure of the *Drosophila* fast potassium channel protein. This schematic shows six transmembrane segments. It is, however, possible that a seventh segment spans the membrane so that the C-terminal is in the extracellular space. If this were the case it would carry the cAMP-mediated phosphorylation site (indicated by an asterisk) into the extracellular compartment. On an analogy with other membrane-embedded proteins this seems unlikely. *N*-glycosylation sites are shown in the usual way; (+) and (−) signs indicate charged side chains. Note that transmembrane segment 4 is strongly positively charged. It is believed to be the voltage sensor. For further explanation see text

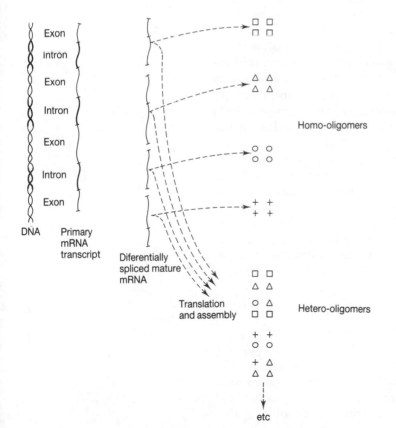

Figure 10.10 Generation of a diversity of A-channels. A variety of homo- and hetero-oligomers of the A-channel protein may be derived by differential splicing of the primary mRNA transcript of *Drosophila* 'shaker' locus. Exons light, introns bold. (After Schwarz *et al.*, 1988, *Nature*, **331**, 137–142.)

channels evolved by gene duplication. It must, however, be borne in mind that it is beginning to seem unlikely that the fast potassium channel consists of just this one unit; it is beginning to look as though the polypeptide isolated from *Drosophila* is a single unit of a multimeric structure (compare the nicotinic acetylcholine receptor).

The likelihood that the structure shown in Figure 10.9 is part of a multimeric structure is increased by the finding that the *Drosophila* 'shaker' gene is a highly complex unit. It appears that it may have multiple promoter sites so that the initiation of transcription may occur at different places in different tissues. Furthermore the primary mRNA once transcribed may be spliced at different points, combining different exons, and thus giving rise to different mature mRNA strands. These would then be translated into subtly different A-channel proteins. These proteins could then assemble to give different homo-oligomers or, even more interestingly, different hetero-oligomers (see Figure 10.10).

10.2.3 Serotonin-dependent potassium channel (S-channel)

It is possible by voltage-clamp experiments to show that a potassium channel distinct from the three mentioned above is present in the membranes of *Aplysia* (sea-hare) neurons. This channel, unlike the slow or fast K^+ channels, is activated at the membrane's resting potential, remains open when the membrane is depolarised and is not affected by Ca^{2+}. The channel is affected, however, by **serotonin**, a common neurotransmitter, and by **cyclic AMP (cAMP)**. It can be shown by patch-clamp analysis that serotonin and cAMP exert their effects by reducing the number of I_{KS} channels open at a given time.

Although S-channels are few and far between their cumulative effect is normally to speed the repolarisation of a neuronal membrane after an action potential. If they are inactivated the flow of K^+ out of a neuron (responsible for this repolarisation) is hindered. Hence the period of depolarisation is lengthened. Hence the period during which Ca^{2+} can flow through its channels to the interior is lengthened. We shall see in Chapter 18 that this could have an important role to play in the molecular basis of memory.

10.2.4 Calcium-dependent channel

Calcium-dependent potassium channels differ from all the channels we have considered so far in that they are sensitive to the **internal** concentration of a modulator: in this case calcium ions. As the Ca^{2+} concentration increases in the cytosol these potassium channels open and allow the escape of K^+. This makes the membrane more difficult to depolarise—any depolarising voltages applied are counteracted by an outward flow of positively charged potassium ions.

In Chapter 9 we noted the possible interaction of these channels with the NMDA Ca^{2+} channel to produce the oscillating membrane potentials underlying pacemaker activity. Calcium-dependent potassium channels are probably also involved in sensory adaptation. All sensory systems adapt to a constant stimulus by a reduction in impulse frequency. It is not difficult to see that this will occur when it is understood (see next section) that each action potential generated leads to the influx of a small amount of calcium through voltage-dependent Ca^{2+} channels. A rapid volley of impulses due to a steady stimulus being turned on will soon increase the internal concentration of Ca^{2+} ions and thus open the Ca^{2+} gates, with the results indicated above.

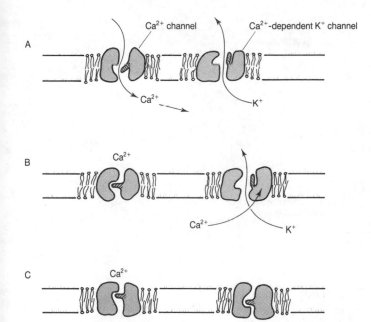

Figure 10.11 Sensory adaptation and Ca^{2+}-dependent K^+ gates. (A) The membrane is depolarised. Ca^{2+} gates and Ca^{2+}-dependent K^+ gates open. (B) The membrane repolarises but unlike the I_K and I_{KA} gates the I_{KCa} gates remain open in the presence of Ca^{2+}. A subsequent depolarising stimulus or transmitter will consequently find it more difficult to depolarise the membrane owing to the countervailing efflux of K^+. (C) Ca^{2+} is removed by intracellular mechanisms and the I_{KCa} channel closes

10.3 CALCIUM CHANNELS

Calcium channels are the last major type of voltage-dependent channel developed in excitable cells. They are to be found in muscle cells (two pharmacologically distinct types) and in several other types of cell as well as in neurons (three distinct varieties). In neurons they play (see Chapter 14) a vital role in the release

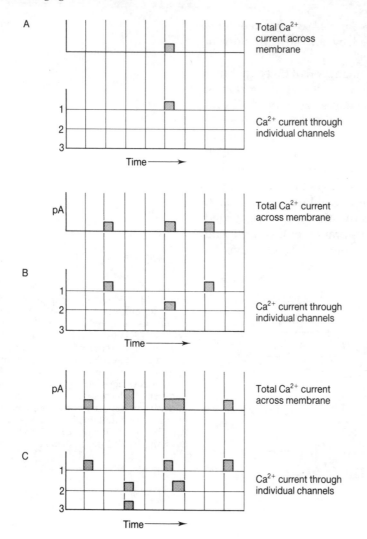

Figure 10.12 Voltage-dependence of Ca^{2+} channels. The schematic shows that when a membrane containing Ca^{2+} channels is progressively depolarised ((A) → (B) → (C)) fresh channels are recruited and the Ca^{2+} current across the membrane increases

of neurotransmitters from synaptic endings. They are also to be found in the membrane of an axon's initial segment where, as we noted above, they can play a part in adaptation. In addition they are found, albeit in smaller numbers, in dendrites, growth cones and cell bodies.

The concentration of calcium ions is very different on the two sides of a neuronal cell membrane. Whereas the extracellular concentration is usually about 3 mM the internal concentration of **free** Ca^{2+} is seldom more than 10^{-4} mM. Opening of channels across the membrane allowing Ca^{2+} ions to cascade in can thus result in a very marked change in the concentration of calcium ions in the cytosol.

Calcium channels are very sensitive to transmembrane voltage.

Studies using the patch-clamp technique show that the channels open and then rapidly close again although, as was the case with all the other channels we have discussed, the mechanism appears to be more complicated than a simple two-stage open/shut cycle. There seem to be intermediate states. Each channel's open/shut cycle has a time-course of about 0.6 ms. The number of channels going through this cycle on a small patch of membrane depends on the transmembrane voltage. As the voltage across the membrane falls, more and more channels are activated. The flow of Ca^{2+} ions consequently increases.

In physiological conditions, when the external concentration of Ca^{2+} is about 3 mM each channel allows the passage of about 0.06 pA of current. It is easy to work out that this means that some 180 000 calcium ions flow through a channel per second. Although the number of Ca^{2+} channels is rather small—ranging from about 4 μm^{-2} in heart muscle to 60 μm^{-2} in snail neurons—the flux is evidently great enough to make a considerable difference to the very low free Ca^{2+} concentration normally present in cytosol. We shall return to this in Chapters 14 and 15, where we consider the neuron as a secretory cell and the release of neurotransmitters by presynaptic terminals.

Calcium channels are **very selective**. This is vital if they are to ensure the influx of calcium ions rather than a mixture of sodium and potassium ions which are both much more common in the extracellular fluid. Compared to a Ca^{2+} concentration of about 3 mM, Na^+ is present at a concentration of about 145 mM. The molecular mechanism underlying this important selectivity is not yet known.

Calcium channels can be affected by a large number of neurotransmitters and drugs. So far all the agents tested have tended to **inactivate ('down-modulate')** the channel. These agents include GABA, serotonin, somatostatin, norepinephrine, enkephalin and 1,4-dihydropyridine (DHP). This last agent has been used to isolate a calcium channel from rabbit skeletal muscle.

A purified DHP–receptor preparation was used to prepare an oligonucleotide probe and this in turn for extracting and cloning the receptor's cDNA. It is found that the protein thus obtained consists of 1873 amino acids, with a molecular weight of approximately 170 kDa.

Examination of this polypeptide shows it to have a striking resemblance to the sodium channel. Like the sodium channel it contains four homologous domains of about 300 amino acids each. Like the sodium channel the amino- and carboxy-terminals are both located on the cytoplasmic side of the membrane. Furthermore if the amino acid sequences of the homologous domains are compared with those in the rat sodium channel protein a strong resemblance is found:

Domain l: 32% identical residues; 62% identical + conservative substitutes

Domain 2: 35% identical residues; 59% identical + conservative substitutes

Domain 3: 37% identical residues; 60% identical + conservative substitutes

Domain 4: 32% identical residues; 61% identical + conservative substitutes

The overall sequence homology is 35% identity or 55% when conservative substitutes are added.

Hydropathic analysis of the polypeptide also shows that it is remarkably similar to the sodium channel. Each of the homologous domains consists of five hydrophobic segments, S1, S2, S3, S5 and S6, and one positively charged segment, S4. All six segments are believed to span the membrane. It is also found that the S4 segment in each homologous domain contains a sequence of positively charged Arg or Lys residues following a regular pattern (Arg(Lys)–X–X–), where X is a non-polar residue. This pattern is also to be found in the S4 segment of every known sodium channel protein. It has been tentatively concluded that, as with the sodium channel, this regular group of positively-charged side-chains forms the voltage sensor.

It is known that the calcium channel has a pore diameter of about 6 Å. It is possible that, as in the Na^+-channel, one or two of the helical transmembrane segments from each homologous domain form the walls of the pore.

Figure 10.13 Structure of the calcium channel. (A) Hydropathy plot of the polypeptide chain. The further above the horizontal line the greater the hydrophobicity. Roman I, II, III and IV indicate the position of the homologous domains while the boxes 1–6 denote the homologous segments within each domain. The rectangles beneath the hydropathicity plot indicate where α-helix and/or β-sheet is predicted and the vertical bars on the line beneath show the position of positively charged residues (lys, arg) (upward) and negatively charged residues (asp, glu) (downward). (B) Putative disposition in the membrane. As with the sodium channel it is likely that in reality the four homologous domains make use of the third dimension to cluster together around a calcium channel. ((A) reprinted with permission from Tanabe *et al.*, 1987, *Nature*, **328**, 313–318. Copyright © 1987, Macmillan Magazines, Ltd.) ⟶

10.4 SODIUM AND POTASSIUM 'LEAK' CHANNELS

In addition to the channels described above, which are either ligand- or voltage-controlled, there are also channels in neuronal cell membranes which allow sodium and potassium ions to 'leak' in or out along their electrochemical gradients. It can be shown that the potassium leak channel is considerably more 'leaky' than the sodium channel. The leakiness of the K^+ channel varies, moreover, in different cells. It is for instance far more leaky in many neuroglial cells than in neurons. We shall see the significance of these non-gated channels in Chapter 11, where we discuss the physical basis of resting potentials and electrotonic conduction.

A

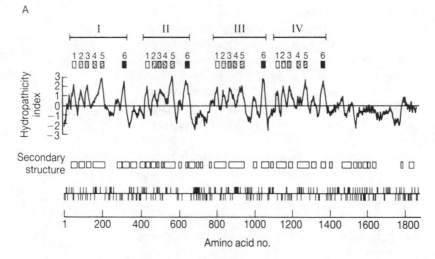

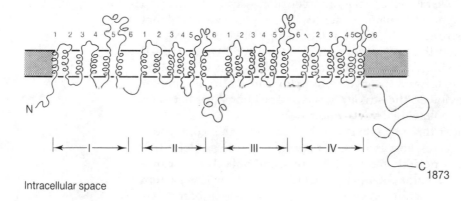

10.5 CONCLUSION

This chapter, like its predecessors, has given us an inkling of the great variety of channels which exist in neuronal membranes. We have seen that there are various physiological subtypes of sodium, potassium and calcium channels. We have also seen that each of these subtypes can exist in several different conditions of openness or shutness. The more we understand about the brain the more infinitely complex it seems.

Yet at the same time that the complexity increases great unifying principles begin to emerge. At root these unifying principles rest on the major unifying theory of all biology: evolution. We have seen in this chapter that the three major voltage-controlled gates—the sodium, potassium and calcium channels—are built according to a common architectural principle. The fast potassium gate consists of a polypeptide of some 616 amino acids with six or seven membrane spanning regions; the sodium and calcium gates consist of a protein some three times as large, with over 1800 amino acids, and consisting of four domains, each of which is rather similar to a single potassium gate. Each of these domains, like the potassium gate, consists of six membrane spanning segments and in each case the fourth segment, like the fourth segment in the potassium gate, is highly polar and suspected of being the voltage sensor. In the sodium and calcium gates the four homologous domains are joined together by stretches of hydrophilic amino acids.

Further still, looking back over chapters 7, 8, 9 and 10, we can begin to see that the multitudinous variety of channels and pumps which abound in neuronal membranes fall into a much smaller number of natural groups. We saw in Chapter 7 that the great variety of G-coupled receptors, β_1 and β_2 AR, mAChR, SKR and the opsins, all showed a remarkably consistent structure, marked by seven membrane-spanning helices. In Chapter 8 we noted that there is a strong evolutionary relationship between the Na^+ + K^+ pump and the Ca^{2+} pump. Next in Chapter 9 we discussed the remarkable family resemblances between nAChRs, the $GABA_A$ receptor and the glycine receptor. Finally in this chapter we have reviewed the striking structural relationships between the various voltage-gated channels.

In the next three chapters we shall see how this complexity of pumps, gates and ion gradients underlies those definitive features of neural biophysics: **resting potentials**, **cable conduction**, **receptor potentials**, and last, but far from least, **action potentials**. The action potential or nerve impulse, in particular, can be understood as arising from the interaction of many of the gated channels which we have just reviewed. Finally, in Chapter 15, we shall broach the equally central topic of synaptic transmission leading on to a discussion of **postsynaptic potentials** in Chapter 16. In these two chapters we shall return once again to many of the channels discussed above and in Chapters 7 and 9. Indeed it is in the study of the molecular structure and function of membrane channels that molecular biology is beginning to unite with biophysics to make a major contribution to neurobiology.

Chapter 11
Resting potentials and cable conduction

That the functioning of the nervous system is accompanied by electrical changes has been known since the work of Galvani and Volta in the late eighteenth century. It was, however, only with the development of mid-twentieth-century electrotechnology (especially electronics) and the discovery of suitable experimental preparations (in particular the cephalopod giant axon) that a genuine understanding of 'animal electricity' became possible.

In this chapter we shall first consider the origin of the 'resting potential' (V_m) which exists across all plasma membranes and in particular across the plasma membranes of neurons. Second, we shall turn our attention to the **'passive'** flows of electrical current and changes of electrical potentials across membranes. We shall deal with 'action potentials' in Chapter 13. We shall see in these two chapters how the electrical phenomena of nervous systems are signs of ion flows controlled by the many gates, channels and pumps which we reviewed in Chapters 8, 9 and 10. The theory of the nervous system at this level begins to take on a coherence and simplicity which would have delighted earlier investigators.

11.1 MEASUREMENT OF THE RESTING POTENTIAL

We noted above that resting potentials are believed to be developed across all cell membranes, whatever the type of cell. Most mammalian neurons, however, have extremely small diameters—seldom more than about 20 μm. The recognition that certain large tubular structures (diameter 500–600 μm) in the squid, *Loligo*, were in fact single **giant axons** was thus of enormous value to electrophysiologists. They were at last able to place fine glass micropipettes filled with an electrolyte inside an axon and measure the resting and action potentials directly. They were also able to squeeze out the axoplasm and subject it to chemical analysis (see Table 8.1). Most of the pioneering work which established the physical basis of membrane potentials was done on this convenient preparation. Once again we are made aware of the great value of non-mammalian preparations in the prosecution of fundamental neuroscience.

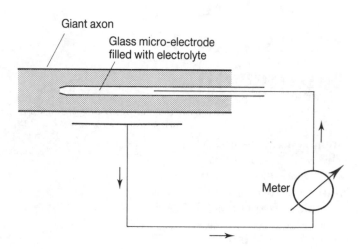

Figure 11.1   Measurement of the resting potential using a squid giant axon preparation. A fine glass micro-electrode is inserted into the giant axon. The potentiometer measures the electrical potential across the membrane. The arrows indicate the direction of current flow

Figure 11.1 shows that when the external electrode is taken to be at 'ground potential' (as is conventional) the internal electrode is found to record a voltage drop of some 50 mV across the membrane. This is the so-called **'resting potential'** (V_m). Our next task is to determine the origin of this ubiquitous potential.

11.2 THE ORIGIN OF THE RESTING POTENTIAL

The giant axon preparation and subsequently other preparations have allowed investigators to determine the ionic concentrations on either side of a neuronal membrane. We have already seen (Chapter 8) how it is possible to calculate the difference in 'free energy' (ΔG) represented by the distribution of a substance on two sides of a membrane. But in that chapter we explicitly put on one side consideration of any electrical forces which might be acting on charged particles such as ions. In this chapter we have to bring these forces into the equation. We have to consider not only the diffusional forces due to concentration differences but also the forces due to differences in electrical potential. For we shall be looking at the distribution of charged ions: Na^+, K^+,

Cl⁻, Ca²⁺, etc. The distribution and movement of ions across membranes is responsible for all the multifarious electrical phenomena which characterise the physiology of nervous systems.

In Chapter 8 we worked out the energetics of a transmembrane system by making use of μ, the chemical potential. In this chapter we introduce another parameter, $\bar{\mu}$, **the electrochemical potential**. This parameter takes into account the electrical forces which ions feel. In effect it is the chemical potential, μ, with an electrical term added.

The magnitude of the electrical force, P, which an ion, I, will feel depends on its valency, Z, and on the electrical potential, ψ, of its surroundings. We can thus write:

$$P = Z_I \psi^\alpha \ldots\ldots\ldots\ldots \qquad 11.1$$

where Z = valency of the ion, I (i.e. $+1$ for Na and K, -1 for Cl, $+2$ for Ca, etc.) and ψ^α = electrical potential of phase α in which ion, I, is located.

Now biologists and biochemists are accustomed to work in moles or gram ions, not single molecules or ions. A mole of univalent ions (i.e. 6×10^{23} ions) carries 96 500 C of electricity, i.e. one faraday (Γ). Hence we can rewrite the preceding equation as.

$$P = Z_I \psi^\alpha F$$

This is the electric force which a mole of ion, I, will experience in phase α.

It will be recalled, from Chapter 8, that the expression for the chemical potential of a substance, A, in phase α, was:

$$\mu_A^\alpha = \mu_A^O + RT \ln C_A^\alpha$$

It follows that the electrochemical potential for an ion, I, in phase α, is given by:

$$\bar{\mu}_I^\alpha = \mu_I^O + RT \ln C_I^\alpha + Z_I \psi^\alpha F \ldots\ldots\ldots \qquad 11.2$$

Next let us remind ourselves of the system we are considering. This is shown in Figure 11.2. The ion, I, is present in both phase α and phase β; the two phases are separated by a **permeable** partition or membrane.

.Now if, as we emphasised above, the membrane between the two solutions is fully permeable to 'I' then microscopic flows will occur

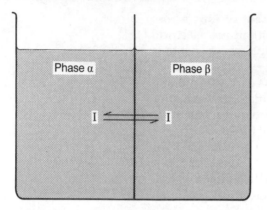

Figure 11.2 Permeable membrane separating two ionic solutions

to ensure that the electrochemical potentials of 'I' on each side of the membrane are identical. The condition for equilibrium is thus:

$$\bar{\mu}_I^{\alpha} = \bar{\mu}_I^{\beta}........ \qquad\qquad 11.3$$

If, next, we expand both sides of eq. 11.3 we have:

$$\mu_I^{\,\circ} + RT \ln C_I^{\alpha} + Z_I\psi^{\alpha}F = \mu_I^{\,\circ} + RT \ln C_I^{\beta} + Z_I\psi^{\beta}F$$

Collecting terms we have:

$$Z_I F(\psi^{\alpha} - \psi^{\beta}) = RT \ln \frac{C_I^{\beta}}{C_I^{\alpha}}$$

Next we take note of two things. First, we can substitute C_O and C_i (the concentrations of I on either side of the membrane) for C_I^{α} and C_I^{β}; second, as any difference in electrical potential between the two phases, α and β, will be felt at the boundary between the phases we can substitute V, the voltage across the membrane, for $(\psi^{\alpha} - \psi^{\beta})$. Hence we may write:

$$V = \frac{RT}{Z_I F} \ln \frac{C_o}{C_i} V.... \qquad\qquad 11.4$$

Eq. 11.4 is the **Nernst equation**, one of the most important equations in neurophysiology.

The Nernst equation relates the electrical potential across a **permeable** membrane to the distribution of charged ions which it separates. Note that the membrane must be permeable to the ion under consideration. This, as we have just seen, is one of the premises on which the derivation of the equation is based. If it holds then it is possible to see that when the system is in equilibrium the electrical potential across the membrane exactly counterbalances any concentration differences.

Let us test the equation by supposing the concentrations of ion 'I' on both sides of the membrane to be identical. If we substitute in eq. 11.4 we see that the logarithmic term becomes unity. The log of unity is zero. Hence the right-hand side of the equation goes to zero. Hence the Nernst equation predicts **no** electrical potential should be developed across the membrane. This, of course, is what is observed. When a cell dies the integrity of its membrane and its pumping mechanisms disappear. Ions flow along their concentration gradients until their concentrations equalise inside and outside the cell. The membrane potential vanishes.

Let us test the equation further by substituting the values for $[K^+]_O$ (i.e 5.5 mM) and $[K^+]_i$ (i.e. 150 mM) which we quoted in Table 8.1.
Then,

$$V_K = \frac{RT}{Z_I F} \ln \frac{5.5}{150}$$

$$= 0.027 \ln 0.036$$

$$= -0.089 \text{ V}$$

or $\qquad$ **−89 mV**

This is known as the **Nernst potassium potential**, V_K. Measurement of the actual resting potential across nerve cell membranes, V_m, usually gives values of −50 to −75 mV. The Nernst potassium potential is evidently markedly larger than this, but not too far out. It does suggest that the membrane potential is caused, as the Nernst equation suggests, by the distribution of ions across it. If, however, values for the concentration of the other ions (Cl^-, Na^+, Ca^{2+}), are substituted in the equation the predicted values for V_m are very far from what is observed. This is especially the case when the values for Na^+ are substituted.

The reasons for this are very simple. As we have seen in previous chapters cell membranes, especially nerve cell membranes, are very complex structures. Their permeability to different ions varies dramatically. And, as we emphasised above, the Nernst equation only works for ions which can pass un-hindered through the membrane in question. It is known, however, that both sodium and chloride ions have very low permeability coefficients.

Furthermore V_m does not depend on the transmembrane distribution of a single ion species but on the distribution of several different types of ion: Na^+ and Cl^- (however low their permeability coefficients), as well as K^+. Thus to gain a fuller understanding of the origin of the electrical potential across nerve cell membranes we must generalise the Nernst equation. We must derive an equation which takes into account the different permeability of the membrane to different ions and the fact that there is not just one ionic species in play but many.

The equation we are looking for was developed by Goldman and is consequently known as the Goldman equation. The equation is also sometimes known as 'the constant field equation' because it assumes that the electric field across the membrane (the electrical potential gradient, V_m) remains constant. This, of course, is a large assumption to make. However the Goldman equation provides a useful first approximation to the biophysical situation. It is written as follows:

$$V = \frac{RT}{F} \ln \frac{P_K[K^+]_o + P_{Na}[Na^+]_o + P_{Cl}[Cl^-]_i}{P_K[K^+]_i + P_{Na}[Na^+]_i + P_{Cl}[Cl^-]_o} \qquad 11.5$$

where P is the permeability constant of the ion concerned, square brackets indicate concentration of the ion either inside (subscript 'i') or outside (subscript 'o') the cell, and R, T and F have their usual connotations.

Note that whereas the external concentrations of the cations K^+ and Na^+ appear in the numerator of the equation, the **internal** concentration of the anion, Cl^-, is placed alongside them in this position.

Let us try some test runs on the Goldman equation. First, if we make the permeability constants of Na^+ and Cl^- equal to zero, i.e. the membrane is completely impermeable to these ions, then the Goldman equation reduces to the Nernst equation for K^+. Similarly if we make $P_K = P_{Cl} = 0$ then the equation reduces to the Nernst equation for Na^+ and predicts V_{Na} as the potential across the membrane.

Now as we noted at the end of Chapter 10, neuronal membranes are not completely impermeable to any of the small inorganic ions found in the extracellular and intracellular compartments. Although cations and anions, being strongly hydrophilic, would find it next to impossible to make their way through the lipid bilayer of a plasma membrane, we saw that there exist 'leak channels' through which they can with difficulty pass.

The molecular nature of these channels is not well known. They are, however, almost certainly proteins—just as were the various channels we examined in Chapters 9 and 10. Moreover, the 'leakiness' of these channels varies markedly from one cell type to another. Neuroglial cells, as we saw, seem to be more permeable to potassium ions than are neurons.

Neurons, as we noted above, resemble other cells in being much more permeable to K^+ than to Cl^- or Na^+:

$$P_K \ggg P_{Cl} \sim P_{Na}$$

Let us put some figures to these relative permeabilities. Measurements of the flow of radiolabelled ions across plasma membranes give the following values:

$$P_K = 1 \times 10^{-7} \text{ cm s}^{-1}$$

$$P_{Cl} = 1 \times 10^{-8} \text{ cm s}^{-1}$$

$$P_{Na} = 1 \times 10^{-8} \text{ cm s}^{-1}$$

Next let us insert these permeability constants and the appropriate ionic concentrations (Table 8.1: cat motor neuron) into the Goldman equation:

$$V_m = 0.027 \ln \frac{(1 \times 10^7 \,[5.51]) + (1 \times 10^8 \,[150]) + (1 \times 10^8 \,[9])}{(1 \times 10^7 \,[150]) + (1 \times 10^8 \,[15]) + (1 \times 10^8 \,[125])}$$

$$= 0.027 \ln \frac{(55 \times 10^8) + (150 \times 10^8) + (9 \times 10^8)}{(1500 \times 10^8) + (15 \times 10^8) + (125 \times 10^8)}$$

$$= -0.055 \text{ V}$$

$$= -55 \text{ mV}$$

The value of -55 mV determined by application of the Goldman equation is quite close to the value of the resting potential across cat motor neurons actually observed by microelectrode recording.

Next, let us see what happens if we increase the potassium permeability by an order of magnitude. If we insert $P_K = 1 \times 10^{-6}$ cm s^{-1} into the equation, keeping all the other permeability constants unchanged we find:

$$V_m = -83 \text{ mV}$$

We have already remarked that the membranes of some glial cells are markedly more permeable to K^+ than the membranes of neurons. Hence we find that the V_m across these membranes is characteristically greater than the customary resting potential of neuronal membranes. Astrocytes, for instance, have V_ms ranging from -70 to -90 mV. This larger than usual K^+ permeability is believed to be of considerable importance in mopping up excess K^+ which diffuses into the brain's intercellular space when neurons are active over appreciable periods of time (see Chapter 13). This mechanism can also be demonstrated to be at work in the retina. Large glial cells, known as Müller cells, take up excess K^+ generated in the nervous part of the retina in response to illumination and discharge it into the vitreous humour. V_m is of course, sensitive to variations in the permeability constants of all the ions distributed across it. In Chapter 13 we shall look closely at what happens when P_{Na} suddenly increases.

Before completing this section it is worth noting that as it is much easier to measure the relative rather than the absolute permeabilities of ions the Goldman equation is often written in a slightly different form:

$$V = \frac{RT}{F} \ln \frac{[K]_o + b[Na]_o + c[Cl]_i}{[K]_i + b[Na]_i + c[Cl]_o} \qquad 11.6$$

where $b = P_{Na}/P_K$ and $c = P_{Cl}/P_K$

We shall see in Chapter 13 that the chloride ion plays little or no part in the generation of action potentials. Hence when considering the ionic bases of action potentials eq. 11.6 is often simplified to:

$$V = \frac{RT}{F} \ln \frac{[K]_o + b[Na]_o}{[K]_i + b[Na]_i} \qquad 11.7$$

We shall see, however, that although the chloride ion is unimportant in action potentials it nevertheless plays a crucial role in the hyperpolarisations of inhibitory synapses. It is important to use the full form of Goldman's equation in these and similar circumstances.

11.3 ELECTROTONIC POTENTIALS AND CABLE CONDUCTION

Not all the electrical signalling in the nervous system is by way of action potentials, or impulses. Indeed it could be argued that some of the most important, if not *the* most important, of the central nervous system's communications depends upon non-impulse signalling. These signals, which are at least one order of magnitude and sometimes two or more orders of magnitude, weaker than action potentials, have been termed **electrotonic potentials**. They are small depolarisations of a nerve process's membrane and are caused by the essentially **passive** spread of electrical current through the conducting fluids inside and outside nerve cells and their processes. Nonetheless, however small electrotonic potentials may be, they can have a very considerable effect on the physiology of neuronal membranes and thus on the large-scale functioning of the brain. To see that this is the case we need only recall the sensitivity of some of the ion channels discussed in Chapter 10 to transmembrane voltage. In later chapters we shall see that the influx of, for instance, Ca^{2+} ions by the opening of voltage-dependent gates may lead to all sorts of dramatic consequences.

Consider Figure 11.3. Here the diagram shows a microelectrode inserted into a neural process and a small amount of current injected. This current flows down the process and leaks out through the membrane back into the bathing fluid to complete the circuit. If the process penetrated by the microelectrode is an axon the amount of current injected will, of course, have to be sufficiently minute not to open the voltage-dependent Na^+ gates (see Chapter 10) and thereby precipitate an action potential. If, however, the process is a dendrite or one of the short axons which are to be found in the brain's local circuit neurons (see Chapter 1) or one of the many types of neuron which are developed between the two plexiform layers in the retina then, because there are very few if any voltage-dependent sodium gates present, the current can be larger.

Because of its considerable importance the spread of electrotonic potentials and the 'electrotonic' or 'cable' conduction upon

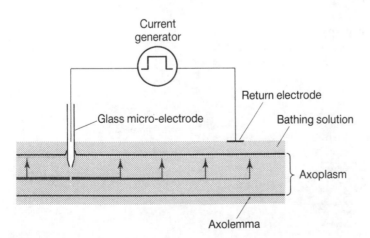

Figure 11.3 Electrotonic conduction in a neuronal process. The current injected by the micro-electrode leaks back out through the axolemma to the return electrode in the bathing fluid

which it depends has been intensively studied. The conduction is often referred to as 'cable conduction' because of its similarity to the transmission of current through long-distance telegraph cables. In both cases the injected current leaks out through the insulating sheath around the conductive core. In consequence some of the mathematical theory developed by telecommunications engineers can be applied to the neurophysiological problem. This theory can be mathematically somewhat fierce. Interested readers will find that titles listed in the bibliography give exhaustive accounts.

Nevertheless some brief account of electrotonic conduction is necessary if the functioning of the nervous system is to be understood. We have already seen in Chapters 9 and 10 how ligand- or voltage-controlled gates in the neuronal membrane allow flows of ions into and out of the cell. These flows carry electric current and depolarise or hyperpolarise the membrane. We shall see in the chapters to come that local circuits spreading from these membrane patches are responsible for switching on or off subsynaptic cells and for the propagation of action potentials.

In order to develop a mathematical framework within which electrotonic conduction can be discussed it is necessary to make some simplifying assumptions at the outset. It is necessary to assume that the following parameters remain constant along the length of the process:

1. r_o: the longitudinal electrical resistance of the extracellular medium.
2. r_i: the longitudinal electrical resistance of the intracellular medium, i.e. the axoplasm.
3. r_m: the transverse electrical resistance of the membrane, i.e. the neurilemma.
4. c_m: the electrical capacity of the membrane.

Next consider Figure 11.4. A current is injected into the neural process at point 'x_0' so that the membrane is depolarised to a

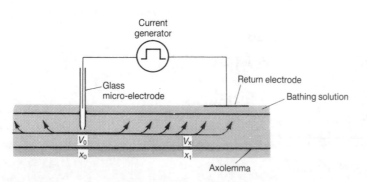

Current
generator

Glass
micro-electrode

Return electrode

Bathing solution

V_0

V_x

x_0

x_1

Axolemma

Figure 11.4 Electrotonic conduction. Current is injected at x_0 to induce a voltage across the membrane of V_0. What is the electrotonic potential, V_x, at some point x_1?

value V_0. Two further simplifying assumptions have to be made here: first, that the injected current remains constant for the duration of the experiment; second, that the process is 'infinitely' long. When these assumptions are made Figure 11.4 shows that the current spreads down the process through the conductive cytosol, leaking out through the neurilemma until it attenuates to zero. Our question is: what is the value of the electrotonic potential, V_x, at some point x_1?

It can be shown that the appropriate cable equation (given the above conditions) is:

$$V = \lambda^2 \frac{d^2V}{dx^2} \qquad \qquad 11.8$$

where λ is (as we shall see below) a 'space constant'.

Eq. 11.8 can be solved to give the following answer to our question:

$$V_x = V_0 \, e^{-x/\lambda} \qquad \qquad 11.9$$

As usual let us test this equation. When $x \to 0$, $e^{-x/\lambda} \to e^0$, and $e^0 = 1$. Hence $V_x = V_0$, as it should.

Next let us give a little attention to the factors responsible for the space constant, λ. If we go back to the derivation of the cable equation (see, for instance, Aidley's text listed in the bibliography) we shall find that it depends on the three electrical resistances mentioned at the beginning of this discussion:

$$\lambda^2 = \frac{r_m}{r_o + r_i} \qquad \qquad 11.10$$

Next, let us put $x = \lambda$ in eq. 11.9. Then

$$V_x = V_0 e^{-1} \qquad \qquad 11.11$$

Eq.11.11 shows that λ is **the distance from the point at which current is injected at which the electrotonic depolarisation has fallen to e^{-1}, i.e. 0.37, of its original value (V_0).**

λ is a useful parameter for comparing the spread of electrotonus along neuronal processes of different types and size. Both the length and the diameter of the process are significant. Let us briefly look at each in turn.

Length. The graph in Figure 11.5 shows how the electrotonic potential falls off with distance from the point at which depolarising current is injected. The lower curve represents the case for a process of 'infinite' length (as in the example we have just discussed). In practice this means any process more than three times longer than λ. This is the solution to the cable conduction equation described above. It is clearly applicable to long undersea telegraph cables. But in many neural instances the process under consideration may be comparatively short. The upper curve in Figure 11.5 shows the case where λ is about the same length as the entire process. When this is the case, as the figure shows, the curve does not in fact fall away asymptotically to the abscissa (as it does for the case of infinite length) but declines much less steeply, perhaps never diminishing by more than 0.75 of the input voltage. This latter instance is of considerable significance for the spread of receptor potentials in receptor cells: a phenomenon we shall discuss in the next chapter.

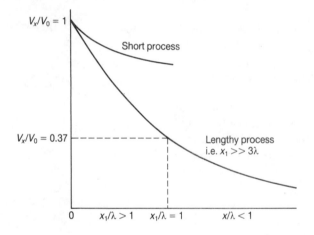

Figure 11.5 Electrotonic conduction in processes of different length. Current is injected at x_0 so that the process is depolarised from a resting potential of -60 mV to V_0 (-40 mV). The length constant, λ, is the distance from x_0 at which the electrotonic potential (V_x) across the membrane has fallen to $1/e$ (i.e 37%) of its value at x_0. For further explanation see text

Diameter. As the diameter of a process increases the magnitude of λ also increases. Let us see why this is the case. First of all we can note that while the longitudinal internal resistance, r_i, decreases as the radius of the process increases the longitudinal external resistance, r_o, remains unaltered. Hence as an approximation we can simplify eq. 11.10 to:

$$\lambda \propto \frac{r_m}{r_i} \qquad\qquad 11.12$$

$$\text{Now } r_m = \frac{R_m \; \Omega \; \text{cm}^2}{2\pi\alpha \; \text{cm}}$$

where R_m is the resistance of unit area of membrane and a is the radius of the neuronal process; and

$$r_i = \frac{R_i \ \Omega \ \text{cm}}{\pi a^2 \ \text{cm}^2}$$

where R_i is the resistivity of unit volume of cytosol. Hence

$$\lambda \propto \sqrt{\left(\frac{R_m}{2\pi a} \times \frac{\pi a^2}{R_i}\right) \ \text{cm}^2}$$

$$\propto \sqrt{\left(\frac{R_m}{R_i} \times \frac{a}{2}\right) \ \text{cm}^2} \qquad\qquad 11.13$$

It is clear from eq. 11.13 that, whilst R_m and R_i remain constant, λ will increase as the diameter of the process increases. In Chapter 13 we shall see that action potentials depend upon underlying cable conduction. Hence we can see from the above analysis why it is that so many invertebrates have developed giant axons. The larger the diameter the greater the spread of the electrotonic conduction and hence, other things being equal, the more rapid the impulse propagation. Invertebrates develop giant fibres in order to respond rapidly to an emergency. Conduction along the squid's giant fibre normally leads to the vigorous tail flexure which propels the cephalopod backwards out of danger. In Chapter 13 we shall see that the vertebrates have evolved a different mechanism for increasing impulse propagation rate—myelination.

The above analysis is also of particular importance to our understanding of the biophysics of dendrites. Let us consider an example. Some of the large apical dendrites springing from the pyramidal cells in the cerebral cortex may be up to 10 μm in diameter. Then taking

$$R_m = 2500 \ \Omega \ \text{cm}^2$$

$$R_i = 70 \ \Omega \ \text{cm}$$

$$a = 0.0005 \ \text{cm}$$

It follows that $\lambda = \sqrt{\left(\dfrac{2500 \ \Omega \ \text{cm}^2}{70 \ \Omega \ \text{cm}} \times \dfrac{0.0005 \ \text{cm}}{2}\right)}$

$$\sim \textbf{0.1 cm or 1 mm}$$

A similar calculation for an extremely fine dendrite ($d = 0.1\ \mu$m) yields a value for λ of about 100 μm or 0.1 mm. In other words a decrease of two orders of magnitude in diameter leads to a decrease of only one order of magnitude in λ. These values for λ are of considerable interest as they fit well with the magnitudes of dendritic processes which neurohistologists observe in the brain.

Before leaving the topics of electrotonic potentials and cable conduction it is worth noting a further important parameter: time. In our discussion so far we have assumed (as noted at the outset) that the depolarising voltage has been constant throughout the experiment. In neurophysiological reality, however, synaptic depolarisations (or hyperpolarisations) are often brief, transient events. In order to study the consequences of such transient electrotonic potentials we have to take into account the electrical capacitance of the membrane. This determines the time taken to build up electrical charge and/or to evacuate that charge. The time taken to reach e^{-1} of the final voltage is called the **charging time constant** or, alternatively, the **whole neuron constant** (τ). If the size and branching characteristics of a dendritic tree are taken into

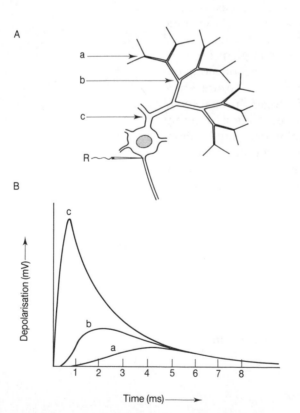

Figure 11.6 Transient electrotonus exhibited at the initial segment of the axon in response to depolarising synaptic events at different points on a dendritic tree. (A) A depolarising current is injected at a, b or c on an idealised dichotomously branching dendritic tree. (C) The graph shows the depolarisation recorded at the initial segment of the axon by recording electrode, R, to each dendritic stimulation. (After Shepherd, 1979, *The Synaptic Organisation of the Brain*, 2nd edition, Oxford: Oxford University Press.)

account it becomes possible to compute the transient electrotonic potentials exhibited by a patch of membrane in the perikaryon or, more significantly, by a patch on the initial segment of the axon, when a synapse is activated on the dendritic tree. The result of one such computation is shown in Figure 11.6.

The figure shows that a synaptic event far out on a dendritic tree has a very different effect on the perikaryon from one close in. Events far out on the tree may not depolarise an initial segment sufficiently to initiate an action potential but they may **bias** that membrane towards activation for tens of milliseconds.

The reader will be aware that the foregoing account describes a detailed mathematical theory the full exposition of which must be left to biophysical texts; he will also be aware that the theory is highly abstract. The mathematician's neuron is very different from the sloppy multitude of variegated forms with which the neurobiologist is familiar. Nevertheless the theory provides a background for investigation of the real brain. Perhaps, indeed, the theory should be compared to Galileo's ideal world of frictionless pulleys and inclined planes which, although very different from our common experience of the nature of things, nevertheless proved indispensable for the development of a genuine physical science.

11.4 CONCLUSION

In this chapter we have examined the biophysical causes of the membrane potentials which the neurophysiologist's micro-electrode detects. We have also looked at the way in which minute electrical currents may spread through neuronal processes in response to tiny membrane depolarisations. In the next chapter we shall consider a selection of sensory cells and note that in all the metazoan cases environmental energies are transduced to alterations in membrane polarity which lead, in turn, to just the sort of electrotonic conduction we have discussed. In Chapter 13 we shall make use of the same biophysical concepts to elucidate the bases of the action potential upon which the nervous system depends for its long-range signalling.

Chapter 12
Sensory transduction

According to the empiricist tradition there is nothing in the mind which was not first in the senses. The detection and transduction of happenings in the environment has always been of great interest to scientists and philosophers. In this chapter we shall look at some representative examples of these processes at the molecular level.

The animal kingdom has developed an overwhelming variety of different sense organs. Let us make a start by looking at two different (but not mutually exclusive) classificatory schemes. Sense organs may be subdivided on the basis of whether they 'look' inside at the internal environment (**enteroreceptors**) or outwards at the external environment (**exteroreceptors**). Or, secondly, they may be classified on the basis of the type of stimulus to which they are most responsive. In this chapter we shall concentrate on the second classification. We shall accordingly look at some examples of **chemoreceptors**, **photoreceptors** and **mechanoreceptors**.

Before we begin it will be well to outline some general features shared by all sensory systems. Sensory cells have the job not only of detecting but also of **transducing** the impinging stimulus into a signal in the organism's internal 'language'. In multicellular forms which have developed a nervous system this signal is ultimately an action potential in a sensory nerve fibre. As all action potentials are very much alike the central nervous system can only tell the type of external energy (chemical, electromagnetic, mechanical) by taking note of *which* fibres are carrying impulses.

The initial transduction is not, however, directly into nerve impulses. The first steps remain firmly in the realm of molecular biology. Indeed in the first example we look at in this chapter they never get further than that level. Bacteria (being small) have no need to develop a nervous system. This does not mean that they lack senses. We shall see that many of them have well developed chemosensory devices. But even in multicellular forms with well-developed nervous systems we shall see that molecular biology still intervenes between signal detection and nerve impulse.

This molecular biology results, as we shall see, in changes in the electrical polarity across the sensory cell's plasma membrane. These changes, which may be hyperpolarisaions or, and more usually, depolarisations, are called **receptor potentials**. In the case of olfactory reception (the second example in this chapter) we shall see that the sensory cell also conducts action potentials. It is a **neurosensory cell**, having the dual function of sensory cell and sensory axon. In this case the receptor potential leads directly to an action potential. It is thus better known as a **generator potential**.

In our final three examples, mammalian gustatory cells, photo-receptor cells and hair cells, the receptor potentials developed in response to the appropriate stimulus do not lead *directly* to action potentials. The sensory nerve fibre, in these cases, is separated by a synapse from the sensory cell. The receptor potentials in these cases thus lead to the release of a neurotransmitter which, falling on the underlying dendrite of the sensory fibres, leads to a generator potential in this latter process. This in turn initiates an action potential in the sensory fibre.

We have noticed throughout the preceding chapters of this book that molecular neurobiologists are slowly uncovering a remarkable uniformity of design at the molecular level. We shall see in this chapter that this underlying unity is also becoming apparent in the structure and function of the sensitive regions of sensory cells.

12.1 CHEMORECEPTORS

12.1.1 Chemosensitivity in prokaryotes

Chemosensitivity probably evolved very early in the history of life on earth. We may speculate that once having hit upon a satisfactory mechanism there was little pressure to change it. It is thus not absurd for neurobiologists to follow their interest into organisms which very definitely lack all vestige of a nervous system: the bacteria.

There is no doubt that motile bacteria are sensitive to the chemical substances in their environment. It has long been known that they will swim up a concentration gradient of an attractant chemical. They can both sense the material in the environment and act on the sensation. How do they do it?

Motile bacteria are propelled by flagella. Prokaryotic flagella are far simpler than those of the eukaryotes. They consist of a single tubular array of flagellin subunits twisted into a helix (Figure 12.1). They also have a very different mechanism for producing motion. Instead of the sliding-filament system believed to be at work in eukaryotic flagella they have the distinction of being the only organic structures so far known to employ a rotary mechanism. The cellular end of the flagellum is rotated at about 100 revolutions per second by a mechanism energised by a transmembrane hydrogen ion gradient.

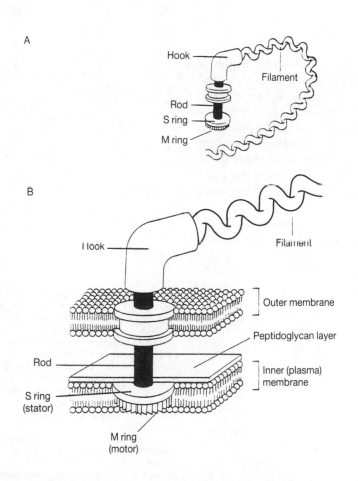

A

Hook
Filament
Rod
S ring
M ring

B

Hook
Filament

Outer membrane

Peptidoglycan layer

Rod

Inner (plasma) membrane

S ring
(stator)

M ring
(motor)

Figure 12.1 Rotary mechanism of a bacterial flagellum. The mechanism penetrates both the outer and inner membrane surrounding the bacterium. Energy derived from a a proton gradient causes the 'M ring' (or motor) to rotate relative to the 'S ring' (or stator) at about 100 revolutions per second. The stator is embedded in the peptidoglycan layer. A rod links the M ring to a hook and then to a helical flagellar filament. A 'bearing' in the outer membrane acts as a seal. (From Adler, in Goldman, Pollard and Rosenbaum, eds, 1976, *Cell Motility*, Cold Spring Harbor, NY: Cold Spring Harbor Laboratory; with permission.)

Most flagellated bacteria have more than one flagellum. *E.coli*, for instance, has eight to ten. When they all rotate in the anti-clockwise direction the bacterium swims forward smoothly. Things, however, are very different if they rotate in the clockwise sense. In this case, because of the helical structure of the flagellum, the flagella all pull outwards, resulting in an irregular 'tumbling' motion (Figure 12.2).

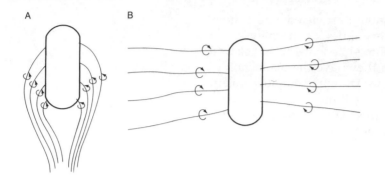

Figure 12.2 Anticlockwise and clockwise rotation of bacterial flagella. (A) Anticlockwise rotation. The flagella stream together as a single bundle which propels the bacterium forwards. (B) Clockwise rotation. The flagella each pull away from the bacterium in the direction of the straight arrows. According to the varying strength of the pull from each flagellum the bacterium veers from side to side and tumbles hither and thither

If the swimming of a bacterial cell is followed under a microscope it will be seen to consist of a series of smooth 'runs' interspersed with episodes of chaotic tumbling. When the cell comes out of its tumble it will set off smoothly again but in a completely random direction. If, however, the cell is placed in a gradient of chemical attractant it is found that when swimming is in the direction of the source fewer tumbles occur than when it is moving in any other direction. The net result is that the bacterium migrates up the concentration gradient towards the source of the attractant.

Clearly this phenomenon provides a valuable system for investigating the general problem of chemoreception. The flagella

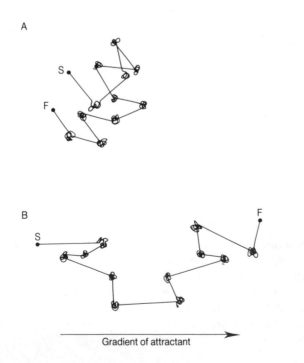

Gradient of attractant

Figure 12.3 Bacterial migration along a concentration gradient of chemical attractant. (A) Bacterial path in the absence of an attractant. The swim alternates between periods when the flagella rotate anticlockwise giving a smooth straight 'run' and short periods when the the flagella rotate clockwise causing 'tumbling'. The direction in which the bracterium is facing when tumbling ceases is completely random hence the next run will be in a random direction. The bacterium makes no progress. S = start; F = finish. (B) Bacterial path in the presence of an attractant. The length of time between tumbles is increased when the bracterium is moving up the gradient and decreased when the it is moving in the opposite direction. Hence although the tumbling episodes still randomise the direction in which the runs occur the bacterium nevertheless swims up towards the source of the attractant. S = start; F = finish

of a bacterium may be attached to a glass slide and the rotation
of the cell observed in response to various chemicals. The genetics
of *E.coli* are, of course, very well known so that the sensory system
may also be examined by genetic techniques.

It has been shown that detection of attractant (or repellant)
molecules is by way of transmembrane proteins. There are two
mechanisms: either an attractant molecule interacts with a
receptor molecule in the bacterium's periplasmic space, causing
a conformational change so that it 'fits' one or other of the
transmembrane receptor proteins; or the attractant interacts with
the transmembrane receptor protein directly. These latter proteins
also have the ability to affect the rotation of the flagella. They are,
in other words, able to transduce the signal represented by the
attractant molecule as well as detect it. In order to distinguish
them from the receptors in the periplasmic space they are known
as **receptor-transducer molecules**.

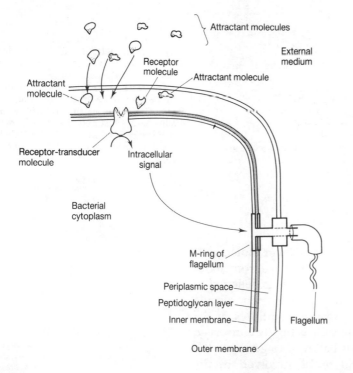

Figure 12.4 Interaction of attractants
with receptor molecules and receptor –
transducer molecules in bacterial
membranes. Chemical attractants (shown
in the external medium) are of two types.
Either they fit the active site of the
receptor – transducer molecule directly or
they are 'adapted' to do so by first fitting
a receptor molecule in the periplasmic
space. The receptor – transducer molecule
is activated so that it generates an
(unknown) intracellular signal which
travels to the flagellar motor. The effect
of this signal is to increase the duration
of the anti-clockwise rotation. For further
explanation see text

This system has one final intriguing feature. It shows **sensory
adaptation**. If *E.coli* is suddenly immersed in an attractant,
tumbling, as expected, is suppressed. But after a time it begins
to be shown again, and after a while, returns to its normal
frequency. This adaptation, moreover, is restricted to the specific
attractant molecule. Addition of a different attractant inhibits the

tumbling in the usual way. The biological significance of adaptation or desensitisation is obvious. But once again it provides a fascinating problem for the molecular biologist.

The genes for a number of the receptor–transducer proteins in *E.coli* have been isolated by the techniques of molecular genetics and their nucleotide sequences determined. The best-known of these genes are the **tar**, **tsr** and **trg** genes. They code respectively for receptor–transducers sensitive to aspartate, serine and to galactose or ribose attached to a receptor.

From the nucleotide sequences the amino acid structure can be determined in the usual way and hydropathic analysis performed to predict membrane-spanning segments. All three of the proteins consist of over 500 amino acids but appear to have only two transmembrane sequences. There is strong homology between the three, especially in the cytoplasmic domain where the processes of sensory adaptation and signalling to the flagellar apparatus occur.

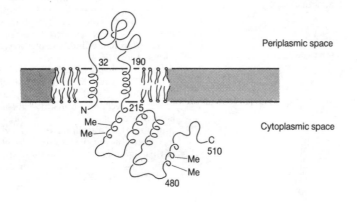

Figure 12.5 Bacterial receptor–transducer molecule. Although all the known receptor–transducer molecules have much the same disposition in the membrane the residue numbers in the figure refer to the *tsr* receptor–transducer molecule. Me = methylation sites: these sites are clustered in two α-helical regions. (After Simon, *et al.*, 1985, *Current Topics in Membranes and Transport*, **23**, 3–15.)

Figure 12.5 suggests that the receptor–transducer molecule is held in the membrane so that an amino acid sequence from about 32 to 190 projects into the periplasmic space. This is believed to form the attractant-binding site. The major part of the molecule from about residue 215 to the carboxy-terminal end lies in the bacterial cytoplasm. This part of the molecule is highly conserved across the three proteins studied and is believed to generate the signal to the flagellar apparatus and to be involved in the adaptation mechanism.

Although the signal to the flagellum remains totally unknown it is believed that adaptation is brought about by methylation of the cytoplasmic domain of the receptor–transducer protein. This occurs when the periplasmic binding site is occupied and, by altering the conformation of the cytoplasmic domain, inhibits the signal to the flagellum. The flagellum can then revert to its old anarchic habits—sometimes rotating clockwise, sometimes anticlockwise.

The great virtue of this system lies in the fact that the genetics of *E.coli* are so well known and easily manipulated. There are good prospects for following up the successful genetic analysis of the receptor–transducer proteins with similar analysis of the molecular mechanisms at work in intracellular signalling and adaptation.

12.1.2 Chemosensitivity in mammals

Let us now turn from chemosensitivity in one of the simplest of living forms to chemoreception in some of the most advanced. In this section we shall look briefly at mammalian olfactory and gustatory reception.

Olfactory reception is carried out by the olfactory epithelium in the nasal cavity. The area which this epithelium covers ranges from a few square centimetres (human) to well over 100 cm^2 (dog). It consists of three types of cell: **supporting (glia-like) cells** which secrete mucus; **neurosensory cells or sensory neurons**; and **basal cells**, which appear to be stem cells capable of dividing and forming new functional neurons throughout life.

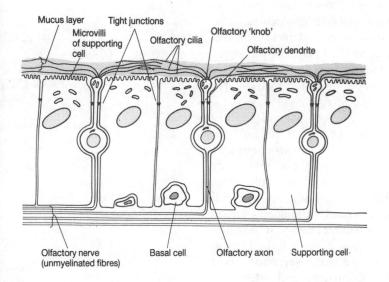

Figure 12.6 Structure of olfactory epithelium. The olfactory cilia are usually very lengthy and lie over the surface of the epithelium embedded in the mucus. Tight junctions between the epithelial cells and between the epithelial cells and the olfactory neurosensory cells prevent any penetration of the intercellular space

Let us concentrate our attention on the **olfactory neurons**. Figure 12.6 shows that they are bipolar cells with a single unbranched dendrite which squeezes up between the supporting cells to end in a small swelling—the olfactory knob. From the knob project up to 20 lengthy cilia. These cilia carry the sensory membrane of the olfactory neuron. Because the olfactory neuron has the dual function of detecting the stimulus and transmitting the nerve impulse into the brain it is in fact a neurosensory cell. Custom and practice, however, ensure that it is normally called a sensory neuron.

The ultrastructure of olfactory cilia is not greatly different from that of other cilia. They contain the usual internal axoneme but are, in mammals at least, non-motile. They are also unusually long and thin, ranging from 30 to 200 μm in length but are often only 0.1–0.2 μm in diameter. This adaptation of a motile organelle, the cilium, to serve a sensory function is also found (as we shall see) in photoreceptors (rod and cone outer segments) and mechanoreceptors (kinocilia of hair cells).

The bunch of thin lengthy cilia springing from an olfactory bulb undoubtedly increases the sensory surface area dramatically. Freeze-fracture electron microscopy shows, furthermore, that the membrane of each cilium contains a high density of globular particles. It is believed that these are the olfactory receptor molecules. This is another point of analogy with the rod and cone cell outer-segments we shall consider in the next section. The membranes of outer-segments are also densely populated with receptor molecules—rhodopsins or iodopsins.

The olfactory system is able to detect and discriminate between a large variety of odorants. It seems probable that one cilium is responsive to a number of different odorant molecules. The sensitivity is also remarkable—humans can detect airborne odorants within the range 10^{-4} M to 10^{-13} M. One of the signs of a bad head cold is a marked falling-away of olfactory sensitivity. This is because the olfactory cilia become engulfed in the extra amount of mucus produced by the supporting cells.

Olfactory receptor molecules have not yet been definitely identified and isolated. It does seem, however, that the globular proteins mentioned above are receptors which can accept one or a small number of similar odorant molecules. The molecular mechanism may not, therefore, be so different (in principle) from that which we discussed in the previous section on bacterial chemosensitivity. It is suggested that the odorant molecule exerts its effect by bringing about a conformational change in a trans-membrane receptor molecule. This in turn may be linked (as in the much better known case of the rod outer-segment) by a 'collison-coupling' mechanism to a G-protein and adenylate cyclase system. There is good evidence for the presence of GTP-binding proteins and adenylate cyclase in olfactory cilia. This hypothetical mechanism is shown in Figure 12.7.

The mechanism shown in Figure 12.7 indicates that on receipt of an odorant molecule the collision-coupling mechanism induces the synthesis of cAMP and/or cGMP. This acts as the second

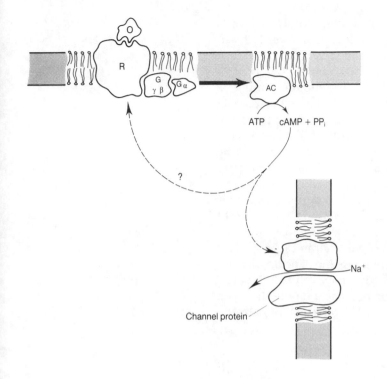

Figure 12.7 Molecular biology of olfactory reception. The figure should be compared with those in Chapter 7. A collision-coupling mechanism results in the synthesis of cAMP. This either acts directly on a channel protein or it acts indirectly by first activating a protein kinase enzyme which subsequently activates the channel protein by phosphorylation. The latter mechanism may also phosphorylate the receptor (R) leading to inactivation and thus to sensory adaptation. Compare the methylation-induced adaptation of bacterial chemosensitivity. O = oderant molecule; R = receptor protein; G = G-protein (α-, β-, and γ-subunits); AC = adenylate cyclase

messenger. This mechanism will be familiar to the reader from earlier chapters of this book. Its great advantage lies in the possibilities for amplification. Many hundreds or thousands of cAMPs may be synthesised in response to the receipt of a single odorant molecule.

Now whereas the effect of the (unknown) second messenger in the bacterial instance was to control the direction of rotation of the flagellum, the second messenger in the olfactory cell can be shown to affect an ion channel. The exceedingly delicate task of patch-clamping an olfactory cilium has been accomplished and conductance channels have been demonstrated which open in response to cAMP. These conductance channels turn out to be tiny. Instead of the pS conductances of the ion channels we met in Chapters 9 and 10 these conductances are to be measured in fS (i.e. 1×10^{-15} S). In this respect they form yet another point of resemblance with the minute conductance channels we shall meet with in rod and cone outer segments. Once again the suspicion is borne in upon us that we are looking at a series of variations of a common underlying theme.

Odorant molecules operating through the second messenger system increase the **number** of these minute channels which are in the open state. The tiny electric current which consequently flows across the ciliary membrane is carried by Na^+ ions.

Whether these Na$^+$ channels are restricted to the cilium's membrane or also operative in the dendrite is not yet known. Analogy with the rod cell and the hair cell stereocilium (see last section of this chapter) suggests that the channels involved in sensory reception are restricted to the cilium, though it must be borne in mind that rod outer segments and hair cell stereocilia are very much bigger than olfactory cilia. Indeed the latter are not true cilia at all but (as we shall shortly see) modified microvilli. It can, however, be calculated that very few channels would be required to produce the observed effect on membrane polarity and this suggests that the channels in olfactory cilia are sufficient.

When the channels open the membrane depolarises. This depolarisation can be observed by microelectrode recording of olfactory neurons. It is observed in response to most odorants and increases with the concentration of the odorant. It is our first example of a receptor/generator potential. As the olfactory neuron is, as we noted above, in fact a neurosensory cell the depolarisation leads directly to the generation of an action potential. The action potential propagates itself along the olfactory fibre to the olfactory bulb in the forebrain.

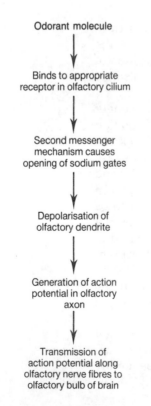

Figure 12.8 Summary of olfactory reception

Finally it should be noted that genetic analysis of the mammalian olfactory system may become possible. Several dozen specific **anosmias** have been detected amongst humans. They are probably due to deficiency in one or another olfactory receptor molecule. Many of these anosmias are inherited in a Mendelian fashion. There is a clear analogy here with human colour blindnesses which are also due to defective receptor proteins—in this case iodopsins. The genetics of human colour blindness are, however, comparatively well known.

Before leaving the topic of chemoreception in mammals it is worth observing that recent investigations of mammalian gustatory cells are beginning to reveal that mechanisms analogous to those operating in olfactory neurons may be at work here also. Gustatory receptor cells are grouped together in the taste buds which are to be found on the tongue and pharynx. Their sensitive ends take the form of microvilli which project into the lumen of the taste bud. Chemicals diffusing in from the buccal cavity stimulate these endings. The mechanism of stimulation is believed to vary from one tastant molecule to another. In a number of cases, however, the receptor molecule in the microvillus membrane is believed to be linked to a collision-coupling second-messenger system. The second messenger may be either inositol triphosphate (see Chapter 16) or cAMP. In the latter case a protein kinase is activated which, with the help of the ATP–ADP system, phosphorylates a K^+ channel protein in the gustatory cell's membrane. The phosphorylation tends to close the K^+ channel and the consequent decrease in K^+ conductivity causes the membrane to depolarise. This depolarisation can be detected by microelectrode techniques. It is a first instance of a receptor potential. For gustatory cells, unlike olfactory neurons, are true receptor cells: depolarisation leads to the release of a transmitter on to the dendrite of a sensory nerve fibre.

12.2 PHOTORECEPTORS

The animal kingdom has developed a great variety of different photoreceptors. The most intensively researched of all these different types are the vertebrate retinal rod and cone cells. We have already met aspects of their molecular physiology several times in this book, especially in Chapter 7, where we discussed the structure and biochemical function of the visual pigments.

It has been calculated that rod cells are able to detect a single photon of light. How do they do it? We shall now try to put together the isolated fragments which we have already discussed to form a picture of the way in which rod and cone cells work.

First let us remind ourselves of the structure of these fascinating cells. Figure 12.9 shows that both rod and cone cells have a very similar design. Both consist of an outer segment, an inner segment, a nuclear region and a synaptic foot, or pedicle.

It is the outer segments of rod and cone cells which contain the visual pigment and are the photosensitive parts of the cell. The figure shows that the outer segments consist of a stack of discs. Electron microscopists have shown that whereas the rod discs are separated from the extracellular space by a continuous boundary membrane, the intradisc space in cones opens into this space.

Figure 12.9 shows that during embryology rod and cone outer segments first appear as cilia springing from their respective cells. This in itself is interesting as we have already seen that the sensitive regions of olfactory cells are also modified cilia. It begins to look as if there is a common design principle at this ultra-structural level. We have already seen evidence of common design at the molecular level. Perhaps evolution has modified an underlying sensory mechanism in several different ways.

A vestige of the ciliary origin of rod and cone outer segments remains in the form of the 'connecting cilium' which joins the outer to the inner segment in the mature cell. This retains the characteristic ring of nine peripheral microtubular doublets of motile cilia but lacks the central pair.

As we noted in Chapter 6, discs are added throughout life to the base of the outer segment and push up to the tip where they are nipped off and digested in the pigment epithelium. The visual pigment—**rhodopsin** in the case of rods—is incorporated into the discs as they are manufactured in the inner segment. Rhodopsin is present in very large amounts—about 70% of outer segment

Figure 12.9   Structure and development of rod and cone cells. (A) Development. Rods and cones originate as ciliated cells lining the ocular ventricle. (i) Each cell bears one cilium. (ii) The cilium grows and its membrane hypertrophies and begins to invaginate. (iii) Hypertrophy of the membrane continues and invagination proceeds at the base of the forming outer segment. The original ultrastructure of internal filaments characteristic of cilia remains in the 'connecting cilium' which runs between the outer and inner segments. (iv) Detail of (iii) to show how the mode of formation of the discs by invagination traps a small fragment of the extracellular compartment as the intradisc space. The space between the discs (the interdisc space) is cytoplasmic. (B) (*facing page*) Structure. (i) Rod; (ii) cone. cc = connecting cilim; e = ellipsoid; f = foot (or pedicle); m = myoid; n = nuclear region; is = inner segment; os = outer segment. (Electron micrographs from Hogan, Alvaredo and Weddel, 1971, *Histology of the Human Eye*, Philadelphia: Saunders; with permission.)

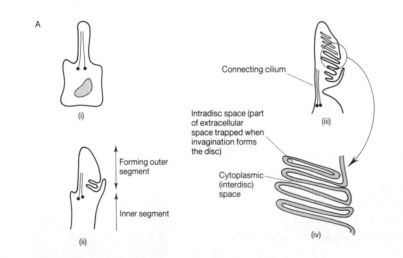

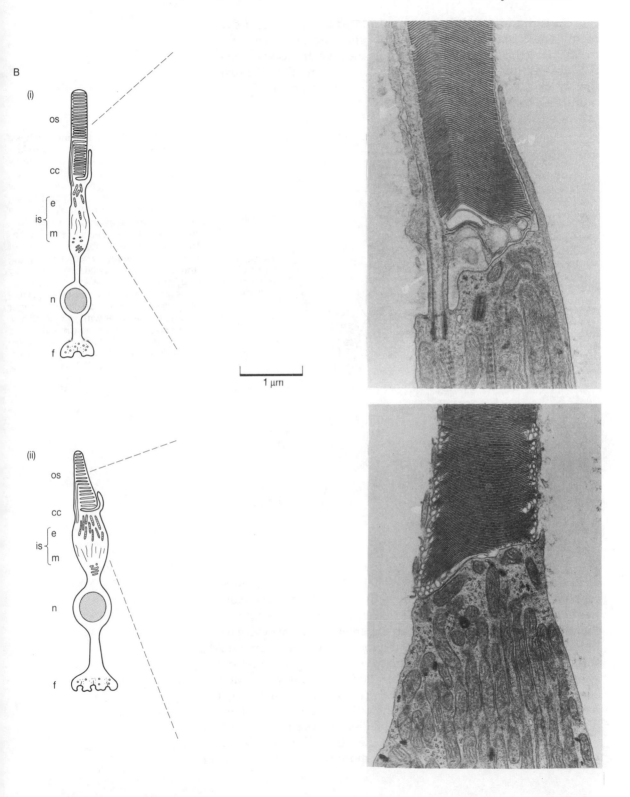

B

(i)

os

cc

is { e

m

n

f

1 µm

(ii)

os

cc

is { e

m

n

f

protein is rhodopsin. It has been calculated that 0.1 μm^2 of disc membrane contains some 2000 rhodopsin molecules. We noted in Chapter 6 that in *Xenopus* disc membrane is synthesised at some 3.2 μm^2 per minute throughout life. This means that approximately 60 000 rhodopsin molecules have to be synthesised every minute—a formidable task.

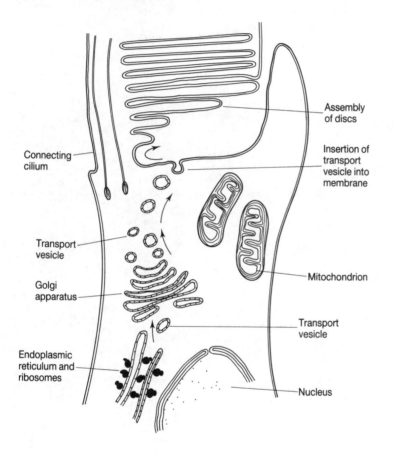

Figure 12.10 Disc membrane synthesis in rod inner-segments. Schematic diagram to show the route of synthesis of visual pigment and rod and cone discs. The pigment is synthesised in the endoplasmic reticulum (ER) and (along with the other phototransduction proteins—see Chapter 7) is inserted into the ER membrane. The latter buds off as transport vesicles to form the *cis* face of the Golgi apparatus. Further packaging and glycosylation occurs in the Golgi body and transport vesicles bud from its *trans* face and move towards the plasma membrane at the top of the inner segment. They fuse with the membrane at this point and create new rod discs. For further details of these processes see Chapter 14, (After Besharse, 1986, in *The Retina: A Model for Cell Biology Studies*, eds. R. Adler and D. Farber, Orlando: Academic Press, pp. 297–352.)

Rhodopsin molecules are packed very close together in outer segment discs. Indeed the distance between rhodopsin molecules has been computed to be no more than about 20 nm. It is obvious that the outer segment provides an extremely effective device for detecting light. Incoming illumination (after having passed through the highly transparent nervous elements of the retina) is presented with a stack of perhaps 20 000 discs in each outer segment. Furthermore those animals (proverbially cats) which have a reflective tapetum behind the outer segments give light a second chance to interact with the piles of rhodopsin molecules.

Let us now focus in on a single disc. This is shown diagrammatically in Figure 12.11. The rhodopsin molecules (see

Chapter 7) are set in the disc membranes so that their carboxy-terminal ends extend into the interdisc (cytoplasmic) space. Although we stated above that the discs are enclosed by a continuous boundary membrane (Figure 12.9) this is not to say that that membrane is totally leak-proof. It is not. It is found to be penetrated by channels which allow the ingress of sodium ions. These channels are analogous to the Na$^+$ channels which have been shown to exist in olfactory cilia. Like those channels they only permit minute current flows—to be measured in fS rather than pS. But unlike those channels they are open when the outer segment is unstimulated, in the dark.

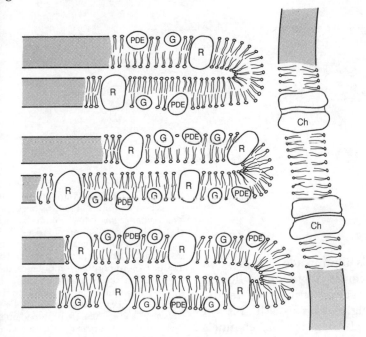

Figure 12.11 Detail of rod discs. Three rod discs are shown abutting the boundary membrane of the outer segment. R = rhodopsin; G = G-protein (or transducin); PDE = phosphodiesterase; Ch = channel protein. Compare with Figure 7.14

The fact that the outer segment boundary membrane is more than usually permeable to sodium ions has important consequences for the resting potential (V_m) of the rod cell. Suppose that P_{Na} is not about 1×10^{-8} cm s^{-1} (as we quoted in Chapter 11) but five times greater, i.e. 5×10^{-7} cm s^{-1}. If we insert this value into the Goldman equation, keeping the permeability coefficients of K$^+$ and Cl$^-$ unchanged, we find that V_m works out at -20 mV.

That the rod cell is depolarised in this way is indeed found when the cell is **unilluminated**. Sodium ions leak into the outer segment and percolate down into the inner segment, where the sodium pump extrudes them. In the dark, therefore, there is a circuit of sodium ions—pumped out of the inner segment only to enter the outer segment.

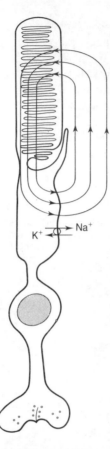

Figure 12.12 Rod cell dark current. Because the outer segment possesses 'leak' channels sodium ions can percolate back into the outer segment. They then flow down to the inner segment where a Na$^+$ + K$^+$ pump extrudes them into the extracellular compartment once again. Hence in the dark a current flows in the direction indicated by the arrows

Figure 12.13 Effect of light on rod cells. (A) When a photon of light is absorbed by an outer segment the sodium channels close. The rod cell hyperpolarises. This may be recorded by a micro-electrode inserted in the inner segment. The amount of hyperpolarisation recorded depends on the intensity of the light flash. This is shown in the graph to the left. (After Penn and Hagins, 1969, *Nature*, **223**, 201–205). (B) (i) A toad outer segment (much larger than mammalian outer segments) is sucked into a glass pipette. As it blocks the end of the pipette all the current which flows into or out of it is supplied from the interior of the pipette and can thus be measured. In the dark this current (as the graph at (iii) shows) is a little over 20 pA. (ii) A pencil beam of light is flashed through the pipette. (iii) The graph shows the effect on the dark current of the flash of light starting at the point marked by the vertical arrow. The reduction in the dark current is dependent on the intensity of the flash stimulus. The bottom line of the graph results from a stimulus 94 times the intensity of flash responsible for the top line. (From Baylor, Lamb and Yau, 1979, *Journal of Physiology*, **288**, 589–611; reproduced by permission of The Physiological Society.) ——▶

All this changes when the cell is illuminated. We saw in Chapter 7 that when rhodopsin receives a photon of light a cascade of biochemical reactions ensues which leads to the transformation of cGMP into the straight-chain 5′-GMP. Now it is found that it is precisely cGMP which keeps the Na$^+$ channels open! Patch-clamp experiments on pieces of rod-cell outer segment membrane have demonstrated that the Na$^+$ channel opening significantly increases in the presence of cGMP. Indeed it can be deduced that three cGMP molecules are required to keep the pore open. The part played by cyclic nucleotides in opening Na$^+$ channels in olfactory cilia should be recalled.

Thus illumination causes the outer segment sodium ion pores to close. The dark current is broken. The boundary membrane of the rod cell begins to hyperpolarise. The same events occur in cone cells when they receive photons of the appropriate wavelength (see Chapter 7). Figure 12.13(A) shows that micro-electrode recording allows this hyperpolarisation to be observed directly. Alternatively, as Figure 12.13(B) shows, rod cell outer segments can be sucked into a micropipette from a piece of detached retina. If a pencil-beam of light is shone though the pipette and the outer segment illuminated the interruption of the dark current can be detected. The greater the intensity of the illuminating beam the more the current is switched off.

A

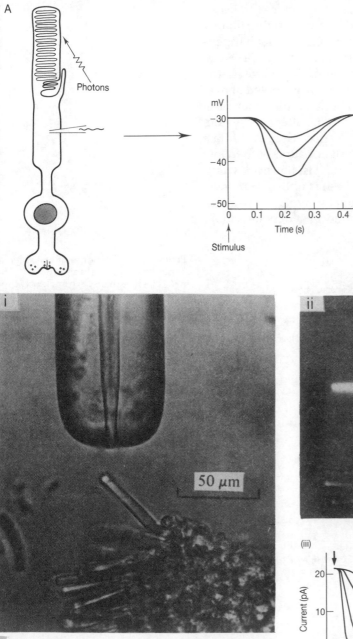

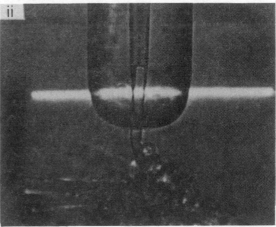

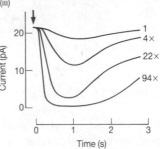

B

We shall see in Chapter 15 that synapses are activated by membrane **depolarisations**. Hyperpolarisations tend to switch synapses off. Hence in the case of rod cells illumination will **reduce** any synaptic activity in their feet. Figure 12.14 shows that in the dark the comparatively depolarised rod cell releases transmitter on to the dendritic ending of the underlying bipolar cell. Illumination inhibits this transmitter release. What happens next depends on the nature of the subsynaptic bipolar cell. There are two cases. In one case, the **hyperpolarising bipolar**, the bipolar cell membrane hyperpolarises. This, as we noted above, tends to inhibit any further action in the cell. In the other case, the **depolarising bipolar**, the reduction of transmitter release from the rod cell causes the bipolar cell to depolarise. This, in contrast to the first case, activates the cell. We shall not attempt to follow the physiology of the retina any further here. It is, however, worth emphasising, in conclusion, that the rod cell is unusual amongst sensory cells in responding to a stimulus by hyperpolarisation. The great majority of sensory cells respond by a depolarisation.

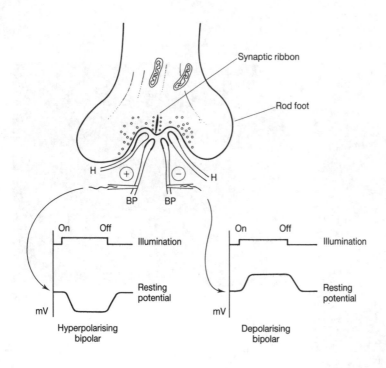

Figure 12.14 Response of rod – bipolar synapses to illumination. The rod – bipolar synapse is complex. The rod foot makes synaptic 'contact' with horizontal cells (H) and bipolar cells (BP). The bipolars are either hyperpolarising, + (sign conserving), or depolarising, – (sign inverting). As the same transmitter is (presumably) employed the difference must be due to different response characteristics of the subsynaptic membranes of the two bipolars. The lower part of the figure shows the responses of the bipolar cells when the rod cell is illuminated. The response is greater the more intense the illumination

12.3 MECHANORECEPTORS

Once again zoologists have discovered an enormous variety of different mechanoreceptors in the animal kingdom. Once again we shall concentrate our attention on one well-researched example—the **hair cell**.

Mechanoreceptive hair cells are found throughout the animal kingdom. They are particularly ubiquitous amongst the vertebrates. They are, for instance, to be found in the lateral line canals of fish and amphibian tadpoles, where they have a function in echolocation, but more importantly, from the human point of view, they are involved in balance and in the detection of sound by the inner ear.

The vertebrate inner ear, like the vertebrate eye, is a very highly evolved organ. Essentially it consists of a complicated membranous structure—the **membranous labyrinth**—held by connective tissues threads within a fluid-filled cavity in the skull's tympanic bone. It consists of three major functional compartments: three **semi-circular canals** which detect the movement of the head; the **utriculus** and **sacculus** which detect the position of the head with respect to gravity and are sensitive to linear acceleration; and lastly (but only in the mammals) a **cochlea**, coiled like a snail's shell, which detects sound. Not only is the membranous labyrinth suspended in an aqueous fluid, the **perilymph**, but it also contains another aqueous fluid, the **endolymph**. These two fluids differ radically in their ionic constitution. Whereas perilymph resembles other extracellular fluids in having a high Na^+ concentration (140 meq l^{-1}) and a low K^+ concentration (5 meq l^{-1}) the endolymph is much more like an intracellular fluid in being rich in K^+ (150 meq l^{-1}) and poor in Na^+ (1–2.5 meq l^{-1}).

At the heart of this intricate structure are to be found groups of hair cells. The tops of these cells and their sensory hairs project into the endolymph whilst the remainder of their boundary membranes are bathed in intercellular fluid which, in turn, is in equilibrium with the perilymph. Because they are interposed in this way between lymphs of such different ionic constitution a very large potential (about 150 mV) is developed across their membranes. Textbooks of physiology explain how these cells are arranged so that movement, gravity or atmospheric pressure variations (the physical basis of sound), will distort, one way or another, their 'hairs'. Figure 12.15 shows the structure of a typical labyrinthine hair cell.

If a scanning electron micrograph of the surface of a single hair cell (Figure 12.16) is examined it can be seen that the hairs tend to stack together into a 'wigwam' structure (preparative artefact cannot be excluded). Each hair cell has up to 50 or 60 'hairs' springing from its surface. Often, as the sectional view of Figure 12.15 shows, they increase in length from one end of the cell to the other. The majority of these 'hairs' are in fact modified (and greatly enlarged) microvilli. They are called **stereocilia**. In addition

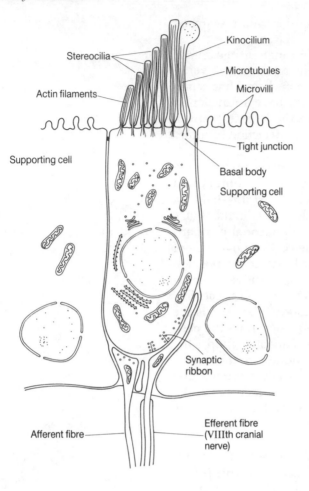

Figure 12.15 Labyrinthine hair cell to show stereocilia and kinocilium. In addition to the primary afferent fibre (a member of the VIIIth cranial nerve) hair cells of the cristae and maculae are also innervated by efferent fibres which give the CNS some control over the sensitivity of the system. Both stereocilia and kinocilia are nipped in at their bases: they are thus both stiff and able to bend at their junction with the cell body. At the base of the cell are numerous synaptic vesicles, many of which are associated (as in rod and cone feet) with synaptic ribbons. (Partly after Hudspeth, 1983, *Scientific American*, **248**, 45–52.)

to the stereocilia a single true cilium, the **kinocilium**, a little taller than the majority of stereocilia and with a bulbous tip, is found at the 'tall' end of the group.

If we increase the magnification yet further and examine a single stereocilium we note first of all that it *is* much larger than a standard microvillus. Instead of being a micrometre or so in length (as is a microvillus) it may be up to 5 μm and sometimes more in extent. Its diameter is also decidedly greater and if the interior is examined it is found to contain a complicated meshwork of actin filaments. Whether this actin network is directly involved in signal detection is not yet known.

It is, however, known that movement of the stereocilium activates the hair cell. Delicate experiments using a glass microprobe to bend the stereocilium this way and that have demonstrated that mechanical distortion leads to changes in the electrical potential across the hair cell's plasma membrane. These

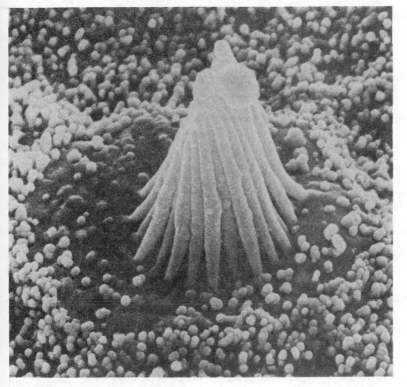

Figure 12.16 Scanning electronmicrograph of hair cells in the labyrinth of toad. The bulbous-ended kinocilium can be clearly seen at the top of the 'wigwam' of stereocilia. (Courtesy of Dr R.A. Jacobs.)

experiments, moreover, show that movement of the stereocilium in one direction produces a different result from movement in the other. Indeed if the stereocilium is moved towards the tall edge of the bundle, towards the kinocilium, a marked **depolarisation** (up to 20 mV) occurs whilst movement of the stereocilium in the opposite direction elicits a **hyperpolarisation** of some 5 mV. Movement at right angles to this axis induces no change in membrane polarity at all.

The transduction process is extremely rapid. Many mammals, members of the Cetacea and the Chiroptera, for example, respond to sound frequencies up to at least 100 khz. There seems to be no time for the elaborate biochemistry of 'collision-coupling' and second messengers which we saw to be at work in chemo- and photoreception. Gated channels in the hair cell membrane must open and shut very rapidly indeed. The electrical response must be due to near-instantaneous flows of ions down their concentration gradients. Where are these gates located?

Again careful experiments have gone far to answer this question. It can be shown that the maximum ionic flows in response to movement occur at the tips of the stereocilia. The response, moreover, is found to be extremely rapid: beginning

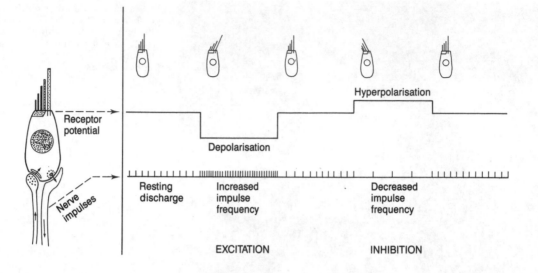

within a few microseconds of stimulus onset and saturating within about 100 μs. The current flows are mostly carried by K$^+$ ions which as we have noted are present in such high concentration in the endolymph. The fact that experiment shows that other cations including some small organic cations, e.g. choline, can pass shows that the channel is fairly wide—perhaps 0.7 nm in diameter. In this respect it differs from the minute channels of olfactory cilia and rod cells.

An interesting model for the action of the stereocilia has been put forward by Hudspeth. Electron microscopic evidence suggests that the stereocilia are connected at their tips by a molecular thread to the next tallest neighbour (Figure 12.18). Random movement will normally open and close the gates at their tips, thus leading

Figure 12.17 The movement of the bundle of stereocilia in one direction causes a depolarisation of the hair cell whilst movement in the opposite direction causes a hyperpolarisation. This is translated into increased and decreased impulse frequency in the sensory fibre. (From Flock, 1965, *Cold Spring Harbor Symposia on Quantitative Biology*, **XXX**, 133–145; with permission.)

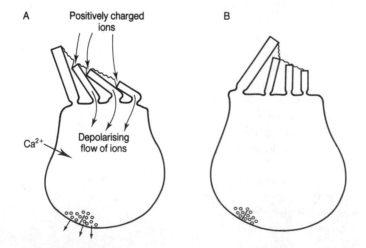

Figure 12.18 Mechanoelectrical transduction by labyrinthine hair cells. (A) The stereocilia are all pushed towards the left and this causes ion channels to open in their tips—perhaps by some mechanical pull. The inward flow of positively charged ions causes a depolarisation which opens Ca^{2+} channels thus leading to release of transmitter on to the dendritic ending of the sensory neuron. (B) When the stereocilia are bent in the other direction the ion channels at their tips are closed. The Ca^{2+} which has flowed in during the depolarising stage is sequestrated or pumped out of the cell, the membrane repolarises, and the release of transmitter ceases. (After Hudspeth, 1985, *Science*, **230**, 745–752.)

to small flows through the channels—this would account for the random background 'noise' which can be detected—as is customary for membrane channels. When a mechanical stimulus bends the group of stereocilia in one direction, however, the gates are pulled open in unison and an inward flow of positively charged ions causes the depolarisation observed. Movement of the stereocilia in the opposite direction tends to close all the gates and hence causes a small hyperpolarisation.

Depolarisation of the hair cell's membrane will open the voltage-dependent Ca^{2+} gates and Ca^{2+} will enter the cell. This, as we shall see more fully in Chapter 14, will lead to the release of transmitter molecules on to the underlying dendrite of an auditory nerve fibre (Figure 12.15).

It should be borne in mind that although this model of the hair cell's mechanism accounts for the **microphonic potentials** which can be detected in the cochlea it does not, on its own, provide an explanation of the ear's ability to discriminate between different frequencies of sound. The hair cell, as we have seen, may be able to respond in a matter of microseconds; synapses and nerve fibres are much more sluggish, generally having response times measured in milliseconds. Nerve fibres, further-more, are restricted by their refractory periods (see next chapter) to conduction rates of less than a thousand impulses per second. Hence it is impossible for single auditory fibres to keep up with the response of a hair cell detecting sound of, say, 15 kHz (human) still less 100 kHz (bat). The explanation of the cochlea's remarkable frequency discrimination ability lies in the differential resonance of different regions of the basilar membrane. This explanation, originally proposed by Helmholtz in the mid-nineteenth century, is set out in textbooks of physiology.

12.4 CONCLUSION

In this chapter we have looked at just a few examples of the innumerable sensory cells found in the living world. We have progressed from a bacterial system which connected sensory detection to action in a very direct way, through neurosensory cells which transduced sensory stimuli into action potentials in the same cell, to sensory cells which detect a stimulus and via complicated biochemistry and biophysics produce receptor potentials to, finally, receptor cells which respond directly to a stimulus by the opening and closing of ion gates. The last two types of sensory cell are incorporated into highly evolved sense organs. The detection of the stimulus in these cases is only the merest beginning of the sensory process.

Chapter 13
The action potential

The **action potential** (= **nerve impulse or 'spike'**) lies at the heart of neurophysiology. It is the element with which the brain scientist builds his theory of brain activity—whether it be the EEG of the association areas, the visual system's 'primal sketch' or the cortical computation which precedes a conscious act. It is the action potential which Sherrington had in mind when he wrote his famous passage describing the brain stirring from slumber:

> Swiftly the head-mass becomes an enchanted loom where millions of flashing shuttles weave a dissolving pattern, always a meaningful pattern though never an abiding one; a shifting harmony of sub-patterns. Now as the waking body rouses, sub-patterns of this great harmony of activity stretch down into the unlit tracts of the stalk piece of the scheme. Strings of flashing and travelling sparks engage the lengths of it. This means that the body is up and rises to meet its waking day. [p.187]

But for the molecular neurobiologist the action potential is itself a point of synthesis—a synthesis of numerous underlying elements: different voltage-gated channels, differential ion flows, the biophysics of cable conduction and electrotonic potentials.

13.1 VOLTAGE-CLAMP ANALYSES

The modern phase of our understanding of the action potential began with the experiments of Hodgkin and Huxley in the early 1950s. Working with the squid giant axon preparation they were able to determine the exact shape of the action potential and the nature of the ion flows responsible for that shape. Figure 13.1 shows a classical recording from this preparation.

Figure 13.1 shows that when a microelectrode is placed within a squid axon a **resting potential** of about -60 mV can be recorded. When an impulse or **action potential** passes over this patch of

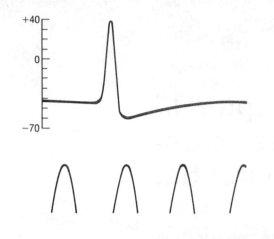

Figure 13.1 Action potential recorded from a squid giant axon. The vertical scale indicates the potential of the internal electrode (mV), the sea-water outside being taken to be at 0 or ground potential. Time marker 500 Hz. This is one of the first pictures of a complete action potential to be published. (Reprinted by permission from Hodgkin and Huxley, 1939, *Nature*, **144**, 710–711; Copyright © 1939, Macmillan Magazines Ltd.)

membrane the potential is reversed so that the internal electrode becomes about $+35$ mV compared to the external. This reversal of polarity is very quickly over. The peak of the action potential is reached about 0.5 ms after onset and the membrane has returned to its resting potential value in about 1.5 ms. The figure shows that the recovery process in fact overshoots the resting potential value. The **afterhyperpolarisation (AHP)** persists for one or two milliseconds before the normal resting potential (V_m) is re-established.

In order to study this extremely rapid voltage change Hodgkin and Huxley developed a device to clamp the voltage across the membrane at any desired value and hold it that value. Figure 13.2 shows a schematic diagram of a **voltage-clamp** circuit.

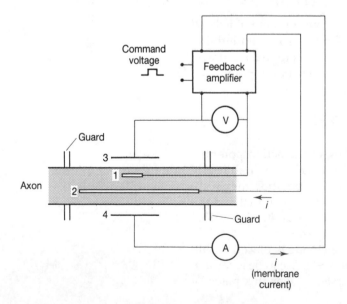

Figure 13.2   Voltage-clamp circuit. In this schematic figure two electrodes are inserted into the axon and two are placed outside. Electrodes 1 and 3 measure the voltage across the membrane. When a command voltage is applied to the feedback amplifier, current is injected (or removed) from the axon by electrode 2. The current flow across the membrane required to maintain it at any specified voltage can then be measured by electrode 4. (After Katz, 1966, *Nerve, Muscle and Synapse*, New York: McGraw Hill.)

In essence a voltage-clamp circuit consists of four electrodes: two inside (1 and 2 in Figure 13.2) and two outside (3 and 4 in Figure 13.2). Electrodes 1 and 3 measure the electrical potential across the axonal membrane. Electrode 2 is used to inject electrons (i.e. current) into or remove them from the axon. If it is required to **depolarise** the membrane then electrons can be removed from the inside of the axon. This removal of negative charge from inside the axonal membrane is monitored by electrodes 1 and 3. The electronic circuitry ensures that just enough current is withdrawn to hold the membrane at the required polarity. This current is obviously identical to the current which ions are carrying across the membrane at that particular depolarisation. Vice versa if it is required to study transmembrane currents when the membrane is hyperpolarised the current flow in electrode 2 may be reversed. Electrons injected into the axon will **hyperpolarise** the membrane.

As Hodgkin and Huxley remarked, the voltage-clamp technique enables one to slow down the millisecond events of the action potential and study them at leisure. It is comparable to taking a movie of a fast-moving event and then studying the action frame by frame under a magnifying glass or, better, using the freeze-frame control on a videorecorder.

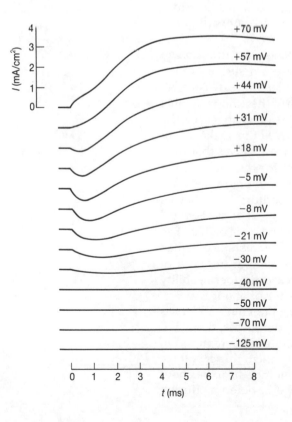

Figure 13.3 Voltage-clamp measurements of currents across a squid giant axon. Currents (mA/cm^2) across the membrane of a squid giant axon clamped at various potentials. Downward deflection indicates inward current. For further explanation see text. (After Hodgkin, Huxley and Katz, 1952, *Journal of Physiology*, **116**, 424–448.)

Figure 13.3 shows the effect of clamping the transmembrane potential at a number of different values. The resting potential is −60 mV and the voltage is stepped upward at discrete intervals. Inward current is represented by a downward deflection of the curve. The figure shows that no transmembrane current can be detected until the membrane is set at −30 mV (a depolarisation of 30 mV). An inward current then begins to show itself, followed by a sustained outward current. The initial inward current becomes more definite as the membrane is stepped to −21 mV, −8 mV, −5 mV, +18 mV but then begins to diminish until it disappears altogether at +57 mV. The outward current, however, grows more and more marked.

The next question, of course, is: exactly which ions are carrying these observed electric currents? This question is also easily tackled with the voltage-clamp technique. There are two complementary approaches. One can remove the suspected ionic carrier and see if that has the expected result on the transmembrane current, or one can block the membrane channels used by the suspected ions and, once again, observe the effect on the current across the voltage-clamped membrane. Both these approaches are shown in Figure 13.4. If the external Na^+ ions are replaced with the impermeant cation, **choline**, the initial inward current is eliminated. If the potassium channels are blocked by **tetraethylammonium chloride (TEA)** then the sustained outward-going current disappears.

The voltage-clamp experiments of the 1950s were thus able to dissect the action potential into two phases: a sudden initial ingress of Na^+ ions followed by a longer lasting egress of K^+ ions. It is clear that the electrical phenomena of the action potential (Figure 13.1) are ultimately based on abrupt changes in the permeability of the membrane to these ions. Let us make use of the Goldman equation (Chapter 11) to assure ourselves that such permeability changes could indeed account for the shape of the impulse. Let us suppose, first, that the membrane becomes suddenly very much more permeable to sodium ions. Let us suppose, in other words, that instead of $P_{Na} \sim 1 \times 10^{-8}$ cm s^{-1} it becomes 1×10^{-6} cm s^{-1}—an increase by a factor of 100. The Goldman equation would then predict a transmembrane potential of about +43 mV—very much what is observed at the peak of the action potential. Similarly if we increase the permeability constant of the potassium ion, P_K, by a factor of about 5 to 5×10^{-7} cm s^{-1} then a transmembrane potential of about −77 mV is predicted—as observed during the afterhyperpolarisation.

It is also possible to work out the number of ions required to flow through unit area of membrane to elicit these voltage changes. If we take the capacitance of the membrane to be about 2 μF cm^{-2} (see Appendix 2) and the change in potential during

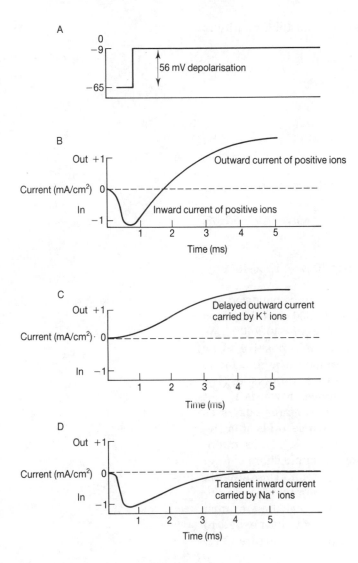

A

0
−9

56 mV depolarisation

−65

B

Out +1

Outward current of positive ions

Current (mA/cm²) 0

In   −1

Inward current of positive ions

1   2   3   4   5

Time (ms)

C

Out +1

Delayed outward current
carried by K⁺ ions

Current (mA/cm²)· 0

In −1

1   2   3   4   5

Time (ms)

D

Out +1

Current (mA/cm²) 0

In −1

Transient inward current
carried by Na⁺ ions

1   2   3   4   5

Time (ms)

Figure 13.4 Na^+ and K^+ are the current carriers in the action potential. (A) The membrane is clamped 56 mV positive to its resting potential. (B) The current flows across the membrane are measured over 5 ms. (C) Na^+ ions are replaced by choline in the external solution. The initial inward current is eliminated. It follows that this transient initial current was carried by Na^+ ions. (D) TEA is added to the extracellular fluid. This is known to block K^+ channels. The sustained outward current is eliminated. It follows that this current was carried by K^+ ions. (Partly after Hodgkin and Huxley, 1952, *Journal of Phsyiology*, **117**, 500–544.)

the rising phase of the action potential to be about 100 mV (i.e from −60 mV to +40 mV) then remembering from elementary physics that

$$Q = VC$$

where Q = quantity of electricity in coulombs (C), V = potential difference across the membrane in volts (V) and C = capacity of membrane in farads (F), we have:

$$Q = 100 \text{ mV} \times 2 \text{ } \mu F \text{ cm}^{-2}$$

$$= (1 \times 10^{-1}) \text{ V} \times (2 \times 10^{-6}) \text{ F cm}^{-2}$$

$$= 2 \times 10^{-7} \text{ C cm}^{-2}$$

Next we note that 1 cm^2 = 1 × 10^8 μm^2, so that the quantity of electricity carried across 1 μm^2 is

$$Q = (2 \times 10^{-7}) \times (1 \times 10^{-8})$$

$$= 2 \times 10^{-15} \text{ C}$$

Then we recall that 96 500 (i.e. approx. 1 × 10^5) C are carried by 1 g ion and it therefore follows that:

2 × 10^{-15} C are carried by 2 × 10^{-15}/1 × 10^5 = 2 × 10^{-20} g ions

Furthermore as 1 g ion consists of 6 × 10^{23} ions (Avogadro's number)

2 × 10^{-15} C are carried by (2 × 10^{-20}) × (6 × 10^{23}) = 12 × 10^3 ions

This calculation emphasises how very delicately balanced the membrane is. It requires only the influx of 12 000 or so Na$^+$ ions to reverse its polarity. Reference back to Chapter 10 will show that when the membrane is clamped at 10 mV positive to its resting potential about 10 000 Na$^+$ ions course through a single channel each **millisecond**. This flow, of course, diminishes ($I = gV$) as the voltage across the membrane moves towards V_{Na}. It is also important to bear in mind that the neurilemma possesses several different types of channel. A few **microseconds** after the opening of the sodium gates the 'delayed' K$^+$ gates open. Rather little Na$^+$ will have flowed through a single channel (e.g. 100 ions in 10 μs) before these I_K channels open. The outward flow of K$^+$ ions tends to repolarise the membrane. Hence the very few Na$^+$ ion gates implied by the above calculation must be multiplied manyfold to achieve the conductivity needed to drive the membrane to its action potential peak (see Figure 13.7).

13.2 PATCH-CLAMP ANALYSES

We looked at the techniques of patch-clamping in Section 9.1.2. We saw that by this means single channels could be studied. We saw, furthermore, in Chapters 9 and 10 that patch-clamping had been extensively used to investigate ion channels. In particular we noted the characteristics of single Na$^+$ and K$^+$ channels. It is the functioning of multiplicities of these voltage-gated channels which underlies the ion flows detected by the Hodgkin–Huxley voltage-clamp analyses.

It will be recalled from Chapter 10 that the sodium channels open in response to a depolarising voltage, stay open for about

0.7 ms, **and then close again**. It will also be recalled that the number of Na$^+$ channels varies widely in different neurons—from ten or so per square micrometre in rat sarcolemma, to 100 μm^{-2} or so in rabbit unmyelinated vagus fibres, up to about 300 μm^{-2} in squid giant axon and several thousand per square micrometre in nodes of Ranvier.

Individual channels in any given membrane population will have slightly different trigger voltages—but, as already noted, once having opened they shut after about 0.7 ms and do not open again. It is easy to see that the effect of this sudden leakiness to sodium ions will be precisely the Na$^+$ current which Hodgkin and Huxley observed in their voltage-clamp experiments.

Once a depolarising stimulus reaches the threshold value, Na$^+$ channels open and sodium ions begin to flood in, thus depolarising the membrane yet further. This has the effect of opening yet more sodium gates and yet more sodium ions cascade in, and so on. This positive feedback loop ensures that the rising phase of the action potential shoots up to its peak in half a millisecond or so.

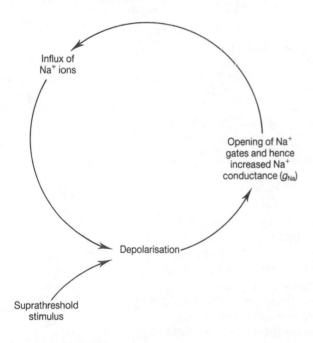

Figure 13.5 Positive feedback loop responsible for the initial phase of the action potential

The patch-clamp technique allows one to examine the channel events underlying an action potential. If a small patch of membrane containing only two or three channels is repeatedly depolarised to threshold at regular intervals the sodium channels can be exercised again and again. Figure 13.6(B) shows three such exercises of the channels in response to 60 mV depolarisations from a 'holding potential' of −110 mV. If the experiment is repeated 144 times and the results summed it is equivalent to depolarising a patch of membrane containing several hundred channels once. The result, shown in the lower part of Figure 13.6, shows a marked similarity in profile to the sodium current curve of Figure 13.4.

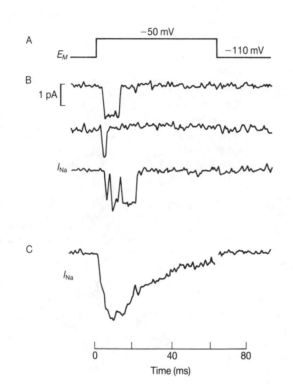

Figure 13.6 Single and summed responses of sodium channels in a patch of myotube membrane to a 60 mV depolarisation from a holding potential of −110 mV. (A) The membrane potential is stepped from a holding potential of −110 mV to −50 mV. (B) Three records showing the opening of sodium gates in the membrane and the inward flux of current carried by Na^+ ions. (C) The sum of 144 trials. (From Hille, 1984, *Ionic Channels of Excitable Membranes*, Sunderland, Mass.: Sinauer; after Patlak and Horn, 1982, *Journal of General Physiology*, **79**, 333−351; with permission.)

We noted in Chapter 10 that each sodium channel allows about 1.6 pA of current to flow. Reference to Figure 13.4, however, shows that the sodium current measured by voltage-clamping entire axons is to be measured not in picoamps but in milliamps. In order to achieve currents in the milliamp range approximately 10^9 channels must be opening. However, it can be easily seen that this is not an unreasonable number. For if we suppose that there are 100 channels per square micrometre then there are 100 $\times$ 10^8 channels per square centimetre—which is an order of magnitude more than the number required. We can also work the calculation the other way and get a feel for the density of sodium channels in the membrane. If we suppose that the diameter of the channel protein is about 10 nm (see Chapter 10) then a square micrometre of membrane (= 1×10^6 nm^2) could contain 10 000 such channels if they were packed tightly edge to edge. But it is found that a square micrometre of membrane only contains about 100 such channels. The packing density is thus only about 1%. In reality, as we have already noted, neurotoxin labelling shows that the packing density is rather higher: several hundred per square micrometre of membrane in squid giant axon. This implies that not all the channels in a patch of membrane open at once.

Let us now turn our attention to the potassium channels. In Chapter 10 we noted that excitable membranes possess a number of different K^+ channels. The channels which are responsible for the sustained outward flux of K^+ ions shown in the voltage-clamp experiments are the so-called **delayed K^+ channels (I_K)**.

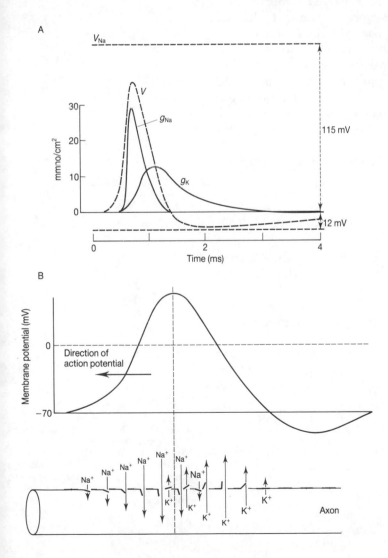

Figure 13.7 Major ion channels and conductances responsible for the action potential. (A) Changes in the sodium and potassium conductances (g_{Na} and g_K) predicted by the Hodgkin/Huxley theory. The left-hand ordinate shows the conductance of the membrane for Na^+ and K^+ ions (mmho/cm^2); the right-hand ordinate shows the voltage across the membrane. The broken line shows the total voltage change across the membrane as the action potential develops. The Nernst sodium (V_{Na}) and potassium (V_K) potentials are shown by horizontal broken lines at top and bottom of the figure. (From Hodgkin and Huxley, 1952, *Journal of Physiology*, **117**, 500–544; reproduced by permission of The Physiological Society.) (B) The upper part of the figure shows the change in voltage across the membrane of an axon (compare with broken line in (A) above). The lower part of the figure shows the flows of sodium and potassium ions which are the major cause of this voltage change. These flows, in turn, are due to the opening and closing of Na^+ and K^+ channels in the axonal membrane

These open rather sluggishly to depolarisation of the membrane—by sluggish is meant about 2 μs! They remain open, moreover, as long as the membrane is depolarised. The greatly increased K$^+$ conductance they confer ensures that the membrane is brought back to the resting potential and beyond, to the AHP. We shall see, later, that this AHP is not a mere detail but has an important neurophysiological consequence.

In addition to the delayed K$^+$ channel practically all neurons (except squid giant axons) possess **fast K$^+$ channels (I_{KA})**. We noted in Figure 13.3 that small depolarisations of the membrane did not initiate an action potential. Only when the depolarisation had reached a threshold 10–20 mV below the resting potential did the sodium gates open and an action potential occur. The neuronal membrane is thus, in a sense, elastic. It 'bounces' back from small, subthreshold, depolarisations. This may be helped by the presence of the fast K$^+$ channels. Although the channels are present in very small numbers their presence allows K$^+$ ions to flow out rapidly in response to small depolarisations and thus quickly repolarise the membrane. Not all workers, it should however be said, accept this mechanism. It has been pointed out that most of the fast K$^+$ channels require the membrane to be hyperpolarised before they open. The significance of this observation will become apparent in the next section of this chapter where we consider the role of the AHP in impulse propagation.

13.3 PROPAGATION OF THE ACTION POTENTIAL

So far we have been considering the ionic movements occurring in a single small patch of axonal membrane. The whole essence of the action potential, however, is that it is a signalling device for tying together the far-flung operations of the brain, for sending messages to the muscles and/or for carrying information from the sense organs to the CNS.

If a depolarising stimulus is delivered at a point midway along an axon it will be found that an action potential starts off in both directions from that point (Figure 13.8). The normal physiological

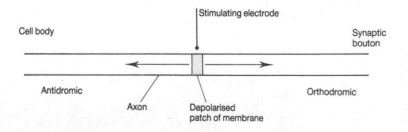

Figure 13.8 Orthodromic and antidromic propagation of an action potential. A membrane is given a depolarising stimulus by a stimulating electrode. The action potential propagates in both directions from the point of stimulation

direction (from the perikaryon to the synaptic bouton) is called the **orthodromic** direction, while the opposite non-physiological direction is termed the **antidromic** direction.

The fact that both antidromic and orthodromic propagation occurs from a stimulus midway down an axon is easily explained in terms of the cable conduction theory we looked at in Chapter 11. It will be recalled that local circuits spread through the axoplasm from a point of depolarisation. In the cases we considered in Chapter 11 these circuits caused small depolarisations (electrotonic depolarisations) at small distances from the point at which the depolarising voltage had been applied. But in an excitable membrane, such as an axon, the small depolarisations are likely to bring the membrane to the threshold required to activate the sodium gates. The positive feedback mechanism described in the preceding section then takes over. An action potential develops on that section of membrane rather than an electrotonic potential.

Once an action potential potential develops on that segment of membrane local circuits will *a fortiori* spread out and depolarise new segments—thus the action potential runs in both directions away from the point of stimulation.

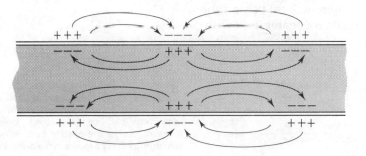

Figure 13.9 Local circuits underlying the propagation of an action potential. Enlargement of Fig. 13.8 to show the local circuits set up by a patch of depolarised membrane

The reader will no doubt have noted a difficulty in the scenario depicted in Figure 13.9. If local circuits spread out in each direction from the region where an action potential has developed how is it that the action potential does not perpetually 'spark back'? Indeed it looks as if the proposed mechanism is altogether a non-starter.

The answer to the conundrum is simple. It has to do with the AHP tacked on to the end of an action potential and with the fact that the sodium channels after having opened during the action potential snap shut and remain shut until the resting potential is re-established. Let us do a little more arithmetic. Figure 13.1 shows that the AHP lasts for at least a millisecond, usually more. Let us suppose that the action potential travels at 20 m s^{-1}—an average value for frog motor nerve fibres. What is the length of fibre left behind the action potential in the AHP state?

$$V = 20 \text{ m s}^{-1}$$

$$= 20 \times (1 \times 10^{6}) \text{ } \mu\text{m s}^{-1}$$

If the AHP state lasts for 1 ms (as we supposed) then the length (l) of axonal membrane left behind the speeding action potential in this state is

$$l = [(2 \times 10^{7}) \text{ } \mu\text{m s}^{-1}] \times (1 \times 10^{-3} \text{ s})$$

$$= 2 \times 10^{4} \text{ } \mu\text{m or 2 cm}$$

This stretch of fibre is populated by tightly closed sodium gates. **The depolarising influence of local circuits cannot open them.** Moreover the fast potassium channels which are especially sensitive when the membrane is hyperpolarised ensure that any incipient depolarisation is quickly reversed by an outflow of K^{+} ions. Thus the local circuits spreading out from the membrane patch carrying the action potential can only affect *fresh* membrane. They will be too attenuated to affect membrane 2 cm behind the action potential. Hence the action potential propagates itself without decrement in one direction only.

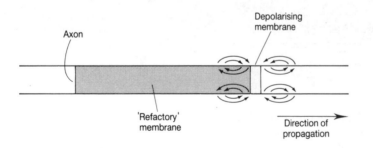

Axon

Depolarising membrane

'Refactory' membrane

Direction of propagation

Figure 13.10   Unidirectional propagation of an action potential. Local circuits spread out from the region of depolarised membrane but can only affect 'fresh' membrane. The membrane over which the impulse has passed is refractory. For further explanation see text

A much-favoured analogy for the propagation of an action potential is that of a train of gunpowder or a line of dominoes. In both cases transmission uses the stored energy of the system. A spark running down the gunpowder trail leaves only ash behind, each domino falls flat in transmitting the impulse to the next in line and has to be stood up on edge again for a further transmission. And so it is with the nerve impulse. It depends on the energy locked in the ion gradients across the membrane. However, unlike the gunpowder trail or the line of dominoes nerve impulses can be repeated many times before all the stored energy is used up. The properties of the ion channel proteins ensure that the transmembrane ionic gradients are not eliminated by one or a few action potentials. But ultimately the ion gradients must be re-established by means of the $Na^+ + K^+$ ion pumps in the membrane. These pumps are at work throughout the neuron's life. Their efforts are swamped when an action potential travels down the axon. They remain hard at work, however, during the quiescent periods between episodes of impulse transmission.

13.4 INITIATION OF THE IMPULSE

Action potentials never normally start up halfway along an axon as was suggested in Figure 13.8. When the neurophysiologist is not playing his tricks action potentials either start at the **initial segment** of the axon (motor or internuncial neurons) or at a **dendritic zone** (sensory neurons). In both cases the initiation is due to local circuits depolarising excitable sections of membrane below their thresholds. The sodium gates begin to open and the action potential takes off.

It is likely that at both regions shown in Figure 13.11 some form of **adaptation** occurs. Adaptation is best known at sensory endings and, indeed, we have already encountered it when discussing sensory cells in Chapter 12. The majority of sensory fibres respond to a stimulus by a rapid burst of impulses, after

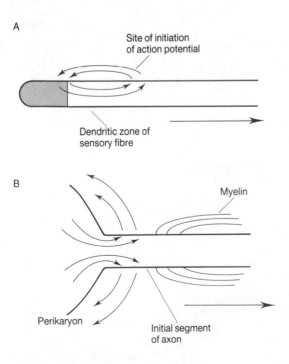

A

Site of initiation
of action potential

Dendritic zone of
sensory fibre

B

Myelin

Perikaryon

Initial segment
of axon

Figure 13.11 Local circuits initiate action potentials at initial segments or dendritic zones. (A) Dendritic ending of a sensory fibre. The ending is depolarised, either directly by environmental energy or by transmitter from an adjacent sensory cell. This depolarisation is termed a generator potential. Local circuits spread from this depolarised region to initiate an action potential in the sensory fibre. (B) Initial segment of an axon. Local circuits spreading from an EPSP (see Chapter 16) on the perikaryon or dendritic tree of a neuron open the sodium gates in the membrane of the axon's initial segment and initiate an action potential

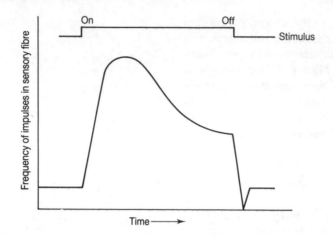

Figure 13.12 Adaptation in a sensory nerve fibre. After an initial burst of impulses in the sensory fibre the frequency falls off to a much lower value—in some cases almost to the pre-stimulus value. This is sensory adaptation

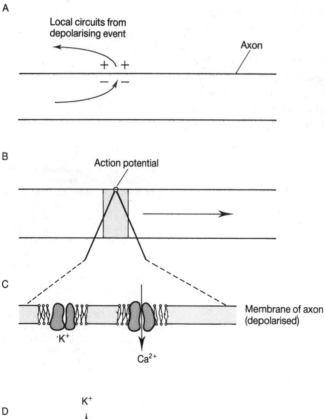

Figure 13.13 An ionic mechanism for sensory adaptation. (A) Local circuits from some depolarising event (either synaptic or sensory) depolarise axon below threshold.(B) An action potential is initiated and propagates away down the axon. (C) Enlargement of the membrane at which the action potential is intiated. Ca^{2+} gates open in response to depolarisation and Ca^{2+} ions flow into the axon. (D) The Ca^{2+} ions affect neighbouring Ca^{2+}-dependent K^+ gates and K^+ ions flow out, thus enhancing the AHP. For further explanation see text

which the frequency decreases. The intensity of the stimulus is conveyed to the central nervous system by the frequency of the initial burst. The subsequent plateau of low-frequency signalling keeps the CNS informed that the stimulus is still present, but is not designed to allow good discrimination between different stimulus intensities. The phenomenon of sensory adaptation is shown in Figure 13.12.

It will be recalled from Chapter 10 that the Ca^{2+}-dependent K^+ channel (I_{KCa}) is believed to be involved in sensory adaptation. It is now possible to see how this may work. Consider Figure 13.13. Local circuits from a depolarised sensory ending act on a patch of excitable membrane to initiate an action potential. It will also be recalled from Chapter 10 that Ca^{2+} gates are strongly voltage-dependent and open when the membrane is depolarised. The membrane is strongly depolarised during an action potential. Hence Ca^{2+} cascades into the fibre. Internal Ca^{2+}, however, tends to open the Ca^{2+}-dependent K^+ gates. K^+, in consequence, flows out. This leads to an increased duration for the AHP. But during the AHP the Na^+ channels are tightly closed—unresponsive to local circuits—and the fast K^+ channels are primed to open in response to depolarising currents. Hence the longer the I_{KCa} current persists the longer the fibre remains unresponsive to generator potentials. Hence sensory adaptation.

13.5 RATE OF PROPAGATION

We noted in Chapter 11 (eq. 11.13) that, other things being equal, the greater the diameter of a process the greater the value of λ, the space constant or **electrotonic length**. In that chapter we were particularly concerned with cable conduction in non-impulse conducting processes. But the analysis applies equally well, of course, to axons. The greater the diameter, the further the local circuits spread down an axon. We saw in that chapter that this physical fact accounts for the evolution of giant fibres in all large invertebrate animals. The rapid signalling which these fibres allow enable the mollusc or annelid or crustacean to respond rapidly to emergencies.

Vertebrate animals have, however, evolved an alternative means for speeding an impulse—**myelination**. Myelinated nerve fibres are seldom above 20 μm in diameter yet, in mammals, they conduct action potentials at well over twice the rate which the 600 μm fibres of the squid can manage. Whilst squid giant fibres seldom conduct at rates much above 50 m s^{-1}, mammalian α fibres can sustain conduction rates of over 120 m s^{-1}. The ability to conduct with great rapidity whilst remaining small is, of course, of great advantage: not only is the message delivered promptly but a large number of small fibres can deliver a great deal more information than one large fibre.

We discussed the nature and formation of the **myelin sheath** around nerve fibres in Section 6.7. We saw there that myelin is formed by glial cells in both the central and peripheral nervous systems. In both cases it is formed by the wrapping of the glial membrane tightly around the axon. In both cases gaps are left between one glial cell and the next in the chain where the axolemma is exposed to the intercellular space. These gaps are called **nodes of Ranvier**.

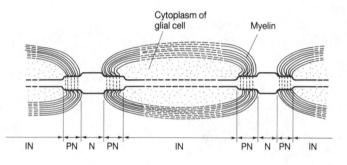

Figure 13.14 Schematic longitudinal section through a myelinated fibre to show the node of Ranvier. N = node of Ranvier; IN = internode; PN = paranode. The stippling on the paranodal membrane represent rows of globular particles which form a firm junction between this part of the axolemma and the myelin. (After Livingstone *et al.*, 1973, *Brain Research*, **58**, 1–24.)

Figure 13.14 shows that region of myelin sheath abutting the node is particularly complex. As the figure shows it is called the **paranode** to distinguish it from the **internode**, which forms the major extent of the myelin sheath. It can be shown that at the paranode the glial cell membrane is firmly anchored to the axolemma. This anchorage is believed not only to weld the myelin firmly to the nerve fibre but also to make a high-resistance seal to electrical current. It also, and importantly, obstructs the movement of membrane-embedded proteins from the node into the internodal region. If myelin is removed from a myelinated axon by diphtheria toxin, or by enzyme attack, the sodium channel and sodium/potassium pump proteins spread out more evenly throughout the axolemma. As there is no evidence that new channels have been synthesised it appears that the paranodal regions of the myelin sheath normally exercise a restraining influence on the movement of these and other membrane proteins. The reader may recall that an analogous situation obtained with sarcolemmal nAChRs after denervation.

Now how does this organisation assist the transmission of action potentials? An answer to this question was proposed many years ago. The tightly wound spirals of the myelin sheath act as a very effective electrical insulator. External current flows cannot penetrate it to affect the ensheathed axolemma. But, of course, the local circuit mechanisms underlying impulse propagation depend on such external current flows. It follows that it is only at the nodes, where the axolemma is exposed, that the local circuits can exert their depolarising effect. Hence the action potential 'jumps' from one node to the next. Technically this is known as **saltatory** conduction. The profound significance of the myelin sheath for the propagation of impulses explains the devastating effects of demyelinating diseases such as multiple sclerosis (see also Section 6.7). It may be that the redistribution of Na^+ channels along demyelinated axon (mentioned above) could account for the uncertain course of the affliction: remissions and exacerbations are a feature of the disease.

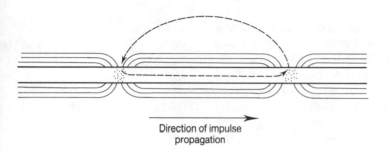

Direction of impulse
propagation

Figure 13.15 Saltatory conduction in myelinated axon. The stippled regions at the nodes indicate where the voltage-dependent gates are located. The broken arrows show the direction of the local circuits when an action potential is travelling down the axon

It might be objected, however, that it is not obvious why this should increase conduction rate. Surely, it might be said, local circuits would anyway spread down axons and depolarise membrane equally far away whether the membrane was insulated by myelin or not? This objection has force. The answer, however, is inherent in eq. 11.12:

$$\lambda \propto \frac{r_m}{r_i}$$

It will be recalled from Chapter 11 that r_m is the transverse resistance of the membrane and r_i the longitudinal resistance of the axoplasm. It is clear that r_m is far greater in a myelinated axon: the electrical resistance of the tightly wound myelin whorls is up to four orders of magnitude greater than neurilemma on its own (see Appendix 2). Hence λ, the space constant, is greatly increased. Hence the influence of local circuits is felt far further down a myelinated than a comparable unmyelinated fibre.

It is also worth remembering that one of the features of the paranodal region of the myelin sheath is that it obstructs the movement of membrane-embedded protein. It is found, in consequence, that there is a very high density of sodium channels at the node—two or three orders of magnitude greater than in the internodal axolemma. This is also the case for the $Na^+ + K^+$ pump proteins.

Now we calculated in Chapter 10 that the quantity of Na^+ flowing into a 12 μm axon during one action potential constituted up to 3% of the Na^+ present beneath that area of membrane. This would place an intolerable strain on the $Na^+ + K^+$ pump if it were to occur all along the membrane and a rapid tattoo of impulses were transmitted. For it has been calculated that a single pump only expels about 200 Na^+ ions per second. In myelinated axons the ion fluxes only occur at the nodes. Intra-axonal diffusion will buffer the concentration build-up of sodium ions. The high concentration of pumps at the node can get rid of the excess during periods of quiescence.

It appears, therefore, that the node allows extra-large current fluxes to occur through the numerous sodium channels so that extra-large local circuits are initiated. This also increases the distance at which electrotonic conduction can exert its effect. Thus the development of myelin whorls around vertebrate axons increases the rate of impulse propagation in several ways: partly by increasing the reach of local circuits; partly by increasing the magnitude of local circuits; partly by buffering the influx and efflux of ions.

The giant fibre systems of invertebrates tackle the buffering problem in a different way. They make use of the mathematical fact that whilst surface area increases as the first power of the radius the volume increases as the second power. Hence although the 600 μm squid axon may develop as many as 500 sodium channels per square micrometre of axolemma the sodium flux when an action potential occurs will only increase the internal sodium concentration by less than 0.01%.

Finally it is worth noting that the high densities of pumps and channels which characterise the axolemma at the nodes are also to be found at the axon's initial segment. This is to be expected for we saw in the last section that this is the membrane where impulses are initiated.

13.6 CONCLUSION

In this chapter we have seen how the major features of the action potential—its initiation, propagation and velocity—all find an explanation at the molecular level. As our understanding of ion channels and pumps increases so will our appreciation of the finer points of impulse transmission. It has already been emphasised that the heterogeneity of their membranes confers different 'personalities' on different neurons. These personalities are expressed in subtly different stimulabilities, adaptabilities and propagation rates. Moreover, like human personalities, neuronal personalities are not fixed and immutable. Neuronal membranes change over time and in response to 'experience'. Although the action potential remains an all-or-nothing event, propagated without decrement from initial segment to telodendria, the comparison of neurons to the units of silicon-based computers becomes ever more strained.

Chapter 14
The neuron as a secretory cell

Science progresses by way of metaphor and analogy. Electricity is likened to a fluid, valency bonds to hooks and eyes, atoms to billiard balls. The science of the brain is no exception to this rule. Descartes in the seventeenth century likened the brain to the intricate hydraulic mechanisms of his day; the nineteenth and early twentieth centuries saw a powerful analogy in the telegraph cable and the telephone exchange; nowadays, in the late twentieth century, the computer metaphor is all-pervasive. Metaphors and analogies both help and bias our understanding. The power of the computer analogy perhaps prevents us seeing the brain from other equally significant viewpoints. In particular it prevents us seeing the brain as if it were an immense gland. Yet this view has much to commend it. Neurons can be seen not so much as relays or on/off valves but as secretory cells. The electrical phenomena of electrotonic and action potentials can, on this analogy, be seen merely as triggers for the release of secretions—the neurotransmitters and modulators.

In this chapter we shall begin to consider this aspect of the nervous system. We shall consider the neuron as a secretory cell. In the next chapter we shall look at the pharmacology of some of the neurotransmitters and neuromodulators which are elaborated by neurons and in the chapter after that we shall consider the action of these secretions on underlying (subsynaptic) membranes and cells.

14.1 NEURONS AND SECRETIONS

Neurons synthesise many different transmitters and modulators. We noted in Chapter 1 that in the 1930s Dale proposed that any given neuron only synthesised one type of transmitter. It followed that all the terminations of that neuron released that same substance. The action of that substance depends, of course, on the nature of the receptors in the subsynaptic membrane. The nACh receptor, as we have already noted, responds to acetylcholine in a very different way from the mACh receptor. **Dale's 'law' or 'principle'** has stood the test of time remarkably well. But like practically all generalisations in biology it is now found to be honoured more in the breach than in the observance. Numerous exceptions, both in the vertebrates and in the invertebrates, are now known. Indeed it begins to seem that a quite common pattern is to find a peptide neuromodulator accompanying a monoamine in a single presynaptic terminal (see Chapter 15).

We shall look in detail at the various transmitter and modulator molecules in Chapter 15. Here, however, we can note that they range from small molecules such as acetylcholine, the catecholamines and individual amino acids, to quite large peptides. We have already considered the structure and evolutionary relationships of some of the latter in Chapters 2, 3 and 4 (see also Table 2.2). The site at which these molecules are synthesised differs. Small transmitters such as acetylcholine are put together (as we shall see) in the terminal. Peptide modulators, in contrast, are synthesised in the perikaryon. However, even the synthesis of acetylcholine requires appropriate enzymes—in particular choline acetyltransferase (CAT)—and these have to be manufactured in the perikaryon. For it is only in the perikaryon that the necessary protein-synthetic equipment—the DNA information tape, the ribosome machine-tools, the endoplasmic reticulum, Golgi apparatus, etc.—exists.

Neurons, thus, are very special types of secretory cell. The secretory membrane (i.e. the presynaptic membrane) can be more than a metre distant from the region where the secretion is synthesised. The connection between the two regions is, of course, provided by the axon. Up till now we have been considering the axon only as if it were a telegraph wire—for conducting nerve impulses. Now we begin to see that it has another and equally important function. It has to act as a conduit for the passage of secretory materials manufactured in the perikaryon and destined for release at the synaptic terminal. Moreover, as we shall see, the transport is not in one direction only. Materials also flow back from the terminal to the perikaryon. **Axoplasmic flows** play crucial roles in the functioning of the nervous system.

It should be mentioned at this point that some neurons have developed their secretory function to the extent of releasing their secretion not across a synaptic gap on to the dendritic membrane of another neuron, but directly into the vascular system. These cells are known straightforwardly as **neurosecretory cells**. Such cells are found in the hypothalamus and pituitary of vertebrates. They are also well developed in many invertebrates.

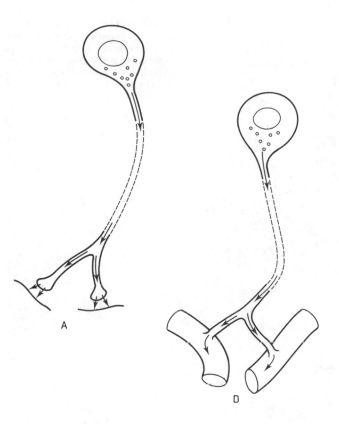

Figure 14.1 Neurons as secretory cells and neurosecretory cells. (A) Typical neuron. The transmitter is released across the synaptic gap and affects the membrane of the cell immediately subjacent. (B) Typical neursecretory cell. The neurosecretion is released into a blood vessel and carried by the blood flow to exert an affect on a distant cell

Readers interested in the topic of neurosecretion, which underlies the vast subject of neuroendocrinology, should consult one of the texts listed in the bibliography. In this chapter we shall deal only with the secretory aspect of 'conventional' neurons.

14.2 SYNTHESIS IN THE PERIKARYON

In Chapter 3 we looked at the molecular biology of protein biosynthesis. We saw that the genetic message held in the structure of DNA is first of all transcribed into mRNA and then translated at the ribosome into the specified amino acid sequence of a protein. This process, we noted, was highly complex, involving many different enzymes and both tRNA and rRNA as well as mRNA. But the molecular biology of protein manufacture does not end there. In secretory cells the protein has to be packaged and transported to its release site.

Electron micrographs of the perikarya of typical nerve cells show all the structural features of a cell employed in intense protein biosynthesis. They possess **large nuclei** with one or more **prominent nucleoli**. Their cytoplasm is richly endowed with

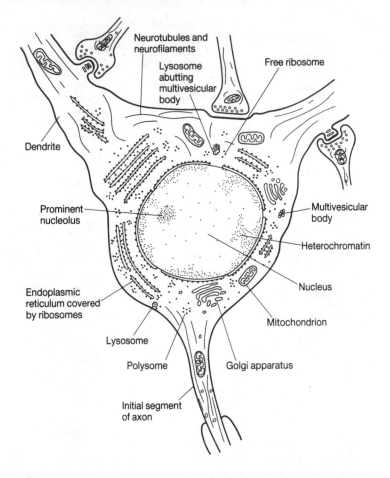

Figure 14.2 Perikaryon of a cortical neuron. Drawing from an electron micrograph of a neuron in the cerebral cortex. Note the massive nucleus, the prominent nucleolus and the complex structure of the cytoplasm

rough endoplasmic reticulum (RER) and there is always one and often a large number of **Golgi bodies**.

Rough endoplasmic reticulum consists of complex stacks of membranes covered by innumerable ribosomes. The latter cause the protuberances or 'roughness' visible in EM pictures. It is these ribosomes which synthesise protein 'for export'.

14.2.1 Co-translational synthesis

It can be shown that the polypeptide chain manufactured at the ribosome is inserted directly into the lumen of the ER. **But how does the ribosome find the ER?** After all, not all the proteins which a neuron manufactures are for export. Some of them will be for the usual 'housekeeping' activities of the perikaryon itself. It would be disastrous if these were to be delivered into the lumen of the ER and sent off for export!

The answer to the question posed above seems to be that the first 30 or so amino acids in the polypeptide chain growing from

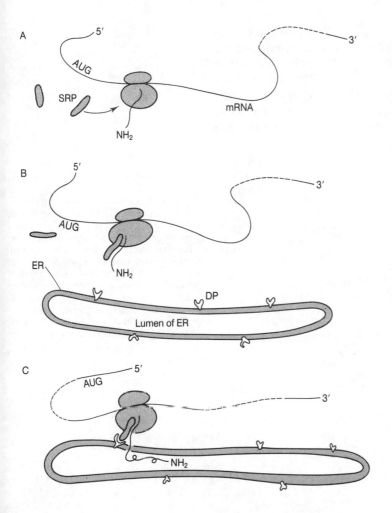

Figure 14.3 Anchorage of a ribosome to the ER. (A) Ribosome attaches to the 5′ end of mRNA and finding a start signal (AUG) commences translation. The initial amino acid sequence is termed the 'signal sequence'. (B) The signal sequence is recognised by a signal recognition protein (SRP) which attaches to it and to the ribosome. (C) The SRP and signal sequence then recognise a 'docking protein (DP) in the ER membrane. A pore opens for the signal sequence, which passes through into the lumen of the ER. Further translation of the mRNA can now commence

the ribosome form a signal sequence which is recognised by a **'signal recognition particle' (SRP)**—see Figure 14.3. This recognition particle is in fact a very complex nucleoprotein consisting of six separate polypeptides and a 300-nucleotide RNA moiety. The recognition particle appears to have two functions. First, it prevents any further translation occurring, thus ensuring that the export protein is not simply dumped in the perikaryal cytoplasm. Second, the SRP is recognised by a 650-residue **'docking protein' (DP)** embedded in the ER membrane. The ribosome, nascent polypeptide chain, and SRP become anchored to the ER.

The story is far from finished at this point. It is found that if the SRP nucleoprotein remains attached to the signal sequence no further translation occurs. It appears, however, that once the ribosome has become anchored to the membrane the signal recognition protein detaches to recycle. This allows the signal-sequence of amino acids, which are generally hydrophobic, to insert themselves into the ER membrane. The ribosome is held in position on the ER by the polypeptide chain protruding through the ER membrane into the lumen. Translation then continues as described in Chapter 3. The polypeptide is thus synthesised and inserted into the lumen of the ER at one and the same time. This is termed **co-translation**. Finally it is found that the N-terminal signal sequence is cut off.

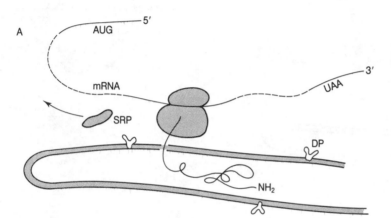

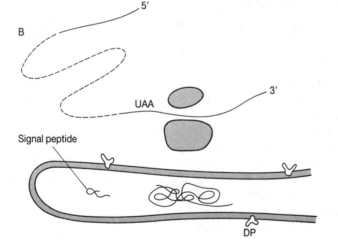

Figure 14.4   Co-translational synthesis of polypeptides at the ER. (A) The signal recognition protein recycles. The polypeptide chain is synthesised at the ribosome and inserted into the lumen of the ER. (B) On reaching a stop signal (e.g. UAA) translation ceases and the two parts of the ribosome separate to recycle. Enzymes within the lumen of the ER remove the signal sequence from the polypeptide and proceed with any appropriate post-translational processing

There are two possible end-results to the process of co-translation. In one case the polypeptide may be secreted entirely into the lumen of the RER. It is found, in fact, that the ribosome is released from the polypeptide before the C-terminal end has passed into the lumen. This happens later. In the second case the polypeptide never gets through into the lumen at all. This is the case with membrane embedded proteins. We have noted in the last few chapters how important these are in molecular neurobiology. These polypeptides, we saw, have one or in many cases more than one hydrophobic sequence which ensure that they remain trapped in the lipid environment of the ER membrane.

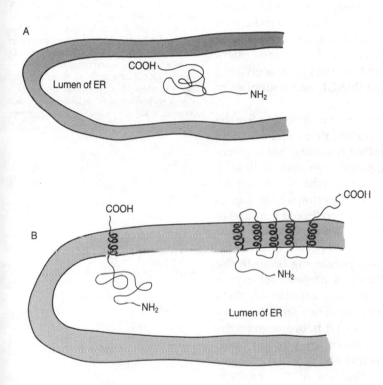

Figure 14.5 Two end results of co-translation. (A) The polypeptide is entirely within the lumen of the ER. (B) Hydrophobic segments (bold) of the polypeptide ensure that it is caught in the ER membrane. In many cases several such hydrophobic segments are trapped in the membrane. The mechanism by which this occurs is not at present clear. It may be that the polypeptide chain is inserted into the membrane as a series of hairpin loops, (cf. Fig. 9.12)

14.2.2 The Golgi body and post-translational modification

We noted in Chapter 3 that post-translational modification of polypeptides and proteins is very common. In particular we saw how some of the peptide neuromodulators—the opioids and tachykinins—are known to be derived from large precursor proteins or polyproteins by post-translational processing. In Chapter 4 we considered the evolutionary implications of this phenomenon. In this section we shall look at where this post-translational processing occurs.

The first steps in post-translational processing occur in the **lumen of the ER**. Here we find that disulphide bonds are made between cysteine residues and the first steps in **glycosylation** are taken. The formation of disulphide bonds is generally regarded as stabilising the three-dimensional structure of a protein, and the process of glycosylation—the adding of carbohydrate chains—is very important for many proteins, as we have noted in preceding chapters and shall note again, especially when we come to consider cell–cell recognition in neuroembryology (Chapter 17).

The initial steps in glycosylation are often called **core glycosylation** to distinguish them from the finishing touches which are carried out later in the Golgi body. These initial steps often involve the addition of a '**core**' **oligosaccharide** to the amino side chain of **asparagine**. Such glycoproteins, as we noted in Chapter 2, are consequently termed N-linked. The core oligosaccharide almost invariably consists of two units of an acetylated monosaccharide, **n-acetylglucosamine (NAG)**, and a number of mannose and glucose units.

Alternatively the carbohydrate moiety may be linked to the the hydroxyl group in the side chains of **serine**, **threonine** or, more rarely, **hydroxylysine** or **hydroxyproline** residues. Such glyco-proteins, as we noted, are consequently termed O-linked. O-linked oligosaccarides are much smaller than the N-linked type. They usually consist of only two, three or perhaps four mono-saccharide units—*n*-acetylglucosamine (again) linked perhaps to galactose and very commonly to *n*-acetylneuraminic acid (= sialic acid).

The next phases of post-translational processing occur in the **Golgi body**. Cells active in the synthesis of proteins for export usually have several, sometimes a very large number of, such bodies. This is the case with many neurons. They are often very well endowed with Golgi complexes. Indeed neurons were the cells in which they were initially discovered, by Camillo Golgi in 1898. An understanding of their structure and function awaited, however, the advent of modern techniques in cell biology. Figure 14.7 shows that Golgi bodies have an intricate structure. They consist of a stack of membranous saccules or cisternae. These saccules are believed to be formed at one face by the fusion of vesicles budding off the ER and to be lost at the other face by their tips budding off to form secretory vesicles. The Golgi body is thus said to have a *cis* or **forming** face and a *trans* or **maturing** face.

As implied in the previous paragraph the precursor proteins in the ER reach the Golgi body in transport vesicles. This also applies to membrane proteins. These travel in the membranes of the transport vesicles and ultimately fuse with the *cis* face of the Golgi body. The static picture which the electron microscope gives of cellular ultrastructure is evidently highly misleading. The 'structural' elements of a cell—its internal membranes and (as we shall see) fibres—are in ceaseless turmoil. Nowhere is this more

Figure 14.6   Glycosylation in the ER and Golgi body. The figure shows N-glycosylation. The initial step is the transfer of an oligosaccharide from dolichol to an asparagine residue in the forming polypeptide chain. Dolichol is a large (75–90 carbon) unsaturated lipid. It is firmly embedded in the ER membrane, which it probably spans three or four times. The subsequent process-ing, as the figure shows, occurs partly in the ER and partly in the Golgi body. D = dolichol; Asn = asparagine; NAG = *N*-acetylglucosamine; Man = mannose; Glc = glucose; Gal = galactose; NANA = *N*-acetylneuraminic acid (also known as sialic acid) $\longrightarrow$

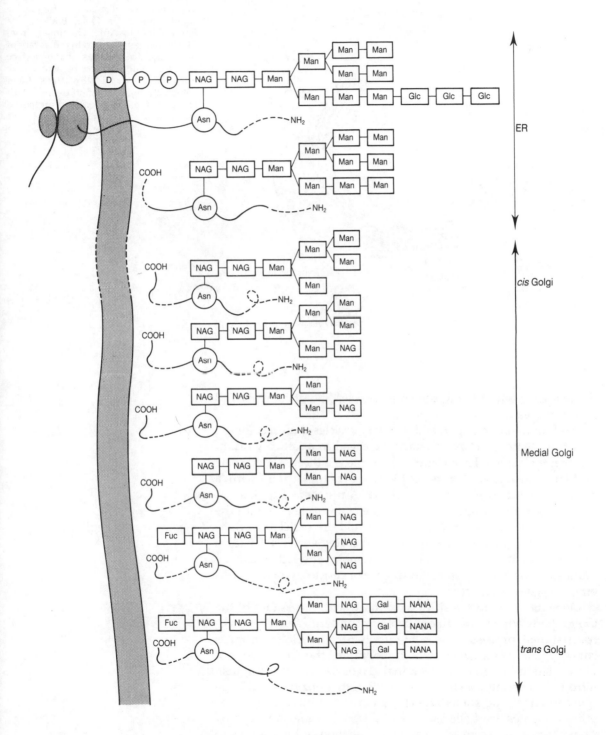

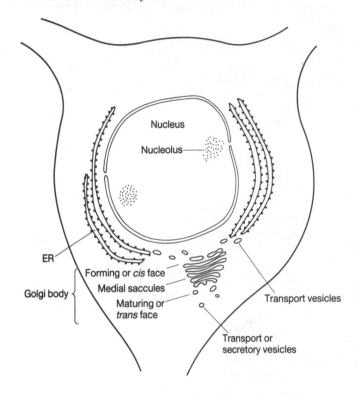

Figure 14.7   Structure of the Golgi body. The perikarya of neurons frequently contain numerous Golgi bodies. The figure shows just one. The flow is from ER via transport vesicles to the *cis* face of the Golgi. The vesicles of the *cis* face coalesce to form saccules and move outwards towards the *trans* face. Ultimately vesicles bud off the *trans* face and carry the fully processed protein to its correct destination

the case than with the ER, transport vesicles, Golgi complex and secretory vesicles.

It is found that transport and secretory vesicles share a common structural feature. They appear to be caged in a lattice work of **clathrin** molecules. Each clathrin molecule is a three-armed ('Isle of Man') structure (Figure 14.8)—called a **triskelion**—with a molecular weight of about 180 000 Da. A number of triskelions form around the lipoprotein membrane of a vesicle and with the aid of several smaller proteins seem to hold the vesicle together. Such clathrin-gripped vesicles are called **coated vesicles**. Clathrin can very easily assemble and disassemble. Indeed it can be induced to assemble even in the absence of vesicles, when it forms empty cage-like structures.

Once the transport vesicles have fused with the *cis* face of the Golgi body their contained proteins undergo further post-translational processing (see Figure 14.6). The Golgi saccules contain many enzymes which continue the processes of glycosylation—often called **terminal glycosylation** to distinguish it from the core glycosylation of the ER. Other enzymes cut large 'polyproteins' into something closer to their ultimate forms. Yet other enzymes are believed to add a signal or tag, perhaps by phosphorylation or by a specific glycosylation, which serves to

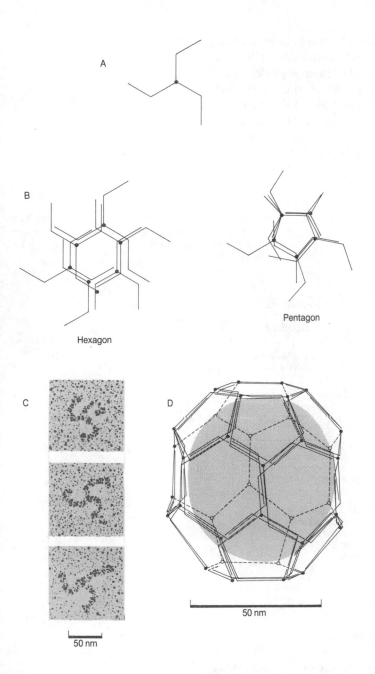

Figure 14.8 Clathrin triskelions and coated vesicles. (A) Clathrin triskelion. (B) Clathrin triskelions spontaneously assemble to form hexagons and pentagons. (C) Thirty-six triskelions organised as a network of twelve pentagons and eight hexagons form the 'coat' surrounding a coated vesicle. The overlapping arms of the triskelions provide strength with flexibility. On the left-hand side are electron micrographs of triskelions. ((C) reprinted by permission from Ungewickell and Branton, 1981, *Nature*, **289**, 420–422., copyright © 1981, Macmillan Magazines Ltd; and from Alberts *et al.*, 1983, *Molecular Biology of the Cell*, New York: Garland Publishing; with permission.)

direct a protein—especially a membrane-bound protein—to its correct destination. Finally the Golgi body carries out an important role in condensing proteins destined for export into highly concentrated packages.

The intricate molecular biology of the perikaryon is now at an end. The proteins are now prepared, packaged and ready for export. In the next section we shall look at what is known about the transport of this material to its final destination. We shall consider, in particular, how it is believed to be moved down the axon. It must, however, be borne in mind that materials, membrane receptors, enzymes, etc., must also be moved out along those other neural proceses—the dendrites. This transport, though far less is known about it, is just as important for the biology of the neuron as is the transport of transmitters and modulators, etc., down the axon.

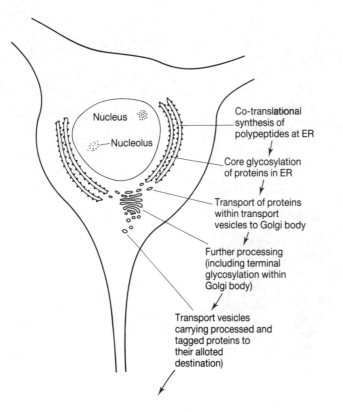

Figure 14.9   Summarising diagram of the pathway of 'export' proteins in neuronal perikarya

14.3 TRANSPORT ALONG THE AXON

The secretory vesicles budding off the *trans* face of the Golgi body have far to go. The recurrent laryngeal nerve fibres of a giraffe stretching all the way down the neck, under the aortic arch, and back up again to the larynx may be several metres in length. Whilst this may be exeptional, axons of over a metre in length are quite common in large animals. The topic of **axoplasmic transport** has thus been one of considerable interest.

Conventional microscopic techniques have revealed, as we

shall shortly see, a complex cytoskeleton within the axon. But as we noted in the preceding section these pictures tend to give the wrong impresssion. The axonal cytoskeleton, like the membranous structures within a perikaryon, is not static like the endoskeleton of the vertebrate body, the exoskeleton of an arthropod or the scaffolding around a building. In vivid contrast it constitutes a scene of dynamic activity.

This dynamism has been revealed both by 'pulse labelling' and by ingenious microscopic techniques. Pulse labelling consists of the introduction of a brief pulse of radioactive label and then finding where the radioactivty has got to in successive intervals of time. When this technique is applied to an axon it reveals waves of radioactive label moving through the axoplasm. Three distinct transport systems appear to be at work. A **fast** system ($1–4$ μm s^{-1}, i.e. $9–36$ cm day^{-1}) and a **slow** system ($0.01–0.04$ μm s^{-1}, i.e. $1–3.5$ mm day^{-1}) transport material from the perikaryon towards the synaptic terminal (**anterograde**), while a system working in the reverse direction at about the same rate as the fast system transports material from the terminal towards the perikaryon (**retrograde**).

The **fast axoplasmic transport** system appears to be responsible for transporting the **secretory vesicles** which we have followed budding off the Golgi apparatus. These vesicles contain neurotransmitters and/or modulators, glycoproteins, enzymes required for neurotransmitter metabolism in the terminal, etc. The **slow system**, on the other hand, is believed to carry elements of the cytoskeleton and to be involved in axonal growth processes. Finally the **retrograde system** carries effete membrane and other used materials, nerve growth factor (NGF), materials taken up from the synaptic cleft, etc., back from the synaptic terminal to the perikaryon.

Biochemical, immunological and electron microscopic techniques have helped identify the fibrous elements responsible for these flows. Such cytoskeletal elements seem pretty generally developed throughout metazoan cells. They have become especially well developed in neurons to carry out what is, at the cellular level, an extraordinary task. It has already been mentioned that many mammalian axons are well over a metre in length. An average diameter for such an axon might be 15 μm. Many are considerably narrower. If we scale things up to a human dimension a water main of diameter 1 m would have to stretch uninterrupted over 66 km to be comparable. It would have to be prepared to bend and crinkle, and carry materials at different speeds in both directions. Axons are indeed remarkable structures.

Cell biologists recognise three major classes of cytoskeletal fibres: **microfilaments** (diameter about 6 nm); **intermediate**

filaments (IFs) (diameter between 7 and 11 nm); and **microtubules** (diameter 22 nm). All three types of fibre are found in
neurons, especially in axons.

Microfilaments are mostly composed of actin. We met this
cytoskeletal component in Chapter 6 when we were considering
the nature of the submembranous cytoskeleton. There it was
believed to play a role in maintaining the shape of the cell. Actin
is also, of course, well known in muscle, where it is crucially
involved in the contractile mechanism. It is likely that it plays a
part in cytoplasmic movements of all types. It is thus not
surprising to find microfilaments well represented in axons. **Actin
fibres (F-actin)** are composed of **globular subunits (G-actin)**. Two
F-actin strands twist around each other to form a **two-stranded
rope**. Numerous cytoplasmic factors are involved in the
polymerisation process whereby G-actin units string together to
form F-actin. Other factors form cross-links between actin fibres,
bundle them together into parallel skeins and/or act as 'spacers'
keeping parallel bundles apart by distances of about 200 nm. The
molecular biology of microfilaments is very intricate and is still
being worked out. In the axon the microfilaments are usually quite
short—seldom more than about 0.5 μm in length.

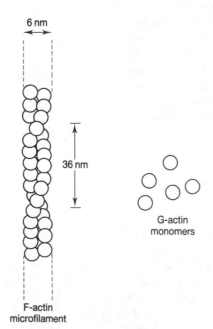

Figure 14.10 Structure of microfilaments. G-actin subunits are in fact more
pear-shaped than spherical. Polymerisation into F-actin is usually
accompanied by the hydrolysis of ATP to
ADP

Intermediate filaments (IFs) unlike either the microfilaments
or the microtubules are biochemically extremely heterogeneous.
Five major classes are recognised. Each class is found in a specific

cell type. In the nervous system glial cells contain glial filaments (a single protein of 51 kDa). In neurons three different IF proteins are recognised: 63 kDa, 160 kDa and 200 kDa.

Although IFs are extremely various they all seem to share a central highly conserved 310 amino-acid rod-like domain. This domain consists of two α-helices wound around each other to

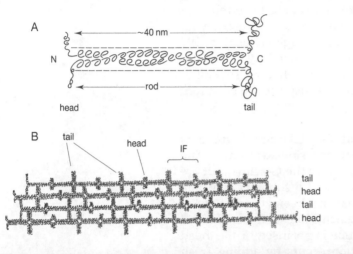

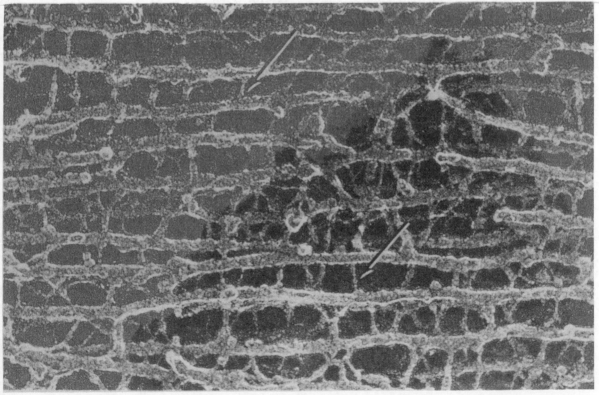

Figure 14.11 Structure of IFs and neurofilaments. (A) An IF consists of a rod-like segment composed of two α-helices wound around each other to form a two-stranded rope. Each rod-like segment ends in a variable region. The C-terminal end (the tail) has a more extensive variable region than the N-terminal end (the head). The whole molecule is about 40 nm in length and 7–11 nm in diameter. (B) The variable entanglements of the heads tend to attach to each other, as do the larger entanglements of the tails. The sideways-spreading tail entanglements also become attached to neighbouring IFs so that bundles, 10 nm or so in diameter, are formed. It is probable (not yet certain) that the IFs in these bundles are arranged in an antiparallel manner. There are no (+) and (-) ends as found in micro-tubules. (C) Neurofilaments observed in the electron microscope using a quick-freeze, deep-etch technique. The arrows indicate cross-bridges between the neurofilaments (×75 000). ((C) from Hirokawa, 1986, *Trends in Neurosciences*, 9, 67–71; with permission.)

form a two-stranded rope. Each α-helix has the characteristic non-polar heptad repeat we discussed in Section 2.1, which ensures that the two-stranded rope structure is stable. At each end of the rod domain there are hypervariable head and tail regions. In the IFs of neurofilaments the tail regions are unusually extensive. It is believed that they may form the cross-linkages which the electron microscopist can see projecting out orthogonally to the neurofilament's long axis. The neurofilament itself is often very lengthy—up to 200 μm. It consists of a number of neural IFs lying parallel to each other and end to end in a staggered fashion. We shall return to discuss neurofilaments further in Chapter 19, where we review some of the ills the brain is heir to: several of these, especially Alzheimer's disease, are suspected to be at root neurofibrillary lesions.

Microtubules (MTs) consist of **tubulin**. Like actin, tubulin is built of globular subunits. But here the similarity ends. The tubulin sub-units are not all alike (as were the G-actins) but are of two sorts—α and β tubulin. The α and β subunits associate together to form dimers and these in turn join end to end to form a 'protofilament'. Finally 13 protofilaments line up in parallel and circle to form a hollow tube. The tube is polarised: it has head (+) and tail (−) end. Polymerisation occurs by adding fresh subunits at the (+) end. 'Treadmilling' has also been observed to occur. In this process units are removed from the (−) end and added to the (+) end. In axons microtubules are aligned so that their (−) ends point to the perikaryon.

Polymerisation requires a number of accessory factors and GTP. Two of the most important accessory factors are the **microtubule accessory proteins (MAPs)** and the **tau** proteins. These accessories appear to be involved both in the poly-merisation process and in the stabilisation of tubulin once it has polymerised. The MAPs may be involved in cross-linking micro-tubules to other cellular structures. There are indications that MAPs differ markedly from cell type to cell type. There is even evidence that the MAPs in dendrites are different from those found in axons. In axons microtubules are comparable in length (about 200 μm) to neurofilaments.

Like actin microfilaments, microtubules are well known to be involved in cell movement. It is the major protein of the axonemes of *eukaryotic* cilia and flagella and in association with another protein, dynein, causes their characteristic beating movements.

The distribution of the fibrous 'skeletal' elements within cells can be studied by **immuno-** and **electron microscopy**. In the first technique the cytoskeletal element of interest is extracted and

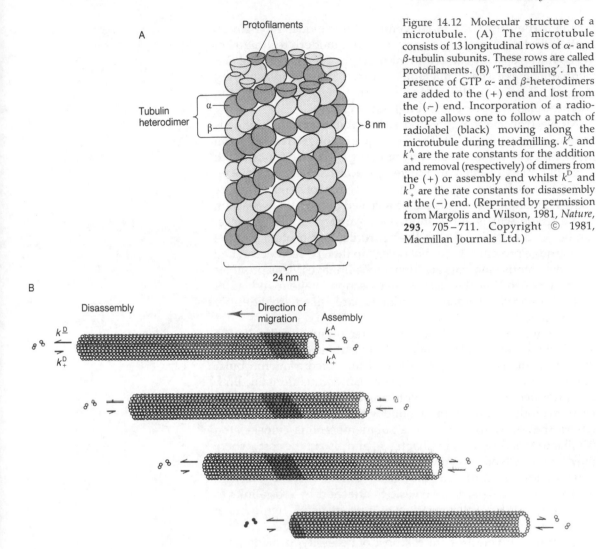

Figure 14.12 Molecular structure of a microtubule. (A) The microtubule consists of 13 longitudinal rows of α- and β-tubulin subunits. These rows are called protofilaments. (B) 'Treadmilling'. In the presence of GTP α- and β-heterodimers are added to the (+) end and lost from the (−) end. Incorporation of a radio-isotope allows one to follow a patch of radiolabel (black) moving along the microtubule during treadmilling. k^A_- and k^A_+ are the rate constants for the addition and removal (respectively) of dimers from the (+) or assembly end whilst k^D_- and k^D_+ are the rate constants for disassembly at the (−) end. (Reprinted by permission from Margolis and Wilson, 1981, *Nature*, **293**, 705–711. Copyright © 1981, Macmillan Journals Ltd.)

purified. An antibody is raised against it and the latter either re-injected into a cell or introduced through an enzymatically weakened plasma membrane. After the antibody has found its cytoskeletal antigen and attached itself another antibody, prepared so that it binds to the first but this time coupled to a fluorescent dye, is introduced. When the cell is exposed to an appropriate wavelength of light the cytoskeletal system under investigation fluoresces.

Electron microscopy has also proved a valuable technique for investigating the cytoskeleton. There are several possible techniques. We shall look at two of the most important. Axons may be either prepared by conventional techniques of chemical fixation and thin sectioning or by the more modern technique of freeze-fracture etching. Electron micrographs prepared by the first technique make the filamentous nature of the axoplasm very evident. It is not difficult to see that neurofilaments and microtubules are present throughout the axon.

An electron micrograph prepared by the second technique is shown in Figure 14.11(C). The technique involves freezing fresh nerve fibres extremely rapidly by bringing them into contact with a copper block cooled to the temperature of liquid nitrogen (-196 °C) or liquid helium (-269 °C). The biochemical nature of the filamentous elements can be revealed by a previous reaction of the tissue with specific antibodies. Antibodies, for instance, can be used to pick out both the neurofilament protein and the cross-bridge protein. These antibodies can then be seen decorating the filamentous elements and their cross-linkages. This provides good evidence that the electron microscope image is indeed of neurofilaments. Similar techniques are used to identify microtubules.

These microscopic and biochemical techniques are beginning to reveal the full complexity of axoplasmic transport. It is believed that the axoplasm can be subdivided into a core microtubular domain and a more peripheral neurofilamentous domain. Both microtubules and neurofilaments are extensively cross-linked. Actin microfilaments are to be found both beneath the axolemma, where they may form part of a submembranous cytoskeleton (similar to that described in Chapter 6), and also in the core, where they are involved in bringing about the axoplasmic flow of neurofilaments and microtubules. Freeze-etched electron micrographs show secretory vesicles attached by cross-links to microtubules. An interpretation of this intricate two-domain system is shown in Figure 14.13.

Immuno- and electron microscopy, of necessity, provide static images. The biologist has to use his imagination to understand the molecular turmoil which these images have caught and frozen. This, however, is not always easy. Indeed the very term 'cytoskeleton' can be deeply misleading. We have already noted that it tends to suggest something stable and enduring: as we regard the skeletons of our own bodies. This analogy may be appropriate for the submembranous cytoskeleton we considered in Chapter 6, but it can easily bias our view of the molecular agitation in the cores of axons.

Fortunately an ingenious new technique has been developed which allows us to glimpse the true molecular dynamism of the 'cytoskeleton'. This technique is called **video-enhanced microscopy** or, more fully (after its inventor), **Allen video-enhanced contrast–differential interference contrast microscopy**

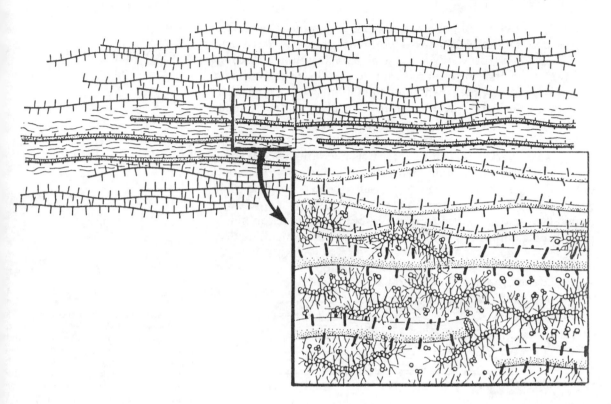

AVEC–DIC. It not only allows the observation of cytoskeletal elements in unfixed living cytoplasm but also, through clever computer techniques, allows the observation of elements far below the limit of resolution of the best optical microscopes. The theoretical limit of resolution of optical microscopy is about 0.25 μm; the AVEC system allows the observation of fibres with a diameter of only 25 nm—an order of magnitude improvement.

In the early 1980s this new methodology was applied to the study of axoplasmic transport. The axon studied was our old friend the giant axon of the squid. Immediately it became apparent that the axoplasm was teeming with activity. Mitochondria were moving along the axon in both directions with a jerky motion; multivesicular bodies (carrying used membrane) and multilamellar bodies (probably mitochondrial remains) were moving toward the perikaryon; dense shoals of transport vesicles were moving in the opposite direction, from the perikaryon to the synaptic terminal.

These observations were followed up by examining the system *in vitro*. We noted in Chapter 11 that one of the great virtues of the squid giant axon was that the axoplasm could be extracted and analysed. It proved possible to sandwich extruded squid

Figure 14.13 Central axonal cytoskeleton. This figure summarises a number of studies on squid giant fibre axoplasm. The major part of the figure shows a microtubule domain surrounded by neurofilaments. The microtubules are associated with numerous short microfilaments. In the higher magnification inset the intricate interweaving of the microtubules and microfilaments is shown. The microfilaments are interwoven with accessory proteins, both globular and filamentous. (Reprinted with permission from Lasek, 1986, *Journal of Cell Science*, Supplement 5, 161–179. Copyright © 1986; The Company of Biologists Ltd.)

axoplasm between two cover-glasses and examine it by AVEC microscopy (Figure 14.14). It was found that organelle movement in the centre of the sandwiched axoplasm was not noticeably different from that in the squid axon itself. The *in vitro* system allows numerous experimental manipulations to be undertaken with a view to establishing the nature of the observed movement, the chemical environment required, the energy source, etc.

In addition to the 'cover-glass sandwich' system of Figure 14.14 it has also proved possible to extract single microtubules and show that in appropriate conditions they will not only transport organelles and indeed carboxylated latex beads, but also glide across cover-slips themselves. AVEC microscopy shows that organelles (and latex beads) move in both directions on single microtubules and pass each other without apparent difficulty.

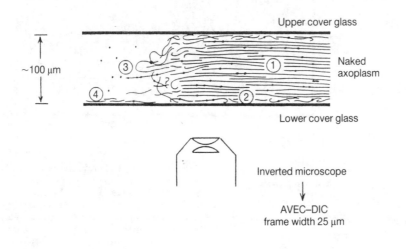

Figure 14.14 *In vitro* examination of extruded squid axoplasm. The axoplasm is sandwiched between two cover glasses and observed by AVEC-DIC microscopy. Organelle movement in the central domain (1) of the axoplasm resembles that seen *in vivo* and is particularly well seen where filaments protrude from the axon surface (3). Microtubules can be clearly observed at the periphery (2) and where they have fallen free from the axoplasm (4). Small particles which become attached to MTs in this last position are transported along their lengths. (Reprinted with permission from Weiss, 1986, *Journal of Cell Science*, Supplement 5, 1–15; Copyright © 1986, The Company of Biologists Ltd.)

The molecular cause of these fascinating movements is a topic of intense research at the present time. A protein of some 110–134 kDa can be extracted from fresh axoplasm which in the presence of ATP enables microtubules to translocate organelles and beads and to writhe, snake and glide over glass substrates. This protein has been named **kinesin**. The rate of translocation and gliding produced by kinesin is strongly dependent on the quantity of ATP provided. It is believed that a pool of kinesin is available in the axoplasm. It is further believed that kinesin induces side-arms of the microtubules to 'row' organelles along the tubule or to 'row' the tubule over the substratum. Whether these arms are permanently attached to the microtubule, or to the translocating organelle, or whether they are in both cases transient or free in the axoplasmic matrix, is not yet known. The production of relative motion by 'rowing' is, however, very familiar to molecular biologists in other contexts. It lies at the root of both muscle movement (myosin) and the movement of eukaryotic flagella and cilia (dynein). It appears, moreover, that different 'force-generating enzymes' are responsible for anterograde and retrograde transport.

Molecular neurobiologists still have far to go before they achieve a full understanding of axoplasmic transport. Nevertheless the progress in the last few years has been remarkable. The development of the new microscopic techniques and the use of the *in vitro* model systems described above have revolutionised the prospects for success. An understanding of the molecular nature of axoplasmic transport is of first rate importance not only for the science of the brain but also (as we have already observed) in that it should allow us to gain insight into the causes of several distressing neuropathologies. We shall return to the latter topic in Chapter 19. Meanwhile Figure 14.15 summarises our present understanding of the process.

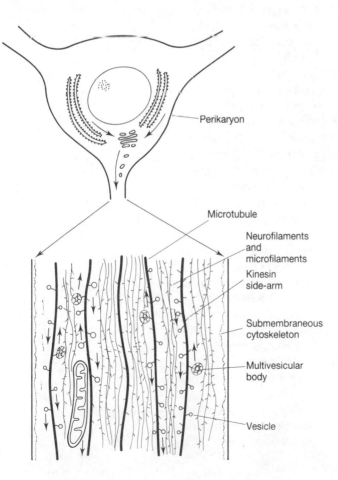

Perikaryon

Microtubule

Neurofilaments and microfilaments

Kinesin side-arm

Submembraneous cytoskeleton

Multivesicular body

Vesicle

Figure 14.15 Axoplasmic transport summarised. The figure schematises the transport mechanisms which are believed to be operating within an axon. Secretory vesicles (containing neurotransmitter or membrane components) are moved outwards in the anterograde direction to the axon terminal. Other material, perhaps used membrane or breakdown products from neurotransmitters, is moved towards the perikaryon (retrograde direction) mostly in the form of multivesicular bodies. These ultimately empty their contents into perikaryal lysosomes for further digestion. Mitochondria are also moved by the microtubular transport system. (Partly after Allen, 1987, *Scientific American*, **256**, 26 – 33.)

Finally it should be noted that the analyses of axoplasmic transport described above have been carried out on peripheral fibres. Although we have no particular reason to suspect that central neurons do it differently the possibility that they do should be borne in mind. In particular it has been suggested that not only secretory vesicles are carried along central axons but also fragments of **smooth endoplasmic reticulum (SER)**. If this is indeed the case the synaptic terminal would be a metabolically more complex place than is usually allowed.

14.4 EXOCYTOSIS AND ENDOCYTOSIS AT THE SYNAPTIC TERMINAL

After days, perhaps weeks, of 'rowing' down the axon the secretory vesicle finally reaches its destination in the synaptic terminal. It now awaits its one brief moment of action. This depends on the arrival of an action potential or, if it is a local circuit neuron, an electrotonic potential at the terminal. When this happens the membrane depolarisation (as we noted in Section 10.3) opens calcium gates. The influx of Ca^{2+} ions triggers release of the vesicle's contents into the synaptic gap.

Let us look in a little more detail at this vital process. Examination of synaptic endings in the electron microscope shows that they contain large numbers of synaptic vesicles. These vesicles vary in shape and size according to their contents. Small spherical translucent vesicles (diameter about 50 nm) contain transmitters such as acetylcholine and glutamate. Other small translucent vesicles assume a more ellipsoidal form and these are believed to contain inhibitory transmitters such as glycine. Larger vesicles (diameter > 60 nm), often with dense cores, contain catecholamines whilst yet larger vesicles (diameter $\sim$ 175 nm) contain peptides.

It should be borne in mind that synaptic vesicles contain much more than just neurotransmitter. Even the small translucent ACh-containing vesicles contain at least 14 distinct proteins ranging in molecular weight from 20 kDa to 160 kDa. The dense cored catecholaminergic vesicles also contain much besides nor-adrenalin. In particular they can be shown to include ATP, ATPase and dopamine-β-hydroxylase. The large vesicles of peptidergic neurons contain ATP, ATPase, adenylate cyclase, Ca^{2+} and perhaps some of the enzymes required for the final stages of post-translational processing.

A great deal of synaptic molecular biology has used the 'honorary' synapse of the **neuromuscular junction**. This junction is conveniently placed for experimental manipulation. It uses ACh as its transmitter.

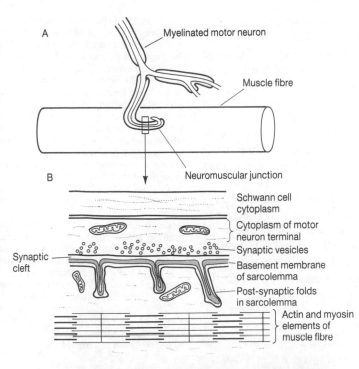

A — Myelinated motor neuron

Muscle fibre

B

Neuromuscular junction

Schwann cell cytoplasm

Cytoplasm of motor neuron terminal

Synaptic vesicles

Synaptic cleft

Basement membrane of sarcolemma

Post-synaptic folds in sarcolemma

Actin and myosin elements of muscle fibre

Figure 14.16 The neuromuscular junction. (A) Motor nerve fibres normally branch to innervate a small group of muscle fibres (the 'motor unit'). Each branch ends on the sarcolemma of a muscle fibre in a tiny spiral. (B) Magnified diagram of portion enclosed in rectangle. The sarcolemma of the muscle fibre immediately beneath the nerve terminal (the motor end plate) is invaginated into a number of post-junctional folds (this is not seen at other synapses). A thick basement membrane is secreted by the sarcolemma. The synaptic cleft between the neuronal membrane and the sarcolemma's basement membrane measures about 4 nm. (C) Electron micrograph of frog neuromuscular junction. The presynaptic terminal of the motor neuron is in the upper left part of the micrograph and the muscle fibre in the lower right. The sarcolemma of the muscle fibre is thrown into junctional folds and the basement membrane is well shown as are the synaptic vesicles in the presynaptic ending. (Micrograph produced by Dr John E. Heuser of Washington University School of Medicine, St Louis, Mo. Reprinted with permission.)

C

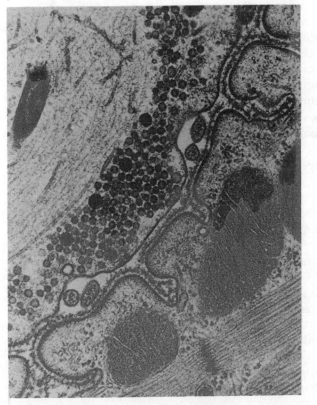

Figure 14.16(C) shows an electron micrograph of the frog neuromuscular junction. The transmitter vesicles are very well shown. Each contains from 1000 to 10 000 molecules of ACh and there may be up to and sometimes more than a million vesicles in a presynaptic terminal. The axoplasm behind the cluster of vesicles can be seen to contain dense accumulations of cytoskeletal elements. This is called the **presynaptic network**.

It can be shown that transmitter vesicles are continuously bumping into the presynaptic membrane and voiding their contents into the synaptic gap. This causes small depolarisations in the subsynaptic membrane. These small depolarisation are called **miniature end-plate potentials (MEPPs)**. This terminology applies only to the neuromuscular junction, where the subsynaptic membrane is called the **motor end plate**. The same phenomenon probably also occurs at central synapses. However, it is only when the presynaptic terminal is depolarised by an action potential that a large population of vesicles fuse with the presynaptic membrane and release their contents. It is only when this occurs that a major effect is exerted on the subsynaptic cell.

Figure 14.17 shows freeze-fracture preparations of the presynaptic membrane of a neuromuscular junction. The specimen has been prepared in such a way that we are looking up at the outer surface of the inner leaflet (PF face) of the terminal as if we were sitting on the postsynaptic membrane. Figure 14.17(A) shows the membrane in the resting state, Figure 14.17(B) 5 ms after stimulation and 14.17(C) several tens of milliseconds later. The interpretation of these remarkable images is as follows. The rows and scatterings of granules in Figure 14.17(A) represent intramembrane proteins—possibly calcium-channel proteins or, alternatively, evidence of internal ridges which guide vesicles to appropriate regions of membrane (see below). The large craters in Figure 14.17(B) indicate where synaptic vesicles have fused and voided their contents into the synaptic gap. The somewhat smaller depressions in Figure 14.17(C) represent regions where membrane is being retrieved after exocytosis has terminated.

These electron micrographs help us visualise the mechanisms at work in the presynaptic terminal. Let us consider them in sequence.

In the previous section we left our synaptic vesicles 'rowing' their way down microtubules to the synaptic terminal. In Section 14.2 we noted that when vesicles were packaged in the perikaryon they often became caged in clathrin basket-works. It has been shown furthermore that clathrin and coated vesicles co-purify with axonal microtubules. It looks as if at least some vesicles are attached to the kinesin 'rowing arms' through their clathrin coats. Clathrin, of course, is not neuron-specific. It is found in most secretory cells. Another 'coat' protein, however, does seem

Figure 14.17   Freeze-fracture replicas of the presynaptic membrane of frog neuromuscular junction. (A) EM shows the membrane 3 ms after the nerve had been stimulated. The double row of particles may represent the undersurface of the dense bars which delimit an 'active zone'. For further explanation see text. (B) EM shows the presynaptic membrane 5 ms after stimulation. Large pits (one of which is arrowed) adjacent to the parallel rows of particles are visible. These are believed to represent the sites where synaptic vesicles have fused with the membrane and voided their contents. (C) EM shows the membrane 50 ms after stimulation. Shallow depressions with large numbers of intramembranous particles are common. These are believed to represent the final stages in the retrieval of the membrane after exocytosis (see Fig. 14.19). The freeze-fracture EMs are of the PF faces of the membrane (see Fig. 6.11). (From Heuser and Reese, 1979, in *The Neurosciences: Fourth Study Program*, eds. F.O. Schmitt and F.G. Worden, Cambridge, Mass.: MIT Press, pp. 573–600; with permission.)

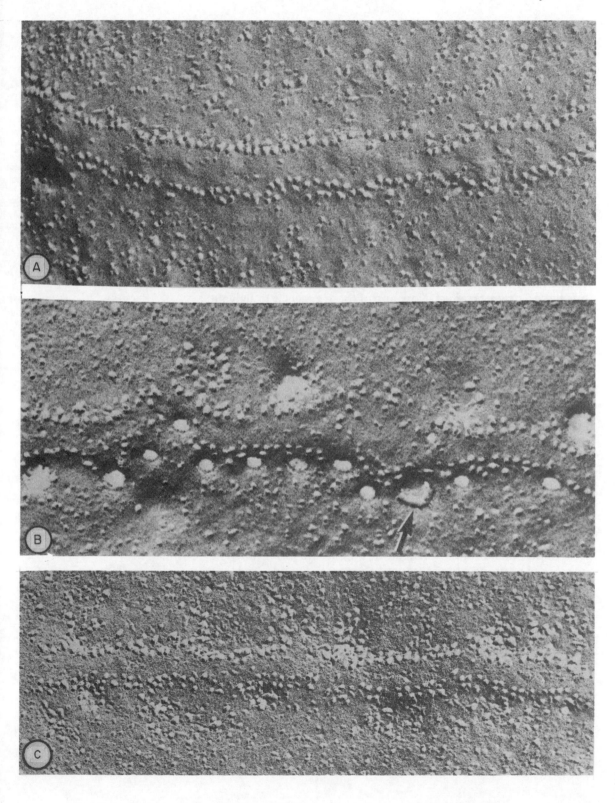

to be restricted to neurons. This is **synapsin 1**. This protein (a dimer of synapsin 1_a (86 kDa) and synapsin 1_b (80 kDa)) appears to form a protein coat specifically around the small (50 nm) vesicles. It is present in large quantites in synaptic terminals.

Now synapsin 1 is biochemically almost identical to the band 4.1 protein of the erythrocyte submembranous cytoskeleton (Figure 6.19). It will be recalled from Chapter 6 that the band 4.1 protein binds both to spectrin and to the intramembranous band 3 protein. We also noted in Chapter 6 that presynaptic terminals contained high concentrations of fodrin, a spectrin-like protein. Could it be that synapsin plays a similar role to that of band 4.1? Could it be, in other words, that it bridges between the lipoprotein wall of the vesicle and one of the cytoskeletal elements which, as we noted above, are so well represented in the terminal?

Next we need to return to the triggering function of calcium ions. We noted in Chapter 10 that free Ca^{2+} ions are in very short supply within cells. Any influx of Ca^{2+} from outside can thus have a dramatic effect. Now one of these effects is to activate several kinase enzymes within the terminal. Two of these Ca^{2+}-dependent kinases are known to phosphorylate synapsin 1. One of these kinases phosphorylates synapsin 1 in such a way that its affinity for vesicle membrane is greatly reduced.

Thus we seem to have a chain of events by which an influx of Ca^{2+} ions leads to the removal of a vesicle's synapsin coat. The disrobed or, at least, 'desynapsinated', vesicle is then free to migrate toward the interior surface of the presynaptic membrane, fuse, and release its contents. At the time of writing this series of events remains speculative. It indicates, however, how research in different parts of molecular biology is beginning to come together and point the way towards an understanding of some of the crucial phenomena of neurobiology.

Let us now turn our attention to this release. Figure 14.16(C) shows the synaptic vesicles thronging close to the P face of the presynaptic membrane. If instead of a neuromuscular junction we were to examine a typical central synapse we would find that the vesicles were ordered by a **presynaptic grid**. This grid is formed of dense projections springing from the presynaptic membrane and pointing inwards into the synaptic interior (Figure 14.18). The projections are bound together by fine filaments and form a highly ordered network on the P face of the presynaptic membrane. The 'design element' seems to be a hexagon. Six triangular spaces surround each projection and these are probably membrane areas specialised for the attachment of synaptic vesicles. Indeed freeze-fracture preparations show hexagonal arrays of intramembranous particles in the P face of the presynaptic membrane. It is tempting to conclude that these particles surround one of the dense projections of the presynaptic

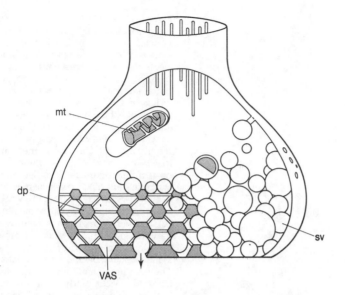

Figure 14.18: Organisation of pre-synaptic grid within a central synapse. The regular hexagonal structure of the presynaptic grid is shown in this diagram. Each triangular space constitutes a 'vesicle attachment site' (VAS) upon which the synaptic vesicles can dock and through which they can void their contents into the synaptic cleft. The triangular spaces surround a regular array of dense projections (dp) in a hexagonal pattern. sv = synaptic vesicle; mt = mitochondrion. (From Akert *et al*, 1972, in *Structure and Function of Synapses*, eds. G.D. Pappas and G.D. Purpura, New York: Raven Press, pp. 67–86; with permission.)

grid and provide points of attachment for transmitter vesicles. In consequence they have been termed **vesicle attachment sites (VAS)**.

Neuromuscular junctions do not show the intricate ultra-structural organisation of central synapses. Instead they sometimes show dense bars opposite the junctional folds of the subsynaptic membrane. The membrane adjacent to these bars is called an **active zone**. It is here that the vesicles fuse to the membrane. It may be, as suggested above, that the lines of intramembranous particles in Figure 14.17(A) represent the foundations of these bars. Figure 14.17(B) appears to show that the exocytotic craters lie alongside these particle lines—as would be expected if the theory of active zones is correct.

The naked vesicle attaches at an appropriate patch of presynaptic membrane—either VAS or active zone. The vesicle's membrane fuses with the presynaptic membrane. This process is also thought to be strongly calcium-dependent. Finally the contents of the vesicle are expelled into the synaptic gap.

It can be shown that the lipoprotein elements of the exocytosing vesicle's membrane mix intimately with the lipoprotein of the presynaptic membrane. Indeed the vesicle's proteins can be shown to diffuse rapidly (diffusion constant $\sim 2 \times 10^{-10}$ cm^2 s^{-1}) away into the presynaptic membrane. However, they are not lost. Within about 10 s after exocytosis **coated pits** begin to appear. This means that the presynaptic membrane begins to invaginate in association with a coat protein—usually synapsin 1, but in other cases probably clathrin. It is believed that the vesicle proteins are recognised by synapsin 1 (or clathrin) and that this induces the endocytosis.

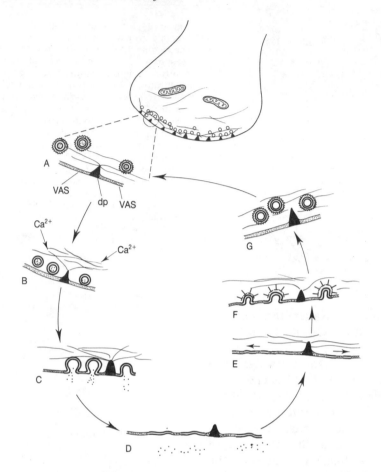

Figure 14.19 Cycle of exocytosis and endocytosis at a synapse. (A) Synaptic vesicles surrounded by clathrin and/or synapsin 'coats' are attached to fibrous elements of the presynaptic grid. (B) Invasion of the terminal by an action potential leads to a sudden transient influx of Ca^{2+} ions. This leads to the 'disrobing' of the synaptic vesicles, which are then free to move to the vesicle attachment sites (VAS) in the presynaptic membrane. (C) The vesicle membranes fuse with the VAS and their neurotransmitter contents are voided into the synaptic cleft. (D) The vesicle membrane begins to diffuse away from the VAS into other parts of the presynaptic membrane. (E) The vesicle membrane continues to move laterally. (F) The vesicle membrane protein is recognised by clathrin and/or synapsin 1 and begins to invaginate. (G) The membrane has fully invaginated as a coated vesicle, ready for reattachment to the presynaptic grid and refilling with neurotransmitter or for transmission back up the axon as a multivesicular body. The reconstituted and refilled vesicle awaits another exocytosis-endocytosis cycle. VAS = vesicle attachment site; dp = dense projection

Once within the presynaptic terminal the vesicle is refilled with neurotransmitter ready for another synaptic event. In other cases, where the transmitter is not synthesised in the terminal but in the perikaryon, the vesicle is moved back along the axon in the retrograde transport stream. Such vesicles normally fuse together to form a **multivesicular body**. Multivesicular bodies can often be seen in the perikarya of active neurons. We shall consider the syntheses of transmitter and modulator molecules in the next chapter.

Although it has taken a long time to describe, the response of a synaptic terminal is in fact extremely rapid. The turning on and off of transmitter release occurs in less than a millisecond. This is because of the extremely efficient mechanisms which the synaptic terminal has for mopping up any free calcium ions. These mechanisms include sequestration in mitochondria, in cisternae of ER (if this is present), and perhaps most importantly by the ubiquitous calcium binding protein, **calmodulin**. Once free calcium ions are removed the trigger for vesicle fusion and exocytosis is eliminated. The synaptic terminal returns to its resting state.

Finally it should be borne in mind that the release of transmitters and modulators from synaptic terminals is quite commonly under the control of so-called **axo-axonic** synapses. These are synapses made by other neurons directly on a synaptic terminal such as we have been considering (Figure 14.20). The operation of such synapses can modulate the release of transmitter by the 'subsynaptic synapse'. This modulation may be brought about through second messenger systems (cAMP, etc.) or directly by depolarising or hyperpolarising the subsynaptic membrane. We shall consider these complexities more fully in Chapter 16, where we examine the structure and functioning of synapses.

Figure 14.20   Axo-axonic synapse

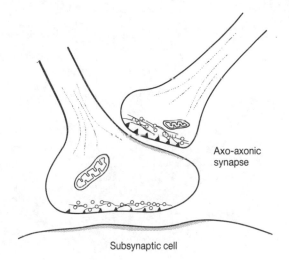

Axo-axonic
synapse

Subsynaptic cell

14.5 CONCLUSION

In this chapter we have seen how material elaborated in neuronal perikarya is moved along axons to their terminal boutons and finally secreted into the synaptic cleft. It should be borne in mind that material will also be moving out along the dendrites. This latter transport is not nearly so well known nor so intense. For the material arriving at the axon terminal has the all-important function of communicating with the subsynaptic cell—neuron or muscle. Our next task, therefore, is to look at the nature of the neurotransmitters, the neuromodulators, their associated enzymes, inhibitors, re-uptake mechanisms etc., which make the presynaptic terminal such a busy and interesting place.

Chapter 15
Neurotransmitters and neuromodulators

In Chapter 14 we noted how secretory and other molecules were synthesised in the neuron's perikaryon and then transported to be released from or incorporated into the synaptic ending. In this chapter we shall look at the nature of some of the secretory molecules which are released into the synaptic gap. It should be noted that far from all such molecules are elaborated in the perikaryon and transported down the axon. Many, as we shall see, are synthesised and resynthesised in the terminal. The enzymes required for this synthesis and the lipoprotein-based mechanisms responsible for their release and re uptake do, however, require the protein synthetic apparatus of the perikaryon. Axoplasmic transport provides a vital communication channel between perikaryon and synapse.

Only a decade or so ago no more than about half a dozen synaptic transmitters were recognised. The old telephone exchange metaphor of the brain predominated (see Chapter 14). The brain was 'seen' as a huge number of 'hard' wires and junctions. The wires were the axons, the junctions the synapses. We noted in Chapter 1 that there are some 10^{11} of the former and some 10^{14} of the latter. It was believed that there was quite sufficient complexity in these numbers to account for the activity of the brain. The synapses only needed to be on/off switches, like the on/off units of the digital computer.

In the late 1980s there has been a dramatic shift in our perceptions. The telephone exchange/computer analogy is now seen to be only (at best) a first approximation. We saw in Chapter 1 how many different types of synaptic apposition are developed in the brain: not only axo-dendritic and axo-somatic, but also axo-axonic, dendro-dendritic and, perhaps most significant of all, axonal 'varicosities' which allow 'en passant' release of neuroactive molecules. The latter substances may diffuse through the brain's intercellular space (perhaps for several millimetres) until they reach an appropriate membrane receptor through which to exert their action. Synapses themselves are, moreover, very far from being simple yes/no logic elements. This recognition has been one of the most important outcomes of work in molecular neurobiology. Finally instead of the half-dozen or so transmitters of a decade ago neurobiologists now recognise **50** or so different molecules and the number is still rising (see Table 15.1).

Neuroactive molecules are often divided into two categories: **neurotransmitters** and **neuromodulators**. The distinction has to do with their synaptic activity. Neurotransmitters have a direct effect on a subsynaptic membrane (this, in the case of varicosities, may be at some distance from the presynaptic membrane) whilst neuromodulators 'modulate' or 'regulate' the action of trans-mitters. This they may do by affecting the transmitter sensitivity of the subsynaptic membrane or by influencing the release of transmitter from the presynaptic terminal. Neurotransmitters, themselves, may be divided into two categories, sometimes called **ionotropic** and **metabotropic** depending on whether they act directly to open ion pores (Chapter 9) or operate through a collision-coupling system in the subsynaptic membrane (Chapter 7).

It must be noted straight away, however, that the distinction between neurotransmitters and neuromodulators is far from sharp. The same synaptically active molecule can at some synapses act as a transmitter and at others as a modulator. The distinction between ionotropic and metabotropic transmitters is also indistinct. A transmitter may have an ionotropic action on one subsynaptic membrane and a metabotropic action on another. We have already met a type example of this in acetylcholine. We saw that its nicotinic action is an extremely rapid ($\sim$ 10 μs) opening of an ion channel leading to a membrane depolarisation, whilst its muscarinic action is much more long-lasting and involves a collision-coupling and cAMP second-messenger system. It is not just the presynaptic ending and its contents which define the nature of the synapse. The subsynaptic membrane is equally, if not more, important.

We shall look at the molecular neurobiology of subsynaptic membranes in Chapter 16. In the present chapter we shall focus our attention on the pharmacology of the more important neuro-transmitters/neuromodulators. We shall find that they fall into a number of natural groups. **Acetylcholine** (the first to be discovered) still stands to an extent in a class of its own; next there is a group of **amino acid** transmitters, some of which are excitatory whilst others are inhibitory; biochemically related to the amino acids are the **indoleamines** such as serotonin and the **catecholamines**, of which noradrenaline is perhaps the best-known example; last, but not least, there is a large (and growing)

Table 15.1   Neurotransmitters and neuromodulators

Acetylcholine (ACh)

Amino acids

Glutamate; aspartate; glycine

Amino acid derivatives

(a) Derived from tryptophan: indoleamines—serotonin

(b) Derived from phenylalanine: catecholamines—dopamine;
norepinephrine; epinephrine, octopamine

(c) Derived from glycine: taurine

(d) Derived from glutamate: γ-Aminobutyric acid (GABA)

(e) Derived from histidine: histamine

Purines

Adenosine

Peptides

(a) Opioid: enkephalins; β-endorphin; dynorphin

(b) Neurohypophyseal: vasopressin, oxytocin, neurophysins

(c) Tachykinins: substance P (SP); substance K (SK) (= neurokinin A
(NKA)); neurokinin B (NKB); kassinin; eledoisin

(d) Gastrins: gastrin; cholecytokinins (CCKs)

(e) Somatostatins: stomatostatin 14; somatostatin 28

(f) Glucagon-related: vasoactive intestinal polypeptide (VIP)

(g) Pancreatic-polypeptide related: neuropeptide Y (NPY)

(h) Miscellaneous: bombesin; neurotensin (NT); bradykinin;
angiotensin; calcitonin gene-related peptide (CGRP)

Partly after Cooper, Bloom and Roth (1985); for formulae of neuropeptides see
Table 2.2

group of neuroactive **peptides**. In addition to these established
transmitters and modulators there are a number of molecules
which are found in the brain and probably have some synaptic
activity. Such molecules include **histamine, purines** such as
adenosine and adenosine triphosphate, some **phenethylamine**

derivatives, for example octamine and tyramine, and so on. We shall not discuss this last group of putative transmitters further.

Before discussing the groups of established transmitters and modulators it is important to list some of the criteria which should be met by any molecule suspected of synaptic activity. For, after all, synaptic endings contain a great variety of substances and there is no reason to suspect that they all play a role at the synaptic junction. A list of appropriate criteria is given in Box 15.1.

Box 15.1 Criteria for neurotransmitters

1. The molecule must be synthesised within the neuron from which it is released. Enzymes and substrates for its synthesis must be found in that neuron

2. The molecule must be stored within the neuron from which it is released

3. Presynaptic stimulation (usually, but not necessarily, electrical) must lead to the release of the molecule

4. Controlled application of the molecule at the appropriate site should elicit the same postsynaptic response as presynaptic stimulation

5. Agents which block the postsynaptic response to presynaptic stimulation should also block the response to exogenously applied putative transmitter

6. The postsynaptic response to the putative transmitter molecule when exogenously applied must be terminated rapidly

7. The suspected molecule must behave identically to the endogenous transmitter with respect to pharmacological potentiation, inhibition, inactivation, etc.

15.1 ACETYLCHOLINE

Acetylcholine is synthesised in synaptic terminals from **choline** and **acetate**. The latter is derived from **acetyl-coenzyme A**. Choline, on the other hand, is partly obtained by re-uptake from the synaptic gap and partly from the blood, where some of it is transported partly as **free choline** and some as the phospholipid **phosphatidylcholine**. Acetyl-coenzyme A is derived from glucose through glycolysis.

The synthesis (as shown in Figure 15.1) is catalysed by **choline acetyltransferase (CAT)**. This enzyme provides a much used marker for cholinergic synapses. One of the ways of detecting

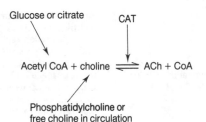

Figure 15.1   Synthesis of acetylcholine.
Explanation see text

CAT within the brain involves the techniques of immunohisto-chemistry. First CAT is extracted and purified. Next antibodies are raised against it in another organism such as a rabbit. This anti-CAT antibody is reacted with CAT in the tissue section. Next it is necessary to produce a marker which can be identified in the microscope. This is usually done by coupling a fluorescent molecule, such as **fluoroscein**, to yet another antibody. This anti-body is prepared by injecting rabbit serum proteins into, say, a goat. The anti-rabbit antibody is then coupled with fluorescein. Finally this fluorescently labelled anti-rabbit antibody is reacted with the tissue section. It attaches itself to the only rabbit protein present in the section, which happens to be the anti-CAT anti-body. The location of CAT in the CNS can then be determined by the fluorescence microscope. Figure 15.2 shows the sequence of steps in this immunohistochemical technique diagrammatically.

There are a number of other ways of determining the presence of cholinergic synapses in the brain. These range from Koelle and Friedenwald's histochemical technique for localising the enzyme acetylcholinesterase, to electrical recording from suspected cells after iontophoretic release of acetylcholine. The cholinergic pathways revealed by these techniques are shown in Figure 15.3. The majority of the cell bodies are located in midbrain nuclei: the **basal nucleus of Meynert**, the **diagonal band nucleus of Broca**, the **nucleus preopticus magnocellularis**. Axons course up from these basal regions to innervate the neocortex and especially the hippocampus. We shall see in Chapter 19 that Alzheimer's disease seems especially to affect cholinergic neurons. The fact that the hippocampus receives such a strong cholinergic input and that this region of the brain has long been regarded as involved in short-term memory may account for one of the most obvious symptoms of Alzheimer's disease: loss of memory.

We have already considered aspects of the cholinergic synapse in previous chapters. In particular we looked in depth at the nature and operation of both nicotinic and muscarinic acetyl-choline receptors. We noted that there were different subtypes of both types of ACh receptor. In Section 2.1 we considered the molecular nature of the acetylcholinesterase enzyme which plays

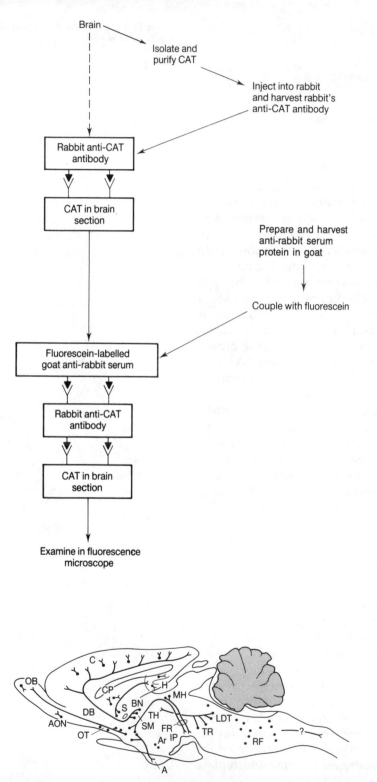

Figure 15.2 An immunohistochemical technique for locating CAT in the CNS. This 'sandwich technique' is just one of many ways of localising CAT in the brain. First an anti-CAT antibody is raised in, for example, a rabbit and reacted with the CAT in the tissue section. This complex, in turn, is reacted with a fluorescein labelled anti-rabbit serum from a goat. The resultant complex can be visualised in the fluorescence microscope

Figure 15.3 Cholinergic pathways in the rat brain (parasagittal section). A = amygdala; AON = anterior olfactory nucleus; Ar = arcuate nucleus; BN = nucleus basalis of Meynert; C = cerebral cortex; CP = caudate putamen; DB = diagonal band nucleus of Broca; FR = fasciculus retroflexus; H = hippocampus; IP = nucleus interpeduncularis; LDT = lateral dorsal tegmental nucleus; MH = medial habenula; OB = olfactory bulb; OT = olfactory tubercle; RF = reticular formation; SM = stria medullaris; TH = thalamus; TR = tegmental reticular formation. (From Cuello and Sofroniew, 1984, *Trends in Neurosciences*, 7 74–78; with permission.)

so vital a role in inactivating ACh once it has exerted its effect on the subsynaptic membrane. It but remains to put these various elements together into an overall picture of the synapse. This is done in Figure 15.4.

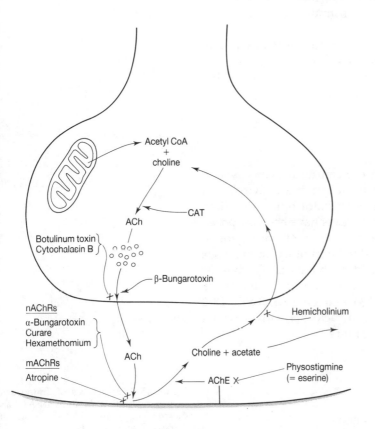

Figure 15.4 Pharmacology of the cholinergic synapse. Acetyl CoA is derived from mitochondrial metabolism. Choline acetyltransferase (CAT) catalyses the formation of ACh. β-Bungarotoxin promotes and botulinum toxin and cytochalasin-B block the release of ACh into the synaptic cleft. α-Bungarotoxin, curare and hexamethomium block nicotinic receptors while atropine blocks muscarinic receptors. Acetylcholinesterase (AChE) breaks ACh into choline and acetate. AChE is inhibited by physostigmine. Whereas acetate escapes ultimately into the circulation choline is taken back into the terminal. This re-uptake is blocked by hemicholinium

Figure 15.4 indicates some of the more important drugs which affect the operation of this synapse. It must be emphasised that very far from all the pharmacological agents which influence cholinergic synapses are shown in the figure. Readers interested in neuropharmacology should consult one of the texts listed in the bibliography for more complete information. The figure shows, however, that drugs can effect (a) the release of ACh from the presynaptic terminal, (b) the subsynaptic ACh receptor (because nicotinic and muscarinic receptors are radically different they have a very different pharmacology), (c) the action of acetylcholinesterase, (d) the re-uptake of choline by the presynaptic terminal.

Figure 15.4 shows the nAChRs and mAChRs on the subsynaptic membrane. In central cholinergic synapses there is evidence that both these receptors are also present on the presynaptic membrane. In particular there is evidence that presynaptic muscarinic receptors work through their G-protein collision-coupling mechanism (see Chapter 7) to down-regulate the release of ACh from the presynaptic terminal. We shall see that feedback control of the release of transmitter is a very general feature of synaptic physiology.

Finally it should be borne in mind that the most intensively investigated cholinergic synapses lie outside the central nervous system, either in the autonomic nervous system or at the neuromuscular junction of skeletal muscle.

15.2 AMINO ACIDS

A number of amino acids found in the central nervous system satisfy at least a majority of the criteria for synaptic activity listed in Box 15.1. In most cases their actions are ionotropic rather than metabotropic. Although some 15 amino acids have been proposed as neurotransmitters only four have so far met with general acceptance. There are two acknowledged excitatory amino acids (EAAs): **glutamic acid** and **aspartic acid**. Both have two carboxylic acid groups. There are two accepted inhibitory amino acids (IAAs): **γ-aminobutyric acid (GABA)** and **glycine**. Table 15.2 shows the other amino acids and amino acid derivatives which have been proposed as neurotransmitters.

Excitatory amino acids (EAAs)

Glutamic acid

$$NH_3^+ - \overset{\displaystyle H}{\underset{\displaystyle CH_2}{C}} - COO^-$$
$$CH_2$$
$$COO^-$$

Aspartic acid

$$NH_3^+ - \overset{\displaystyle H}{\underset{\displaystyle CH_2}{C}} - COO^-$$
$$COO^-$$

Inhibitory amino acids (IAAs)

γ-Amino butyric acid (GABA)

$$NH_3^+ - CH_2 - CH_2 - CH_2 - COO^-$$

Glycine

$$NH_3^+ - CH_2 - COO^-$$

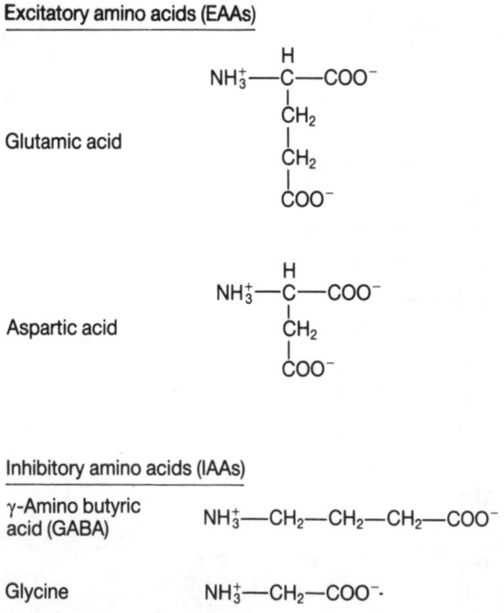

Figure 15.5 Structures of amino acid neurotransmitters. Note that EAAs are dicarboxylic whilst IAAs are monocarboxylic amino acids

Table 15.2 Amino acid neurotransmitters

Excitatory	Inhibitory
Glutamic acid	γ-Aminobutyric acid (GABA)
Aspartic acid	Glycine
- - - - - - - - - - - - - -	- - - - - - - - - - - - - - -
Cysteine	Taurine
Cysteine – sulphonic acid	β-Alanine

Amino acids below the broken line have yet to satisfy all the criteria of Box 15.1. Nevertheless there is some evidence that they have a transmitter activity

15.2.1 Excitatory amino acids (EAAs): glutamic acid and aspartic acid

Both glutamic and aspartic acids are non-essential amino acids which are synthesised from glucose and other precursors in the Krebs cycle. This cycle takes place in synaptic mitochondria. It is from one of the intermediates in the cycle—either oxaloacetate or α-ketoglutarate—that aspartate and glutamate are derived.

Both aspartate and glutamate are widely distributed in the central nervous system. Iontophoretic application of very small amounts of either amino acid (10^{-15} M in the case of glutamate; aspartate is somewhat less potent) leads to an almost instantaneous depolarisation of the subsynaptic membranes of virtually all neurons. Reference to section 9.4 shows that the membrane receptors for these ionotropic responses are classified by means of their pharmacological agonists and antagonists. We saw that K (kainate) and Q (quisqualate) receptors were the two most important.

We also noted in Chapter 9 that another type of glutamate receptor existed in the brain: the NMDA receptor. We saw that this, although an ionotropic receptor, has a slower and more complicated response to activation by EAAs. NMDA receptors are particularly strongly represented in the hippocampus and the cerebellum. We shall consider their putative significance in these regions in Chapter 18.

It appears that aspartate and glutamate, once released into the synapse, are rapidly taken up by a high-affinity transport system in the aspartaminergic and glutaminergic nerve endings and also by adjacent glial cells. Within glial cells glutamate is transformed into glutamine by glutamine synthetase and then transferred back

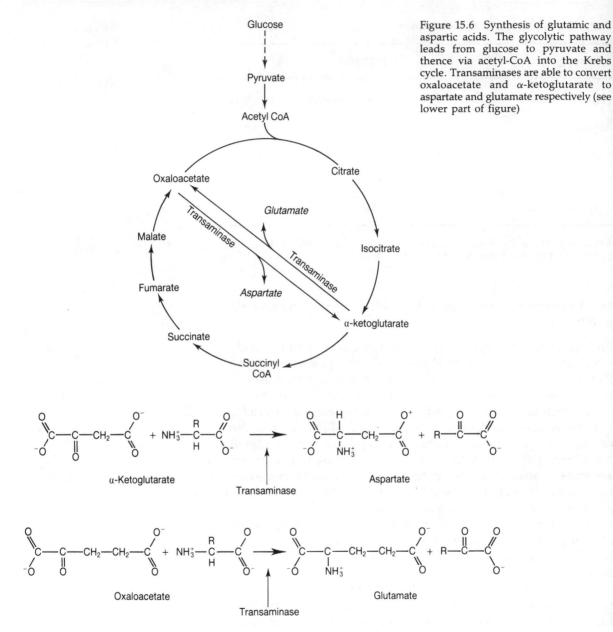

Figure 15.6 Synthesis of glutamic and aspartic acids. The glycolytic pathway leads from glucose to pyruvate and thence via acetyl-CoA into the Krebs cycle. Transaminases are able to convert oxaloacetate and α-ketoglutarate to aspartate and glutamate respectively (see lower part of figure)

into the glutaminergic nerve ending, where it is deaminated once more to glutamate. This pathway is shown in Figure 15.7. A similar biochemistry obtains for aspartate, which appears to share the same uptake system.

Because of their seemingly ubiquitous distribution in the brain it has been difficult to locate specifically glutaminergic or aspartatergic pathways. It is, however, possible to home in on aspartatergic neurons by making use of the fact that its high-

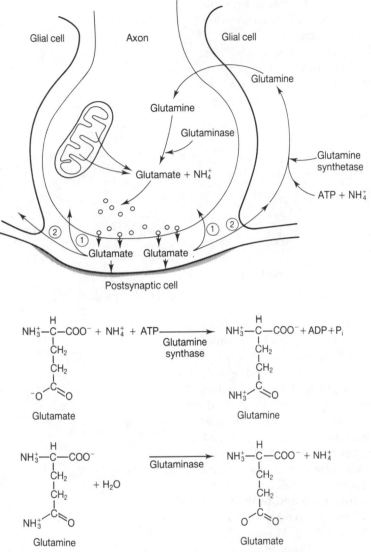

Figure 15.7 Glutaminergic synapse. Glutamate is released from synaptic vesicles into the synaptic cleft. Two re-uptake paths are shown: (1) back into the synaptic terminal; (2) into neighbouring glial cells. In glial cells glutamine synthetase forms glutamine from the glutamate and this then passes back into the synaptic terminal. Here glutaminase reforms glutamate and this forms a pool of free glutamate with fresh glutamate derived from Krebs cycle activity in mitochondria. The free glutamate is sequestrated into synaptic vesicles to await the arrival of the next action potential. The reactions catalysed by glutamine synthetase and glutaminase are shown in the lower part of the figure

affinity uptake system will carry *d-aspartate*, which once in the cell is not further metabolised. Radiolabelled *d*-aspartate can thus be used to locate aspartatergic synapses. Sectioning of nerve pathways coupled with observations of the loss of this high-affinity uptake system and the diminution of aspartate and/or glutamate has thus been used to trace EAA pathways.

15.2.2 Inhibitory amino acids: γ-aminobutyric acid and glycine

γ-aminobutyric acid (GABA). GABA is found throughout the CNS of both vertebrates and invertebrates. In the vertebrates its concentration is greater than the perhaps better known neurotransmitters acetylcholine and noradrenaline. Perhaps 25–45% of all nerve terminals contain this transmitter.

GABA is formed by the decarboxylation of glutamate by **glutamic acid decarboxylase (GAD)**. The enzyme is present in the cytosol of GABA-ergic terminals. The reaction is shown in Figure 15.8.

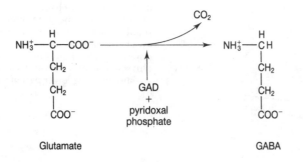

Figure 15.8 Synthesis of GABA from glutamate. GAD (glutamic acid decarboxylase) requires pyridoxal phosphate as a co-enzyme

GAD allows the synaptic terminals of GABA-ergic neurons to be identified histologically. The technique is, in essence, the same as that described above for CAT-containing terminals. Antibodies raised against the enzyme can be coupled with markers which can then be located in thin or ultra-thin sections of the CNS either with the light or the electron microscope. Again, as with cholinergic synapses, iontophoretic release of GABA and electrophysiological recording of the response have also been employed to complement the immunohistochemistry.

GABA-ergic synapses have been identified in many regions of the brain. They are found in the retina, cerebellum, cerebral cortex, hippocampus, thalamus, olfactory bulb and in the basal ganglia. Indeed there is evidence that loss of GABA synapses in the brain's basal ganglia is one of the factors in **Huntingdon's chorea**. We shall see later that other transmitters may also be involved. The symptoms of the condition—sudden uncontrollable movements of the body, especially the limbs—is likely to be due to the development of imbalances between excitatory and inhibitory synapses in some of the basal ganglia. For it is known that in some instances (see later) these ganglia contain the motor programs which control bodily movements.

Turning to the GABA-ergic synapse itself it can be demonstrated that release of GABA into the synaptic cleft results in a hyperpolarisation of the subsynaptic membrane. Pharmacological evidence shows that there are two types of GABA receptor: **GABA$_A$** and **GABA$_B$** receptors. The GABA$_A$ receptor is blocked by bicuculline and picrotoxin. These blockers have, in contrast, no effect on GABA_B receptors. Instead, another agent, baclofen, is found to act as a selective agonist of these receptors. We discussed the GABA_A receptor in detail in Chapter 9. We noted that it had a strong affinity for the benzodiazepines. These so-called 'anxiolytic' (i.e anxiety-reducing) drugs enhance the activity of GABA-ergic synapses by increasing (in some as yet unknown way) the ability of GABA to open its chloride channel. It is believed that the GABA_A receptors are found on the **subsynaptic** membranes of 'classical' inhibitory synapses. In contrast there is evidence that in many cases (not all) GABA_B receptors are located on **presynaptic** membranes.

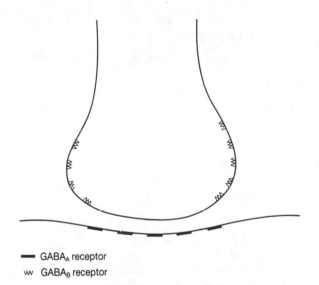

Figure 15.9 Differential location of GABA_A and GABA_B receptors

— GABA_A receptor
w GABA_B receptor

The presynaptic location of the GABA_B receptor suggests that it is involved in presynaptic inhibition. There is also evidence that unlike the GABA_A receptor it is metabotropic in action. It is believed to work through a G-protein collision-coupling mechanism to **inhibit** membrane-bound adenylate cyclase. The consequent reduction in intraterminal cAMP is in turn believed to reduce the amount of GABA released when the terminal is invaded by an action potential. We have already noted that an analogous feedback control of transmitter release is found in central cholinergic synapses and we shall see that similar mechanisms are at work in other well-known types of synapse.

Re-uptake of GABA is similar to that of the excitatory amino acids mentioned above. There are powerful uptake systems (Na⁺-dependent) in both GABA nerve terminals and in surrounding glial cells. Much of the recycled GABA is probably directly re-usable. A proportion, however, is converted to succinic semialdehyde by the mitochondrial enzyme **GABA aminotransferase (GABA-T)**. As Figure 15.10 shows this is believed to occur in both synaptic terminals and glia. The succinic semialdehyde enters the Krebs cycle from which GABA can once again be obtained via oxaloacetic and glutamic acid.

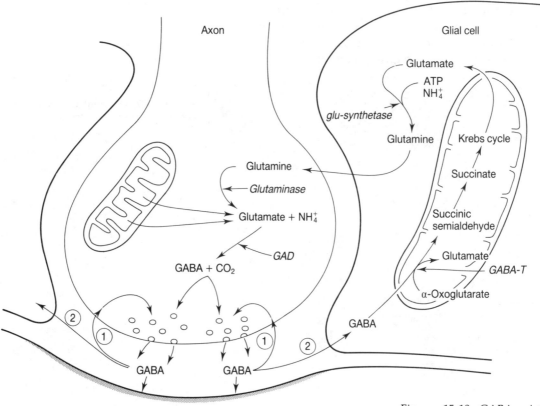

Postsynaptic cell

Figure 15.10 GABAergic synapse. GABA is released from synaptic vesicles into the synaptic cleft. Two re-uptake paths are shown: (1) back into the synaptic terminal; (2) into neighbouring glial cells. In the mitochondria of glial cells GABA is converted by GABA aminotransferase (GABA-T) to succinic semialdehyde. This enters the Krebs cycle, from which glutamate (Fig. 15.6) emerges. Glutamine synthetase (glu-synthetase) convertes glutamate to glutamine and this is taken up by the synaptic terminal. Under the influence of glutaminase and GAD glutamine is converted first to glutamate and then to GABA, which is sequestered once again in vesicles. Further supplies of glutamate are available from Krebs cycle intermediates in presynaptic mitochondria

Glycine. Glycine is the other well-established inhibitory amino acid transmitter. Unlike GABA, glycine is mostly restricted to the **spinal cord** and **brain stem**. Glycine is, of course, one of the commonest of amino acids and its small size ensures that it can pass the blood – brain barrier with ease. In the CNS it is derived from serine by the action of serine transhydroxymethylase.

Glycine is probably stored (like GABA) in small elliptical vesicles in presynaptic terminals. Release of the transmitter induces rapid hyperpolarisation of the subsynaptic membrane. A high-affinity Na^+-dependent re-uptake system exists which pumps glycine back from the synaptic cleft into nerve terminals and glial cells.

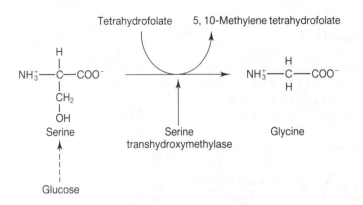

Figure 15.11 Synthesis of glycine. Most neural glycine is formed from serine by a folate-dependent reaction catalysed by serine transhydroxymethylase. Serine itself is derived from glucose via 3-phospho-*d*-glycerate and 3-phospho-serine; glycine may, in addition, be formed from neural peptides and proteins

We discussed the molecular structure of the glycine receptor in Section 9.3 and noted that it is competitively blocked by **strychnine**. Small doses of strychnine thus cause enhanced reflex responses whilst large doses result in generalised motor dis-inhibition and general convulsions. Death is caused by dis-inhibition of the respiratory muscles and hence asphyxia.

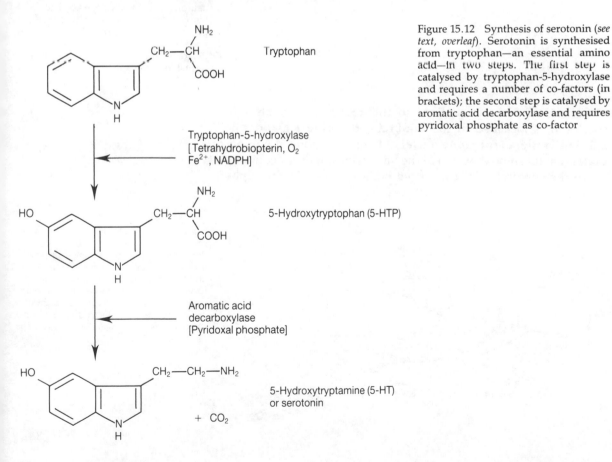

Figure 15.12 Synthesis of serotonin (*see text, overleaf*). Serotonin is synthesised from tryptophan—an essential amino acid—in two steps. The first step is catalysed by tryptophan-5-hydroxylase and requires a number of co-factors (in brackets); the second step is catalysed by aromatic acid decarboxylase and requires pyridoxal phosphate as co-factor

15.3 SEROTONIN
(= 5-HYDROXYTRYPTAMINE, 5-HT)

Figure 15.12 shows that serotonin is synthesised from tryptophan via the intermediate 5-hydroxytryptophan. The synthesis requires two enzymes—**tryptophan hydroxylase** and **aromatic amino acid decarboxylase**. The first step in the sequence is rate-limiting.

Serotonin can be localised in the brain by reacting the tissue with formaldehyde vapour. Serotonin is converted into 6-hydroxy-3,4-dihydrocarboline which, when illuminated in the ultraviolet (λ = 390 nm), gives a strong yellow-green fluorescence (λ = 520 nm). The reaction is shown in Figure 15.13. The technique can be made yet more specific by eliminating any fluorescence from catecholaminergic neurons by the prior application of the catecholaminergic-specific neurotoxin 6-hydroxydopamine (6-OHDA).

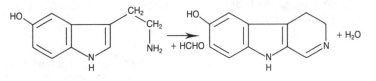

Serotonin + Formaldehyde → 3,4-Dihydro-β-carboline + Water

(Yellow fluorescence)

Figure 15.13 Reaction of serotonin with formaldehyde vapour. This technique for detecting the presence of serotoninergic neurons was first developed by Falck and his co-workers in the early 1960s. To prevent the diffusion and enhance the reaction the tissue is normally freeze-dried before exposing it to dry formaldehyde vapour

Subjection of brain sections to this technique reveals that serotonin is localised in the **midbrain**, the **pineal gland**, the **substantia nigra** and **raphe nuclei** of brain stem, and the **hypothalamus**. It can be detected in the varicosities of fibres coursing up to the cerebral cortex from cell bodies located in the raphe nuclei.

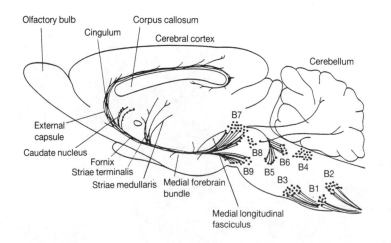

Figure 15.14 Serotoninergic pathways in rat brain (parasagittal section). Serotoninergic neurons are grouped in nine or so nuclei in the brain stem, pons and midbrain. The nuclei B5 to B9 project forward to the diencephalon and telencephalon, whilst the more caudal groups project to the medulla and spinal cord. (After Cooper, Bloom and Roth, 1985, *The Biochemical Basis of Neuropharmacology*, New York: Oxford University Press.)

Serotonin is stored in vesicles in at least some serotoninergic terminals. Release of serotonin does not result in the rapid response (depolarisation or hyperpolarisation) of the subsynaptic membrane which is characteristic of the amino acids and nicotinic acetylcholine. We shall see in Chapter 16 that its action is more like the muscarinic action of acetylcholine or the action of noradrenaline at the β-adrenergic receptor: in other words it acts through a collision-coupling second-messenger system. The response, moreover, may be quite widespread as release from varicosities results in diffusion of the transmitter over many subsynaptic cells. In this instance there is no sharp localisation of pre- and subsynaptic membranes, one 'above' the other. We shall see below that the type of response elicited may be either inhibitory or excitatory.

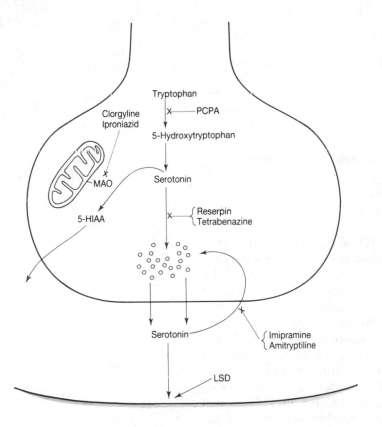

Figure 15.15 Pharmacology of the serotoninergic synapse. The synthetic step from tryptophan to 5-hydroxytryptophan is blocked by *p*-chlorophenylalanine (PCPA); the sequestration of serotonin into vesicles is blocked by both reserpine and tetrabenazine. Any free serotonin in the terminal is in danger of being deaminated by monoamine oxidase (MAO) on the outside of mitochondria to 5-hydroxyindoleacetic acid (5-HIAA). This deamination may be blocked by MAO inhibitors such as clorgyline and iproniazid. Powerful re-uptake mechanisms in the presynaptic membrane are inhibited by imipamine and amytryptilline, whilst lysergic acid diethlyamide (LSD) partially potentiates subsynaptic serotonin receptors

Three classes of serotonin receptors are nowadays recognised: 5-HT$_1$, 5-HT$_2$ and 5-HT$_3$. The classification depends on differential response to a number of agonists and antagonists. These classes have been further subdivided into subclasses. Thus the 5-HT$_1$ receptor is subdivided into three subclasses—5-HT$_{1A}$,

5-HT_{1B} and 5-HT_{1C}—and the 5-HT_3 receptor is similarly subdivided into 5-HT_{3A}, 5-HT_{3B} and 5-HT_{3C}. The pharmacological agents used to make this intricate classification are shown in Table 15.3.

Table 15.3 Pharmacological classification of 5-HT receptors

Receptor	Agonist	Antagonist
5-HT_{1A}	8-OH DPAT	Spiperone
5-HT_{1B}	5-Carboxy-AT	ICS 21 – 009
5-HT_{1C}	$(+)S\text{-}\alpha\text{-Methyl-5-HT}$	Mesulergine
5-HT_2	$(+)S\text{-}\alpha\text{-Methyl-5-HT}$	Ketanserin
5-HT_3*	2-Methyl-5-HT	ICS 205 – 930 Cocaine

*5-HT_3 is divided into three subgroups (a, b and c) by the relative binding strengths of a number of antagonists. Selective agonists and antagonists for these subtypes are not yet available

8-OH DPAT = 8-hydroxy-2(di-*n*-propylamino)tetraline; 5-carboxy-AT = 5-carboxyamidotryptamine

Adapted from Richardson and Engel (1986)

Whereas all the subclasses of 5-HT_1 and 5-HT_2 receptor have been found in the brain (as well as elsewhere) the three subclasses of the 5-HT_3 receptor have so far only been found in the peripheral nervous system. **5-HT_1 receptors** are usually located in the presynaptic membrane. They are coupled to a G-protein system, leading to increased adenylate cyclase activity. Activation of the system by 5-HT leads to **presynaptic inhibition**. As in the GABA system described above there is evidently a negative feedback loop controlling the release of serotonin from serotoninergic terminals. In contrast **5-HT_2 receptors** are located post-synaptically and, although similarly coupled to a G-protein mechanism, lead to depolarisation and thus **excitation of the subsynaptic cell**.

5-HT is quickly removed from serotoninergic synapses by a high-affinity re-uptake system. Once back inside the terminal it is sequestered once again into vesicles. Any serotonin not in vesicles tends to be deaminated by **monoamine oxidase (MAO)** into **5-hydroxyindoleacetic acid (5-HIAA)**.

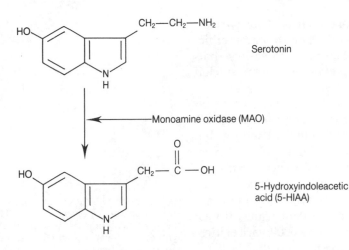

Figure 15.16   Deamination of serotonin by MAO

15.4 CATECHOLAMINES

We noted in Chapter 7 that a group of important neurotransmitters share a common ring structure—catechol. The two most important neuroactive catecholamines are **dopamine (DA)** and **noradrenaline (= norepinephrine, NE)**. Figure 15.17 shows the synthetic pathway from phenylalanine.

Tyrosine hydroxylase is the rate-limiting enzyme. As Figure 15.17 indicates it requires **tetrahydrobiopterin (BH4)** as a co-factor and is sensitive to oxygen concentration. **α-Methyl-*p*-tyrosine (AMPT)** competitively inhibits tyrosine hydroxylase and consequently blocks the synthesis of all catecholamines. The figure also shows that norepinephrine can be converted into epinephrine by a methylation of the amino group. This reaction occurs in a few nerve cells in the brain stem. In general, however, noradrenaline is the transmitter at adrenergic synapses.

The location of dopamine and noradrenaline in the brain can be determined in much the same way as we noted for serotonin. Formaldehyde vapour transforms both noradrenaline and dopamine into quinonoids, which fluoresce with a green colour ($\lambda = 470$ nm) when illuminated with light of $\lambda = 405$ nm. This technique shows that both dopaminergic and noradrenergic neurons have their cell bodies in the brain stem. Dopaminergic cell bodies are located principally in **substantia nigra** and **ventral tegmentum**. Noradrenergic cell bodies are found in various nuclei in the medulla and in the **locus coeruleus** beneath the cerebellum. We noted in the previous section that a neurotoxin, **6-hydroxydopamine (6-OHDA)**, selectively destroys catecholaminergic neurons. This selectivity can be made specific for dopaminergic neurons by using an agent such as **desipramine** to protect noradrenergic cells from the attentions of 6-OHDA. Thus we can establish the pathways of noradrenergic and dopaminergic neurons by a process of elimination. Figure 15.18 shows that catecholaminergic brain fibres sweep up from brain stem nuclei to innervate large parts of the cortex.

Both dopaminergic and noradrenergic fibres resemble serotoninergic fibres in developing varicosities along their lengths. These varicosities are of considerable importance in setting the level of activity over large regions of cortex. Figure 15.19 shows the pathway of noradrenergic fibres from the **locus coeruleus**. The fibres enter the neocortex anteriorly and course backwards in layer six. They send branches up into the upper layers of the cortex at regular intervals and develop many varicosities. It has been computed that in the rat cerebrum some 6000 varicosities are present in each cubic millimetre of cortex and that in con-

Figure 15.17 Synthesis of catecholamines from phenylalanine. The enzymes catalysing each step of the synthetic pathway are shown and their co-factors are bracketed

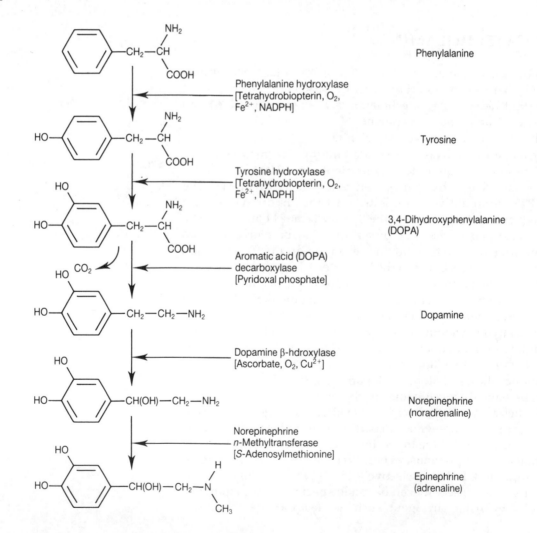

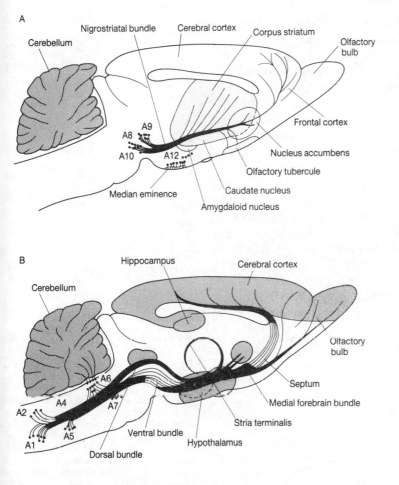

A

Cerebellum

Nigrostriatal bundle   Cerebral cortex   Corpus striatum

Olfactory bulb

A9
A8
A10   A12

Frontal cortex

Nucleus accumbens

Olfactory tubercule

Median eminence   Caudate nucleus

Amygdaloid nucleus

B

Hippocampus   Cerebral cortex

Cerebellum

Olfactory bulb

A6
A4   A7
A2   Septum

Medial forebrain bundle

A5   Stria terminalis

A1   Ventral bundle   Hypothalamus

Dorsal bundle

Figure 15.18 Dopaminergic and noradrenergic pathways in rat brain (parasagittal section). (A) Dopaminergic pathways. The major pathway (the nigrostriatal bundle) originates in the substantia nigra (A8, A9) and courses forwards to innervate the corpus striatum. (B) Noradrenergic pathways. A major pathway originates in the locus coeruleus (A6) and projects forwards as a number of distinct fibre bundles giving off branches to many brain regions. Other noradrenergic nuclei are in the ventral part of the brain stem (A1, A2, A5 and A7) and these send a few fibres back down the cord, although most mingle with coerulean fibres ascending to the forebrain. (After Bradford, 1986, *Chemical Neurobiology*, New York: Freeman.)

sequence no neuron in the cortex is more than 30 μm distant from this source of noradrenaline. Activity in coerulean fibres is thus considered to release a 'mist' of transmitter which percolates through the extracellular space of the cortex until it is either sequestrated or finds an appropriate receptor.

Let us next look briefly at the pharmacology of each of the two catecholamines.

Dopamine (DA). This catecholamine is stored in large dense cored vesicles in dopaminergic terminals. It is released in the usual calcium-dependent manner. **Amphetamine** (and some similar molecules) also bring about the release of dopamine into the synaptic cleft. There appear to be at least **four** pharmacologically distinguishable types of dopamine receptor. The best known type is the D_1 **receptor**. This operates by a collision-coupling mechanism, leading ultimately to the synthesis of cAMP. A second type of dopamine receptor, D_2, does not act through a cAMP mechanism and can be distinguished from the first by a special sensitivity to **haloperidol** and **spiperone**.

The activity of dopamine in the synaptic cleft is terminated by a powerful re-uptake system in the presynaptic membranes of dopaminergic neurons. Dopamine is then sequestered into vesicles along with ATP and some inorganic ions such as Mg^{2+} and Ca^{2+}. Any dopamine not so sequestered is liable to attack by **monamine oxidase (MAO)** and **catechol-*o*-methyltransferase (COMT)**. These enzymes convert dopamine to 3,4-dihydroxy-phenylacetic acid (DOPAC) and 3-methoxytyramine, respectively. Both the latter compounds lack synaptic activity. It should be noted, however, that the enzymic degradation of catecholamines is significantly slower than the degradation of acetylcholine by acetylcholinesterase. It should also be noted that there are at least **two distinct forms of MAO**. These forms are distinguishable by their substrate specificity and by their sensitivity to inhibitors. **MAO-A** has a substrate preference for catecholamines and serotonin and is inhibited by clorgyline, whilst **MAO-B** prefers β-phenylethylamine and benzylamine and is inhibited by deprenyl.

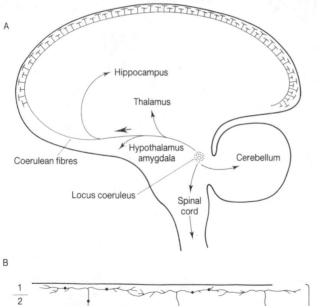

Figure 15.19 Schematic to show the major route of coerulean fibres in the human brain. (A) The locus coeruleus is a small nucleus (c. 20 000 neurons) in the central grey matter of the metencephalon. A major tract of fibres from cells in this nucleus courses forwards and enters the bottom layer of the cerebral cortex anteriorly and then runs towards the posterior. (B) Section through the cerebral cortex to show the disposition of branches from coerulean fibres. The major ramifications are in layers 5, 4(B) and 1. Varicosities are well developed in all regions. (After Morrison, Molliver and Grzanna, 1979, *Science*, **205**, 313–316.)

A

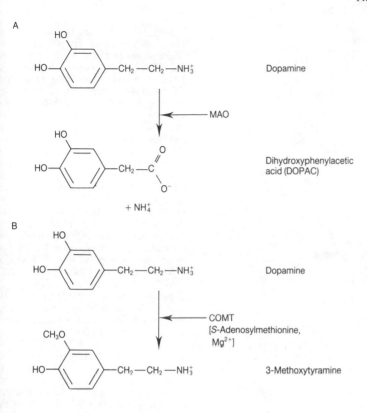

Dopamine

MAO

Dihydroxyphenylacetic
acid (DOPAC)

$+ NH_4^+$

B

Dopamine

COMT
[*S*-Adenosylmethionine,
Mg^{2+}]

3-Methoxytyramine

Figure 15.20 Inactivation of dopamine by MAO and COMT. (A) Monoamine oxidase (MAO) removes the terminal amino group from dopamine to form dihydroxyphenylacetic acid (DOPAC). (B) Catechol-*O*-methyl transferase (COMT) adds a methyl group from *S*-adenosylmethionine to dopamine to form 3-methoxytyramine. Mg^{2+} is required as a co-factor. 3-Methoxytyramine may be further transformed to homovanillic acid (HVA) by the action of MAO and this, in turn, is acted on by COMT to form DOPAC

Finally, it should be mentioned in this section that **Parkinsonism**, a pathology which affects the elderly, is due to a deterioration of the dopaminergic pathways from the substantia nigra to the corpus striatum. The symptoms can be ameliorated by oral administration of L-dopa. This molecule, unlike dopamine itself which is not sufficiently lipid-soluble, is able to pass the blood–brain barrier. Once in the brain it is decarboxylated to dopamine and goes some way to making up for the lack of the endogenous molecule. We shall return to Parkinsonism in Chapter 19.

Noradrenaline (= norepinephrine, NE). Noradrenaline, like dopamine, is stored in large, dense-cored vesicles. These vesicles contain ATP and a number of proteins and divalent metal ions in addition to noradrenaline. Release of noradrenaline into the synaptic cleft occurs in a calcium-dependent manner, as described in Chapter 14. Once again a number of drugs, including **amphetamine**, facilitate the release, whereas others, for example **guanethidine**, have the opposite effect and block it.

The subsynaptic membrane possesses two main types of adrenergic receptor: **α-adrenoceptors** and **β-adrenoceptors** (both

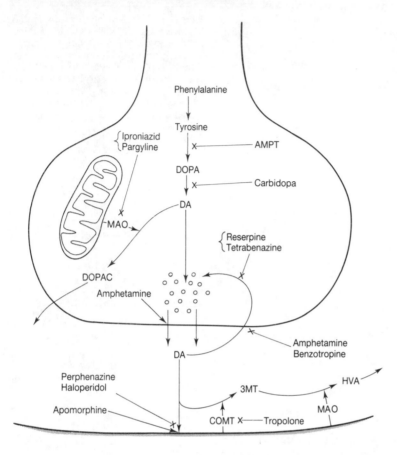

Figure 15.21 Dopaminergic synapse. The synthetic step from tyrosine to DOPA is blocked by α-methyl-p-tyrosine (AMPT). a competitive inhibitor of tyrosine hydroxylase. The step from DOPA to dopamine (DA) is blocked by carbidopa which inhibits DOPA decarboxylase. The sequestration of DA into vesicles is blocked by reserpine and tetrabenazine. Monoamine oxidase (MAO) (believed to be bound to the exterior of motochondria) converts free DA to dihydroxyphenylacetic acid (DOPAC). MAO is inhibited by pargyline (an inhibitor of MAO-B) and iproniazid (an inhibitor of both MAO-A and MAO-B). The release of DA into the synaptic cleft is potentiated by amphetamine (probably mainly because of its effect on re-uptake). Once in the cleft DA is exposed to both COMT and MAO. COMT converts DA to 3-methoxytyramine (MT) and MAO converts MT to homovanillic acid (HVA). Amphetamine and benzotropine block the re-uptake of DA back into the presynaptic terminal; reserpine and tetrabenazine block resequestration once DA gets back into the terminal. Apomophine is a DA agonist at both post- and presynaptic sites. Perphenazine and haloperidol are antagonists at the postsynaptic membrane. Tropolone blocks the postsynaptic action of COMT

of which have two subtypes—α_1 and α_2, β_1 and β_2). The pharmacological distinction between these different receptor types is shown in Table 15.4. We discussed the β_2-adrenoceptor in depth in Chapter 7. It will be recalled that it is linked via a collision-coupling mechanism to the synthesis of cAMP. This also seems to be the case with the α_1-receptor. The α_2-receptor, in contrast, does not seem to be linked to adenylate cyclase and is believed to be located on the presynaptic membrane, where it causes an inhibitory response in that membrane. Once again we meet the same negative feedback design principle: release of the transmitter acts as its own shut-off.

The feedback control of the adrenergic synapse is more complex than has yet been demonstrated in other types of synapse. A build-up of noradrenaline in the synaptic cleft is detected by the α_2-receptor and the consequent of the presynaptic membrane hyperpolarisation (i.e. inhibition) effectively prevents the release of any further transmitter. But there is more. For the β_2-receptor, which is also located in the

Table 15.4 Pharmacological distinction between adrenoreceptors

Receptor	Agonist	Antagonist
α_1-Adrenoceptor	Phenylephrine	Prazosin
α_2-Adrenoceptor	Clonidine	Yohimbine
β_1-Adrenoceptor	Dobutamine	Practolol
β_2-Adrenoceptor	Procaterol	Butoxamine

After McIlwain and Bachelard (1985); Minneman *et al*. (1986)

presynaptic membrane, is activated only when low concentrations of noradrenaline are present in the cleft and leads to increased transmitter release. Thus there is a two-way, a negative and a positive feedback, control of the release of NE from adrenergic terminals. The 'push–pull' action of these two types of pre-synaptic receptor modulate the amount of noradrenaline present in the synaptic cleft.

Noradrenaline is removed from the synaptic cleft by an Na^+-dependent ATPase. This pump is very efficient and removes all but a very low concentration of noradrenaline from the cleft. Once back in the terminal the noradrenaline (like dopamine) is sequestered into dense-cored vesicles. This sequestration process depends on Mg^{2+} ions. Agents which chelate Mg^{2+}, such as **reserpine**, inhibit this storage process. As any free noradrenaline is inactivated by MAO or COMT adrenergic terminals subjected to reserpine become depleted in the transmitter. Reserpine acts in the same way at the dopaminergic synapse.

It was found many years ago that MAO inhibitors (**MAOIs**) (e.g. iproniazid, nialamide, pargyline) lifted psychological states of depression. This observation led to what has been called **the biogenic amine theory of depression**. It was suggested that endogenous depression was caused by a deficiency in biogenic, especially catechol, amines. This idea received support from the finding that reserpine tends to cause sedation in experimental animals and depression in humans. Further support was provided by the finding that tricyclic compounds such as desipramine, imipramine and amitriptyline, which are known to block re-uptake of noradrenaline and serotonin into presynaptic terminals, are powerful antidepressants. The biogenic amine theory thus argues that depressive states result from a paucity of catecholamines and/or serotonin in the synaptic cleft. In this

A

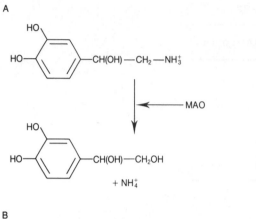

Norepinephrine
(noradrenaline)

MAO

Dihydroxyphenylglycol
(DOPEG)

B

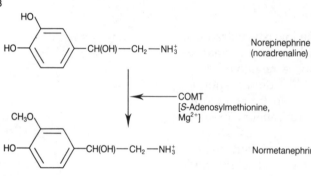

Norepinephrine
(noradrenaline)

COMT
[*S*-Adenosylmethionine,
Mg^{2+}]

Normetanephrine (NM)

Figure 15.22 Inactivation of noradrenaline by MAO and COMT. (A) MAO deaminates norepinephrine to 3,4-dihydoxyphenylglycol (DOPEG). (B) COMT methylates norepinephrine to noremetanephrine (NM). *S*-Adenosylmethionine and Mg^{2+} are required as cofactors. NM may be further metabolised by MAO and aldehyde reductase to 3-methoxy-4-phenylglycol (MHPG)

Desipramine

Imipramine

Amitriptyline

Figure 15.23 Structures of tricyclic antidepressants

simple form the theory is, no doubt, simplistic. The brain is a very complicated place. The biogenic amine theory of depression can, however, be developed, and is being developed, into a more sophisticated theory which has much to commend it. We shall return to consider depressive illness further in Chapter 19.

The pharmacology of the noradrenergic synapse is extremely intricate. Large numbers of drugs have been shown to affect various aspects of its operation. Once again the interested reader must consult one of the neuropharmacology texts listed in the bibliography for full details. Figure 15.24, however, shows some of the major features of the synapse.

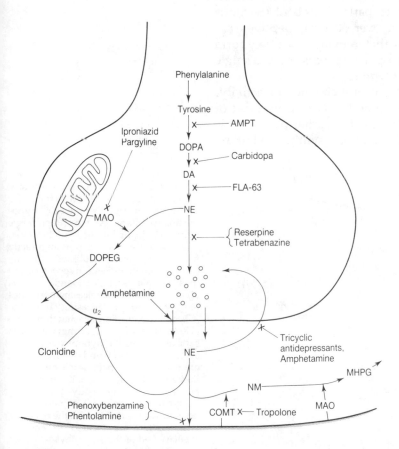

Figure 15.24 The noradrenergic synapse. The pharmacology of the adrenergic synapse is similar to that of the dopaminergic synapse. Only additional features will be described here. The synthetic step from dopamine (DA) to norepinephrine (NE) can be blocked by bis-(1-methyl-4-homopiperazinyl-thiocarbonyl)-disulphide (FLA-63). Mitochondrion-bound MAO converts unsequestered NE to 3,4-dihydroxy-phenylglycol (DOPEG). The tricyclic antidepressants and amphetamine block re-uptake of NE released into the synaptic cleft. Clonidine is a powerful agonist at presynaptic α_2 receptors and has a lesser effect on postsynaptic receptors. Phenoxybenzamine and phetolamine are powerful blockers of postsynaptic receptors. COMT in the synaptic cleft converts NE to normetanephrine (NM) (blocked by tropolone) and MAO converts NM to 3-methoxy-4-phenyl-glycol (MHPG)

It should be borne in mind, when considering Figure 15.24, that the four subtypes of adrenergic receptor have different pharmacologies (Table 15.4). This is consistent with the situation obtaining with the other receptors considered in this chapter (with the possible exception of the glycine receptor). It is clear that synaptic membranes are bewilderingly complex. Nonetheless some broad principles are beginning to emerge from the thicket of detail—principles which have to do with release and re-uptake, with sequestration and enzymic degradation, and with the feedback control of transmitter release. We shall now leave our consideration of 'classical' transmitters and venture into the new and rapidly developing topic of neuroactive peptides.

15.5 PEPTIDES

We have already considered the structure, synthesis, post-transcriptional and post-translational modification of the better-known neuroactive peptides in earlier parts of this book (Sections 2.1, 3.2 and 4.3). We noted that over 50 such peptides are nowadays recognised and we saw that in many cases they form families, derived by the post-transcriptional processing of a single mother protein (pre-protein or polyprotein).

In this chapter we shall briefly look at their synaptic activity. First it should be noted that neuropeptides differ from most of the smaller molecules we have discussed in earlier parts of this Chapter in that they are not recycled and/or resynthesised in the

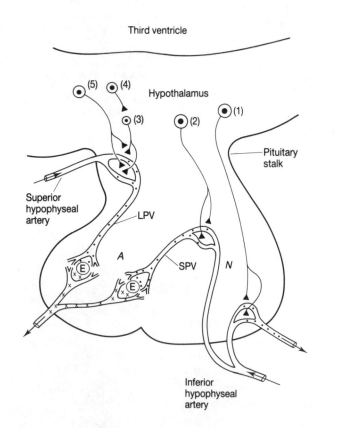

Figure 15.25 Hypothalamo-pituitary system. The figure schematises the major pathways in the peptidergic hypothalamo-pituitary system. Peptidergic neuron (1), located in the hypothalamus, releases oxytocin or vasopressin directly into the general circulation via the capillary bed in the neurohypophysis (N) (posterior pituitary). Peptidergic neurons (2) and (3) synthesise releasing hormones (e.g. corticotropin-releasing hormone (CRH), thyrotropin-releasing hormone (TRH), etc.) and secrete them into the capillary bed of the hypophyseal portal system. Neurons (4) and (5) link the rest of the brain to the peptidergic neurons—they act with 'conventional' transmitters either on the cell body (4) or the presynaptic endings (5) of peptidergic neurons. The cells (E) which the releasing factors affect are located in another capillary bed of the hypophyseal portal system in the adenohypophysis (A). LPV = long portal vessel; SPV = short portal vessel. (After Kandel and Schwartz, 1985, *Principles of Neural Science*, New York: Elsevier.)

presynaptic terminal. Neuropeptides are synthesised by the processes described in Chapter 14 in the neuronal perikaryon and are transported to the presynaptic terminal in the axoplasmic flow. As axons can be lengthy it is consequently possible for an overworked neuron to run out of presynaptic neuropeptide.

Second, it must be borne in mind that neuropeptides function in other ways than as neurotransmitters/modulators. They may, for instance, make use of the vascular system for distribution. This is particularly the case in the **hypothalamo-pituitary** system. In this respect they are closer to hormones than neurotransmitters and should indeed be regarded as 'local hormones'. In yet other cases the vascular system may distribute them to distant parts of the body, outside the nervous system altogether. We noted in Chapter 14 that this leads into the large and diverse subject of neuroendocrinology, which we shall not attempt to enter. Biology, unfortunately, has scant regard for the tidy classificatory schemes of the scientist!

Table 15.5 Distribution of some neuroactive peptides

Peptide	H	B-H	SC	N	GI	Pa	Sk	Pi
Enkephalin	+	+	+	+	+			
Substance P	+	+	+	+	+	+	+	+
Neurotensin	+	+	+		+		+	
VIP	+	+			+	+		
Gastrin	+	+			+	+		

H = hypothalamus; B-H = brain minus hypothalamus; SC = spinal cord; N = peripheral nerve; GI = gastrointestinal tract; Pa = pancreas; Sk = skin; Pi = pituitary

Partly modified from Samuelson (1979)

It would clearly be impossible to discuss 50 or more different neuroactive peptides in one short section. We shall therefore concentrate on just a few comparatively well-known examples. We shall look at a family of peptides which are found both in the central nervous system and in the gastrointestinal (GI) tract, the so-called 'gut–brain axis'. We shall, however, only consider their actions in the central nervous system. This family, as Table 15.5 shows, includes the opioids (especially the enkaphalins) and substance P (SP), as well as vasoactive intestinal peptide

(VIP), cholescystokinin (CCK), neurotensin (NT), gastrin, bombesin and a few others. Of this large and diverse goup of peptides we shall only consider the best known members: substance P and the enkephalins.

Substance P. We saw in Table 2.2 that SP is an 11-residue peptide related to two decapeptides (substance K (= neurokinin A) and neuromedin K (neurokinin B)). SP is found in the **dorsal horn** of the mammalian spinal cord and in a number of regions of the brain, especially the **substantia nigra** of the midbrain. It has also been shown to exist in significant quantities in the **inferior mesenteric ganglia**. This ganglion has provided a convenient experimental preparation.

Stimulation of preganglionic fibres elicits long-lasting depolarisation in the ganglion. This slow EPSP is not blocked by cholinergic antagonists but can be mimicked by the application of SP. Furthermore if **capsaicin**, derived from red pepper, is applied to the ganglion SP is known to be released. When pre-ganglionic stimulation is applied to these SP-depleted ganglia the slow EPSP is not developed. These various approaches suggest, therefore, that the slow EPSP, which may last from 20 seconds to 4 minutes, is due to substance P.

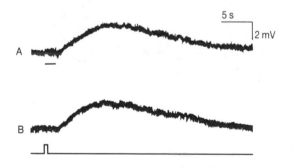

Figure 15.26 SP-induced 'slow' EPSP. (A) Response of a neuron in the inferior mesenteric ganglion to stimulation in the presence of cholinergic blockers hexamethonium (400 μM) and atropine (4 μM). The response was induced by stimulation of the lumbar splanchnic nerves (10 Hz, 2 s) shown by the horizontal bar. (B) Response of the same neuron in the presence of the same cholinergic blockers to application of SP (5 μM) by a micropipette (shown by the blip in the lower horizontal line). (From Tsunoo, Konishi and Otsuka, 1982, *Neuroscience*, 7, 2025–2037; with permission.)

In the spinal cord substance P has been found to be associated with small-diameter primary afferent fibres. These fibres are the **C fibres** which are implicated in **pain** sensations. This observation does not, however, exclude SP from other afferent pathways—it may also, for instance, be involved in pathways carrying information from **baroreceptors**.

Enkephalins. Table 2.2 showed that two pentapeptide enkephalins—met-enkephalin and leu-enkephalin—have been identified. Another endogenous opioid has been detected in the pituitary and in extracts of the duodenum. This is **dynorphin** and

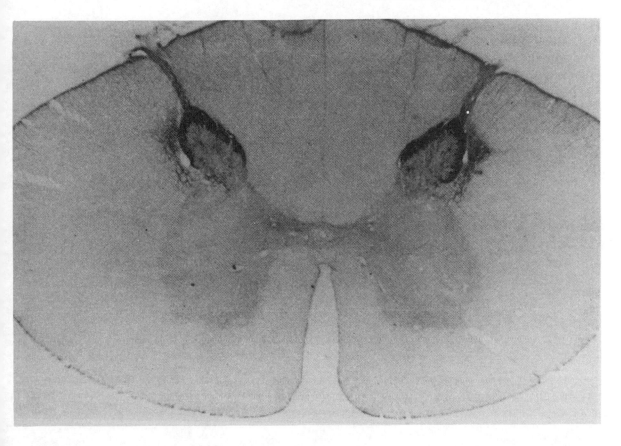

is leu-enkephalin extended at the C-terminal end by -tyr-gly-gly-phe-leu-arg-arg-ile-arg-pro-lys-leu-lys-trp-asp-asn-glu.

Enkephalins are distributed widely throughout the brain. On average met-enkephalin is about three times more prevalent than leu-enkephalin. The heaviest concentrations are to be found in the **dorsal horn** of the spinal cord, the **periaqueductal grey matter** (around the central canal and cerebral ventricles), the **limbic system** and the **basal ganglia**—especially the **globus pallidus**. This distribution is interesting as the dorsal horn of grey matter and periaqueductal grey matter contain the multisynaptic **spino-thalamic tract**. This tract is believed to be responsible for our sensation of dull aching pains (in contrast to sharp pricking pains). The limbic system has been implicated in emotional response whilst the globus pallidus is part of the system which controls motor output (see Section 15.2 above). It is worth noting that in cases of **Huntingdon's chorea** the concentration of met-enkephalin in the globus pallidus diminishes to a third of normal—from 1.5 ng g^{-1} to 0.5 ng g^{-1}.

The discovery in the early 1970s that enkephalins bind to the same sites as opium, morphine, codeine, etc., was one of the most

Figure 15.27   Location of SP synapses in the substantia gelatinosa of the spinal cord. The darkly stained regions in the dorsal horn of this transverse section of monkey spinal cord indicate where substance P is concentrated. (Courtesy of Dr S. Hunt.)

exciting events in the history of neuropharmacology. It promised that at long last we should have some insight into both the neural events underlying pain and the way in which various exogenous opiates can relieve pain; it promised also some insight into the mechanisms of addiction, which have for millennia provided such anguish for addicts and problems for society.

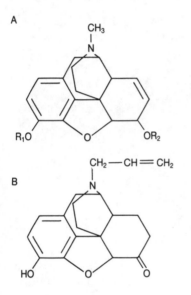

A

Morphine $R_1 = R_2 = H$
Codeine $R_1 = CH_3$; $R_2 = H$
Heroin $R_1 = R_2 = COCH_3$

B

Naxolone

Figure 15.28 Structures of morphine and related drugs

Opioid receptors have been subdivided into a number of types. The most important of these have been designated μ, δ and κ. The **μ-receptor** responds to agonists in the following order: β-endorphin > morphine > met-enkephalin > leu-enkephalin; the **δ-receptor** responds to leu-enkephalin > met-enkephalin > β-endorphin > morphine; the **κ-receptor** has a different set of agonists which include pentazocine, ethylketocyclazocine and butorphanol.

The three types of opioid receptor are distributed somewhat differently in the brain. The μ-receptors have a widespread distribution but are especially dense in the thalamus and amygdala. It is believed that they may be involved in pain regulation and in sensorimotor co-ordination. The δ-receptors, in contrast, have a more restricted distribution. They are especially heavily concentrated in olfactory regions of the brain such as the caudate putamen and the nucleus accumbens. Finally the κ-receptors are once again rather sparsely distributed but are found especially in the hypothalamus and preoptic area. It is likely that they are involved in water balance and food intake as well as in pain perception.

It is believed that enkephalinergic neurons involved in the regulation of the sensation of pain exert their effects by releasing their transmitter on to the presynaptic terminals of pain pathway neurons. It was indicated above that the spinal cord and brain stem pain pathways are multisynaptic routes. There is thus much opportunity for enkephalinergic interneurons to modulate the flow of messages. Indeed some have suggested that this is *one* of the ways in which the CNS keeps the pathway damped down during the heat of the battle or game. Only afterwards do we feel our bumps and bruises, or worse. The putative interneuronal action of enkephalinergic neurons is shown in Figure 15.29.

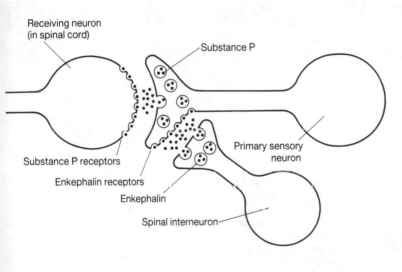

Receiving neuron
(in spinal cord)

Substance P

Substance P receptors

Enkephalin receptors

Enkephalin

Spinal interneuron

Primary sensory
neuron

Figure 15.29   Enkephalinergic control of primary pain fibre in substantia gelatinosa. A primary sensory neuron using SP as its transmitter synapses with a neuron of the spinothalamic tract. Its input into the 'pain pathway' is controlled by the enkephalinergic interneuron which is shown acting presynaptically to inhibit the release of SP. (After Iverson, 1979, *Scientific American*, **241**, 118–129. Copyright © 1979, by Scientific American Inc. All rights reserved.)

The molecular mechanism by which enkephalins are able to damp down activity in spinothalamic tract neurons remains to be discovered. There is circumstantial evidence that enkephalins occupying μ-receptors lead to membrane hyperpolarisation. If the μ-receptors are on the presynaptic terminals of spinothalamic tract neurons or, as in Figure 15.29, primary 'pain' neurons, it is clear that the depolarisation required for transmitter release would be less likely to occur. Other investigations have shown that in some tissues enkephalins inhibit the action of adenylate cyclase.

It is likely that the painful symptoms experienced by addicts when an exogenous opiate is withdrawn are due to a type of **'denervation supersensitivity'**. It can be argued that the continuous presence of the opiate in the addict's pain pathways leads to a compensatory increase in synaptic sensitivity 'downstream' in the pathway. This is known in other cases of diminished impulse traffic in a multisynaptic pathway. It seems that the number of receptors on subsynaptic membranes increases to balance the low level of activity. Hence (returning to the pain pathway) when the drug is removed, downstream synapses will respond to activity which would not normally be transmitted. The addict's 'drying-out' phase can thus be accompanied by extremely distressing withdrawal pains.

15.6 COHABITATION OF PEPTIDES AND NON-PEPTIDES

We have already noted that 'Dale's principle' (one neuron—one transmitter) is now known to have many exceptions. It has recently become apparent that neuroactive peptides frequently share a neuron with a non-peptide transmitter. Table 15.6 shows that practically all combinations of peptide and non-peptide transmitter have been found. As these cohabitations have been

Table 15.6 Cohabitation of neuroactive peptides and non-peptides

Non-peptide transmitter	Peptide	Tissue (species)
Dopamine	Enkephalin	Carotid body (cat)
	CCK	Brain (rat, human)
Noradrenaline	Somatostatin	Sympathetic ganglia (guinea pig)
	Enkephalin	Sympathetic ganglia (rat, ox)
		Adrenal medulla (several species)
		Locus coeruleus (cat)
	Neurotensin	Adrenal medulla (cat)
Serotonin	Substance P	Medulla (rat)
	Enkephalin	Medulla (rat, cat)
Acetylcholine	VIP	Autonomic ganglia (cat)
	Enkephalin	Preganglionic nerves (cat)
		Cochlear nerve (guinea pig)
	Neurotensin	Preganglionic nerves (cat)
	Somatostatin	Heart (toad)
	Substance P	Ciliary ganglion (bird)
GABA	Somatostatin	Thalamus (cat)

Modified from Lundberg and Hokfelt (1983)

largely established by immuno-histochemical techniques which are sometimes not absolutely specific for neuropeptides there remain some uncertainties in the identifications. Table 15.6, nevertheless, shows the very widespread nature of this phenomenon.

The exact significance of cohabitation remains to be determined. It may be that the peptide and the non-peptide act synergistically or, in contrast, it could be that the peptide or the non-peptide act **presynaptically** to inhibit the release of their companion. One might imagine, for example, that because of the different geography of synthesis (see Section 15.5) the neuropeptide in a hard-working neuron might run out before the non-peptide. If the former acted to inhibit or potentiate the release of the latter, interesting control circuits may be possible.

Alternatively one may modulate the **subsynaptic** effects of the other. The peptide, for instance, may work through a second-messenger system on the underlying cell's biochemistry. This may result in the ion channels in the subsynaptic membrane being 'up' or 'down' modulated. The subsynaptic response to the cohabiting non-peptide transmitter (such as ACh or one of the amino acids) could thus be controlled. Finally, it is always possible that the two cohabitants have quite distinct and independent roles.

These are just a few of the possibilities which our contemporary understanding suggests. The molecular complexity at the synapse is evidently far greater than was suspected even a few years ago.

15.7 CONCLUSION

At the outset of Chapter 14 we noted that the brain might be seen as an immense gland rather than as an intricate electronic computer. We are now in a position to feel the force of this analogy and also to recognise the import of Freeman's proposition (Chapter 1) that the flow of activity in the brain could best be likened to the 'continuum of a chemical reaction'. Unlike the majority of chemical reactions, however, the brain's activity occurs not in just one or at most a few phase-spaces but in billions of interconnected compartments.

It is often asked: why are there so many neurotransmitters and neuromodulators? The question betrays a misconstrual of the brain. An inappropriate analogy is at work. The brain is once again being likened, probably unconsciously, to a telephone exchange or electronic computer. But we have seen that this is not the way things are in the brain. Its operation is far more subtle. At a certain generality of definition no doubt the brain is a computer. But, so far as its hardware, its operating system, is concerned, it is a chemical computer.

Thus the answer to the question posed above is easy. The brain does not operate by 'yes/no' gates, 'on/off' switches, but by fluxes of chemicals affecting diverse receptors which in turn often modulate intracellular biochemical processes. Only at a very first analysis can synapses by classified straightforwardly into 'excitatory' and 'inhibitory'; deeper investigation almost always shows a host of subtle variations, mostly at the molecular level. Only at a first analysis does the brain consist of discrete synaptic appositions. Further research shows that many synapses are made 'en passant', many transmitters and modulators are released from 'varicosities' to percolate through the extracellular space to exert 'long-range' influence. The biochemical environment in which neurons work is subtle and ever-changing. In the next chapter we shall see that subtlety is also very much a feature of the subsynaptic cell and its responses.

Chapter 16
The subsynaptic membrane

In Chapter 15 we reviewed some of the transmitters and modulators which the presynaptic terminal releases into the synaptic gap. In this chapter we shall look at what happens next. What effect do these substances have on the subsynaptic membrane? We shall see that, just as action potentials result from the activity of a variety of membrane-embedded voltage-gated channels, so the response of sub- or postsynaptic membranes reflects the underlying activity of a multiplicity of G-coupled and ligand-coupled receptors (see Chapters 7 and 9).

We saw something of the morphological variety of synapses in Section 1.2 and we also noted the major features of the 'classical' chemical synapse (Figure 1.16). We saw that the presynaptic and the post- or subsynaptic membrane were separated from each other by a gap or **cleft** of some 30–40 nm. That this gap is not 'empty' is shown by the structure of **synaptosomes**.

Synaptosomes can be obtained from the central nervous system by homogenisation in buffered sucrose solutions and subsequent density-gradient centrifugation. One of the fractions in the centrifuge tube contains broken-off nerve endings or synaptosomes. Microscopic examination shows that they consist not only of the presynaptic terminal but a portion of adhering subsynaptic membrane also. This provides good evidence that there is some adhesive material between the two membranes.

Synaptosomes have proved of considerable importance in brain research. Although they are broken-off boutons their boundary membrane reseals to form a tiny (1–2 μm) sac containing mitochondria, vesicles, neurotransmitters, enzymes and the other elements of synaptic terminals. When incubated in appropriate physiological media they can be shown to respire and an active $Na^+ + K^+$ pump ensures that a resting potential (-30 to -60 mV) is maintained across their membrane. Finally, when electrically depolarised or treated with depolarising agents (e.g.

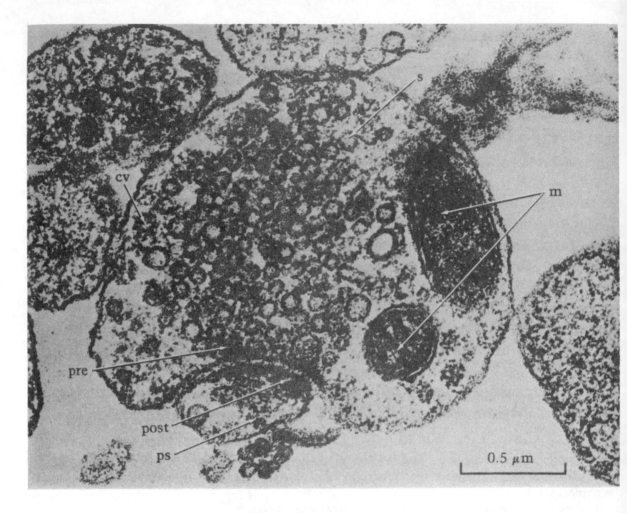

veratridine) synaptosomes can be shown to release neurotransmitters into the incubating medium. Because synaptosome preparations are obtained from the homogenisation of a large number of terminals a cocktail of neurotransmitters is released. The nature of this cocktail varies according to the brain region from which the synaptosomes were obtained. Thus cerebral-cortical synaptosomes release GABA, glycine, glutamate, aspartate; synaptosomes derived from the corpus striatum are enriched in dopamine; those derived from the spinal cord are enriched in glycine.

Figure 16.1 shows not only that a portion of subsynaptic membrane adheres to the presynaptic terminal but also that it carries with it the **subsynaptic density**. We noted in Chapter 1 that this density was a characteristic of chemically conducting synapses. It has proved possible to isolate this density from the synaptosome. If synaptosomes are exposed to the strong

Figure 16.1 Synaptosome from rat cerebral cortex after incubation in physiological saline for 10 min. cv = coated vesicle; m = mitochondria; post = post (i.e. sub-) synaptic density; pre = presynaptic grid element; ps = postsynaptic 'bag'. (From Csillag and Hajós, 1980, *J. Neurochem.*, **34**, 495–503; with permission.)

detergent *n*-lauroyl sarcosinate (NLS) the subsynaptic density is detached and can then be examined on its own. We shall return to consider this structure in more detail at the end of this chapter. First, however, let us consider the physiology and biochemistry of the subsynaptic membrane.

16.1 ELECTROPHYSIOLOGY OF THE SUBSYNAPTIC MEMBRANE

A decade or so ago, when things were simpler, neuro-physiologists divided synapses into two functional types: **excitatory** and **inhibitory**. We have already seen and we shall see further below that in the late 1980s the plot has thickened. Nevertheless it will be sensible to start with the simple picture and add complications later.

16.1.1 The excitatory synapse

The type example of the excitatory synapse is the vertebrate cholinergic neuromuscular junction. We have already looked at the nature of the nicotinic acetylcholine receptor in depth (Chapter 9) and we considered its pharmacology in Chapter 15. Here we can note, first of all, that when ACh is released from the presynaptic terminal and lands on the nAChR a flux of both Na^+ and K^+ ions traverses the subsynaptic membrane. The two ions pass through the nAChR channel with approximately equal ease.

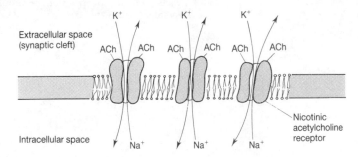

Figure 16.2 Fluxes of Na^+ and K^+ ions across the subsynaptic membrane of a cholinergic synapse

Figure 16.2 shows that both Na^+ and K^+ flow down their electrochemical gradients. The force behind both ions is simply the difference between the membrane potential (V_m) and their respective Nernst potentials (V_{Na} and V_K). If we suppose that the permeability constant of K^+ increases tenfold and that the permeability constant of Na^+ increases until it approaches 0.75 that of K^+ (i.e. much more than tenfold) and insert these values into Goldman's equation (eq. 11.5) we obtain $V_m \sim -7$ **mV**.

And this is very much what is observed. In the case of the neuro-muscular junction this depolarisation is called an **end-plate potential (EPP)**. In the central nervous synapses it is known as a **postsynaptic potential (PSP)**. Moreover as it leads, as we shall see, to excitation of the postsynaptic cell it is called an **excitatory post-synaptic potential (EPSP)**.

If we now recall our discussion of electrotonic potentials and cable conduction in Chapter 11 we can see that we have the classical condition for the spread of local circuits. In the neuromuscular junction these spread from the EPP to other parts of the sarcolemma where, if they find voltage-dependent Na$^+$ gates, they will initiate an action potential. Similarly in central synapses local circuits spreading from the EPSP will open any sodium channels embedded in the neuronal membrane. Now we have seen that, in general, sodium channels are not found in dendritic membrane but only in axolemma. We saw in Chapter 13, moreover, that voltage-dependent sodium gates are particularly densely distributed on the initial segment of the axon (see also Appendix 2). This, then, is where the local circuits spreading out from the EPSP make their influence felt.

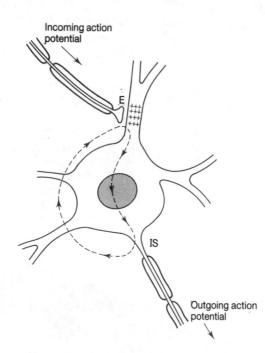

Figure 16.3   Spread of local circuits from an EPSP. The activation of an excitatory synapse (E) leads to the depolarisation of the subsynaptic membrane. Local circuits spread from this region (arrows) and affect the initial segment (IS) of the axon. If the circuits are sufficiently strong then the IS will be depolarised to threshold and an action potential will be initiated which will be propagated without decrement down the axon

Referring back to Chapter 11 again we can see that the position at which the EPSP occurs on the neuron's soma (i.e. perikayron + dendritic tree) is very important. EPSPs occurring far out on the dendritic tree may only exert a 'biasing' affect on the initial egment, never bringing it below the threshold necessary to initiate an action potential. This biasing effect may, however, be quite long lasting. Although the EPSP may endure for only a few milliseconds, the bias on the initial segment may persist for tens of milliseconds. In contrast EPSPs occurring close to or actually in the perikaryon will exert a rapid and decisive effect. Local circuits will open sodium gates on the initial segment and set off the action potential. Finally it is worth noting that the area of the synaptic contact is also very significant. Clearly a large synapse will depolarise a comparatively large patch of subsynaptic membrane, resulting in comparatively large current fluxes along the local circuits.

We noted above that the EPSP seldom endures for more than a few milliseconds. This is because, as we saw in Chapter 15, there are always mechanisms in the synaptic cleft which inactivate the transmitter. In the case of the cholinergic synapse, we saw that this mechanism takes the form of an enzyme, **acetylcholinesterase (AChE)**, which splits ACh into two parts—acetate and choline. The choline is pumped back into the presynaptic ending and used again for the synthesis of fresh ACh. The phenomenon is quite general. Excitatory transmitters are not allowed to hang around in the synaptic cleft. They are either inactivated by a specific enzyme (or enzymes) or pumped back into the presynaptic terminal.

Finally it is important to recognise that EPSPs (unlike action potentials) are not 'all-or-nothing' events. The magnitude of an EPSP (i.e. the magnitude of the depolarisation) depends on the quantity of excitatory transmitter released into the synaptic cleft. This fact makes possible the phenomenon of **temporal summation**. If a rapid 'tattoo' of impulses arrives at the presynaptic terminal fresh ACh is released into the cleft before ACh from the earlier impulses has been inactivated by AChE. More nAChRs are opened, more Na^+ and K^+ ions flux down their electrochemical gradients, and the greater is the membrane depolarisation.

In addition to temporal summation excitatory synapses also show **spatial summation**. If two or more EPSPs occur at the same time on different parts of a neuron's soma the local circuits will sum together. It could thus well be that while one EPSP on its own would not be sufficient to initiate an action potential, two acting together would be adequate to depolarise the initial segment membrane beyond the required threshold.

6.1.2 The inhibitory synapse

There are as many, if not more, inhibitory synapses in the CNS as there are excitatory synapses. We noted in Chapter 15 that the best-known inhibitory transmitters are γ-aminobutyric acid (GABA) and glycine. These transmitters are sequestered in small translucent vesicles in the presynaptic ending. There is some evidence that the vesicles are elliptical rather than spherical.

When an action potential arrives at an inhibitory terminal the usual molecular events occur which result in the transmitter being voided into the synaptic cleft. Once it reaches the synaptic membrane, however, a **hyperpolarisation** rather than a depolarisation ensues. This is known as an **inhibitory postsynaptic potential (IPSP)**. Let us examine the ionic mechanisms underlying this potential.

We saw in Chapter 9 that inhibitory transmitters open very narrow channels in the membrane—channels which will only allow ions with a hydrated radius less than or equal to that of the **chloride ion** to flux through. Table 16.1 shows that all the naturally occurring ions in and around neurons in fact have greater hydrated radii than Cl^-. It can be shown that both glycine-activated and GABA-activated channels have the following relative conductance sequence: $Cl^- > Br^- > I^- > F^-$. Not only do the channels select ions with a small hydrated radius but they also select anions.

We discussed the molecular nature of both the GABA and the glycine receptor (GlyR) in Section 9.3. We saw that the GlyR was an oligomeric transmembrane complex of which a 48 kDa transmembrane protein is believed to form the channel for chloride ions. An associated 98 kDa submembrane protein is, perhaps,

Table 16.1 Hydrated radii of some physiological ions

Ion	Non-hydrated radius (Å)	Hydrated radius (Å)	Molecules of water 'carried'
Cl^-	1.81	3.6	4.0
K^+	1.33	3.8	5.4
Na^+	0.95	5.6	8.0
Ca^{2+}	0.99	9.6	16.6
Mg^{2+}	0.65	10.8	22.2

The concept of a 'hydrated radius' is, as Hille (1984) puts it, somewhat 'fuzzy'. It should not be thought that a given ion is associated with a specific set of water molecules. Because no covalent bonds are involved the time for which any given water molecule is associated with a specific ion can be measured in nanoseconds. The 'hydrated radius' is best thought of as giving an indication of the strength of attraction between an ion and the surrounding aqueous solvent.

part of the cytoskeletal meshwork of the subsynaptic density. We saw that it could be located at central subsynaptic sites by both immunofluorescence light microscopy and immunogold electron microscopy (Figure 9.14).

Next let us look at the consequence for the subsynaptic membrane when this channel is activated. We can use the same procedure as in the previous section. We can test the effect of opening a Cl$^-$ channel by inserting a greatly increased value for chloride's permeability constant in the Goldman equation. Let us suppose that instead of P_{Cl} being about 1×10^{-8} cm s^{-1} it increases a hundredfold to 1×10^{-6} cm s^{-1}. Keeping the values for all the other permeability constants unchanged the Goldman equation predicts a $V_m \sim -69$ mV. This is a **hyperpolarisation** of some 14 mV compared to the resting potential of -55 mV worked out in Section 11.2.

The membrane patch carrying the IPSP clearly acts as a source of local circuits. The direction of the currents is, however, in the opposite direction to that associated with the EPSP. Instead of tending to depolarise the initial segment these circuits tend to hyperpolarise it. They tend, in other words, to make it more difficult to bring the initial segment membrane to the threshold potential required to spark an action potential.

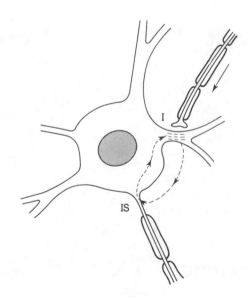

Figure 16.4   Spread of local circuits from an IPSP. The inhibitory synapse (I) hyperpolarises the dendritic membrane immediately beneath. Local circuits run in the opposite sense to those in Fig. 15.3 and the initial segment (IS) is consequently hyperpolarised (inhibited)

Other aspects of the IPSP are analogous to the EPSP. There is **temporal** and **spatial** summation. The position of the synapse on the subsynaptic neuron's soma and the area of synaptic contact has the same significance for inhibitory as it had for excitatory synapses.

16.1.3 Interaction of EPSPs and IPSPs

We have already noted that central neurons customarily have thousands (sometimes hundreds of thousands) of synaptic contacts dotted over their perikarya and dendritic arborisations. In the general case we can assume that half of these will be excitatory and half inhibitory. It is likely, also, that some members of both types will be active at the same time. It follows that local circuits will spread from IPSPs and EPSPs through the cell ultimately to the axon's initial segment. Here they will summate in an **algebraic** fashion. Whether the axon fires off an action potential depends on which type of postsynaptic potential predominates.

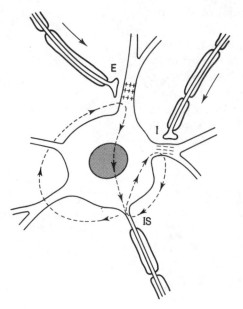

Figure 16.5   Algebraic summation at the initial segment of local circuits engendered by excitatory and inhibitory synapses. E = excitatory synapse; I = inhibitory synapse; IS = initial segment

Clearly the situation in the neuron is richly complex. Unfortunately for the neuroscientist this is only the beginning. We shall see in the next sections that further intricacies are built upon what may already seem intricate enough.

16.2 ION CHANNELS IN THE SUBSYNAPTIC MEMBRANE

We have noted in several earlier chapters the importance of the patch-clamp technique for studying the operation of single membrane channels. We also noted that much evidence has accumulated which suggests that channels can exist in more than just 'open' and 'shut' states—that, in other words, there are a number of intermediate conditions. Finally we saw that to account for the millivolt shifts in membrane potential which constitute action potentials, EPSPs and IPSPs, populations of channels must be at work. The individuals in these populations open, generally speaking, in a random fashion.

In earlier chapters of this book we have used a straightforward formulation of Ohm's law ($I = gV$) to describe the movement of ions through channels. Let us develop this formulation a little to take into account the complexity of the situation obtaining in biological membranes. McBurney (1983) has provided a useful analysis of a population of channels. Their operation can be described by eq. 16.1:

$$nT + nR(\gamma_c) \underset{\beta}{\overset{\alpha}{\rightleftharpoons}} nTR(\gamma_o) \quad \dots \qquad 16.1$$

where T = transmitter molecules, R = receptor sites, γ_c = closed channel conductance, γ_o = open channel conductance, and n is the number of transmitter molecules which must bind to the receptor sites to open the channel with a rate constant β. When the channel is opened the conductance across the membrane increases by ($\gamma_o - \gamma_c$). Channel-closing occurs with a rate constant of α when the transmitter detaches or is otherwise inactivated.

The magnitude of the current carried through the channel will, as usual, be the product of the **conductivity** of the channel, γ (usually measured in picoSiemens) and the driving force across the membrane. The latter is the electrochemical potential gradient for the ion (I) across the membrane. This is given by the difference between the membrane potential (V_m) and the null (or reversal) potential of the ion—i.e. the Nernst potential (V_I) for the ion. The driving force may thus be expressed as ($\boldsymbol{V_m - V_I}$).

The time for which each channel stays open depends on α, the rate constant for transmitter unbinding, in eq. 16.1. This will depend on numerous factors in the immediate environment of the channel protein. The greater the value of α the smaller will be the value of τ, the *average* channel opening constant. Figure 16.6 shows in (A) the opening of one channel over a time of some tens of milliseconds, in (B) the opening of a population of such channels and in (C) the summated effect of such a population on a membrane such as the subsynaptic membrane.

Note the difference between this analysis and the response of populations of voltage-gated channels in excitable membranes (Section 13.2). The difference is, of course, due to the fact that voltage-gates are, in a sense, co-operative. The opening of one of these gates and the consequent flow of current depolarises the

(A) One channel, one opening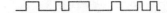

(B) One channel, many openings

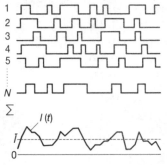

(C) Many channels, many openings

Figure 16.6 Summated effect of a population of ion channels in a subsynaptic membrane. (A) The opening and 'open-time' (t) of a single channel depends on numerous factors in its biochemical environment (see text). When it opens a brief pulse of current (i) is carried through. (B) In the presence of a constant concentration of agonist the channel will open many times. This opening will be random depending, as it does, on random collisions of the agonist with the receptor. (C) A subsynaptic membrane will usually contain many activatable ion channels. The summated effect of the random openings of these numerous channels gives the fluctuating current ($I(t)$) shown at the bottom of the figure. This current will fluctuate about a mean level $\bar{I}$. For further explanation see text. (After McBurney, 1983; *Trends in Neurosciences*, 6, 297–302; with permission.)

membrane and hence increases the probability that neighbouring channels will open.

The diagram in Figure 16.6 still assumes, however, that a membrane gate exists in just two states—open and closed—although the duration of the open state varies about a mean. This simple picture has now been complicated by the recognition that single gates can exist in several different conductance states. It has also been found that a gate may oscillate or 'flicker' between open and shut states. Finally there is evidence that in some conditions a single channel may open in 'bursts' and 'clusters' of bursts. These findings imply that the comparatively simple

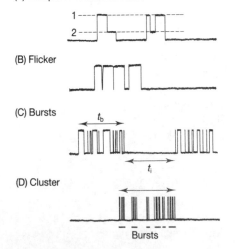

Figure 16.7 Conductance characteristics of single ACh-activated channels. The diagrams show some of the features exhibited by single ACh-activated channels. Time base for records (A) and (B) about 50 ms, for records (C) and (D) about 2 and 20 s, respectively. (A) A single channel can exist in more than one conductance state. (B) A channel may flicker rapidly between open and closed states. (C) A channel may open in 'bursts' lasting for up to a second (t_b) followed by a quiescent interval (t_i) before the next burst. (D) The bursts may be grouped in 'clusters'. (From McBurney, 1983, *Trends in Neurosciences*, 6, 297–302; with permission.)

scheme of Figure 16.6 does not represent the full complexity of ion fluxes in the subsynaptic membrane.

Returning, however, to our analysis of eq. 16.1 and Figure 16.6 we can see that different transmitters, different agonists, different antagonists, may exert their effects in different ways. It may be that an effect is produced by increasing the number of channels open over any given time, or it may be that the synaptically-active agent affects τ, the average open time or, finally, it may be that γ, the conductivity of the channel, is affected. Evidently there is great scope for transmitters to elicit subtly different subsynaptic events.

Perhaps this is another of the reasons for the nervous system developing such a bewildering variety of transmitters. It can, for instance, be shown that whereas GABA opens channels in cultured spinal neurons with $\tau = 30.4$ ms, taurine (which as we saw in Chapter 15 is a 'doubtful' transmitter) gives a $\tau = 2.3$ ms; glutamate on crab muscle gives a $\tau = 1.4$ ms whilst aspartate on the same preparation causes channel-opening with $\tau = 0.8$ ms.

16.3 MODULATION OF ION CHANNELS BY SECOND-MESSENGER SYSTEMS

So far in this chapter we have been considering very rapid events (usually less than 5 ms) in the subsynaptic membrane. We have seen how they may 'switch on' or 'switch off' the subsynaptic neuron. The next thing we have to do is to remind ourselves that many transmitters do not directly open ion gates at all but work through **collision-coupling second-messenger systems**. The outcome of these second-messenger systems may be to affect the conductivity of ion gates elsewhere in the subsynaptic membrane or, indeed, in other parts of the subsynaptic cell's neurilemma. Thus we add another layer of complexity on top of an already intricate enough situation.

We have already looked at some of these modulated channels in Chapter 10. One of the best known instances is the **Ca^{2+} channel (I_{Ca}-channel)**. It can be shown that this is modulated by a second-messenger system initiated by noradrenaline. The sequence of events is shown in Figure 16.8. The increased synthesis of cAMP following activation of the β-adrenergic receptor (β-AR) (see Section 7.1) leads to activation of a cAMP-dependent protein kinase. The latter phosphorylates the I_{Ca} channel. Phosphorylation (as we have seen in previous chapters) affects a channel's conductivity. In this case there appears to be 'down-modulation'. The flux of Ca^{2+} through the channel is decreased. Although these channels are probably rather few and far between the effect is nonetheless important. For instance it will be remembered from Chapter 14 that Ca^{2+} plays a crucial role in the exocytosis of transmitters and other material from presynaptic terminals. It follows that if the subsynaptic membrane happens to be that of a synaptic bouton (see Figure 14.20) then the release of NE on to β-AR receptors can have very significant consequences.

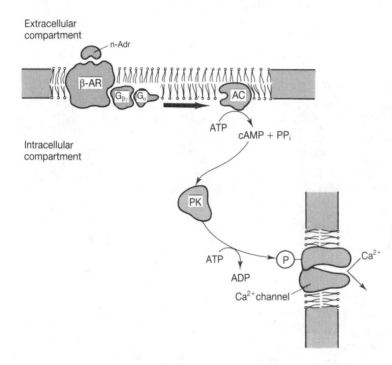

Figure 16.8 Adrenergic-activated second-messenger system on presynaptic terminals. The β-AR collision-coupling mechanism results in the generation of cAMP in the presynaptic ending; this activates a cAMP-dependent protein-kinase to phosphorylate (and thus down-modulate) a calcium channel. For further explanation see text. n-Adr = nor-adrenalin; β-AR = β-adrenergic receptor; G(γβα) = G-protein and its subunits; AC = adenylate cyclase; PK = protein kinase

Another interesting second-messenger system is that connected to the **muscarinic cholinergic receptor (mAChR)**. Once again we discussed the molecular biology of this receptor in Chapter 7. We saw that it resembled the β-adrenergic receptor in being connected via a collision-coupling mechanism to adenylate cyclase. It has been shown that the cAMP generated by this mechanism affects a particular set of K^+ channels in the subsynaptic membrane. These channels are quite distinct from the nAChR channels and from the K^+ channels which underly the action potential. Because they are affected (switched off) by activation of the muscarinic receptor they have been called **M channels (I_{KM})**.

The **M channels** normally allow K^+ to flux out of the cell. They are strongly voltage-dependent. As the membrane depolarises during an EPSP they progressively open. This increases the K^+ conductance across the membrane. If this increased conductance is inserted into the Goldman equation it can be seen that it has the effect of bringing the membrane back towards its resting potential. If, however, these channels are inactivated the

EPSP lasts considerably longer. This is exactly what happens when the mAChR is activated. Hence by this indirect route the muscarinic receptor can exert a very noticeable effect on spike initiation at the initial segment.

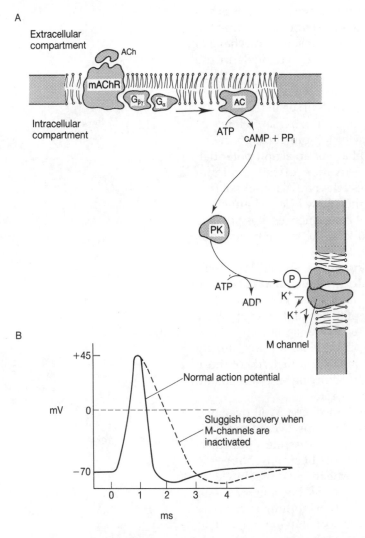

A

B

Figure 16.9 The influence of mAChR activation on impulse initiation. (A) The collision-coupling mechanism generates cAMP which activates a cAMP-dependent protein-kinase to phosphorylate and thus close the I_{KM} channel. Compare Fig. 7.5. (B) Because the I_{KM} channel has been blocked the K$^+$-induced recovery phase of the action potential is retarded. The membrane is thus refractory for longer than normal. When this occurs on an initial segment or dendritic zone the initiation of subsequent impulses is delayed. Abbreviations are as in Fig. 16.8. For further explanation see text

Let us look at one final instance of this receptor-mediated modulation of ion conductivity. This is the **serotonin-dependent potassium channel (I_{KS}).** We saw in Chapter 10 that this channel had been studied in the convenient preparation provided by the sea-hare *Aplysia*. It is also to be found in the less readily accessible vertebrate nervous system. The I_{KS} channel in *Aplysia* enables K$^+$ ions to flux through the membrane to the outside. It will be recalled that the resting potential (V_m) is very sensitive to the concentrations of K^+ inside and outside. If this flow is blocked the external concentration will slowly fall and the internal concentration will slowly rise. If this occurs the potential across the membrane will slowly fall. In other words a long, slowly increasing EPSP develops.

It can be shown that activation of serotoninergic synapses has just this result. Patch-clamp recording, moreover, shows that the effect is mediated through a cAMP second-messenger mechanism which results, as usual, in the **number** of I_{KS} channels in the open state being reduced, not a reduction in conductivity of those which are open.

Serotoninergic synapses are also, as we shall see in Chapter 18, found on some presynaptic terminals in *Aplysia*. Here, as mentioned in Chapter 10, the outflow of K^+ ions through the I_{KS} channels help to establish the AHP phase of an action potential. If these channels are reduced by activation of the serotonin receptor the onset of the AHP will be delayed. We shall see that the increased length of time which this allows Ca^{2+} channels to remain open may have very important consequences. It is possible that similar mechanisms are at work in mammalian nervous systems.

In mammalian systems serotonin can be shown to down-modulate yet another channel: the **calcium-dependent potassium channel (I_{KCa})**. The precise mechanism at work here remains to be discovered. Reference back to Chapter 10 will, however, show that modulation of this channel could have significant neuro-physiological consequences. The I_{KCa} channel is, we saw, deeply implicated in **adaptation**. Reduction in the conductivity of these channels could thus prevent adaptation occurring and thus ensure that a neuron kept on firing at a rapid rate.

We have only discussed the tip of an iceberg. Well over two dozen modulators of ion channels have been discovered and their properties analysed. The old picture of discrete, punctate, synaptic events—either IPSPs or EPSPs—is beginning to recede into history. Nevertheless it must be borne in mind that however complicated the neurochemical interactions become, the end result, the action potential, remains an all-or-nothing event. The outcome of all the interactions, chemical, spatial, temporal, is 'felt' at the **initial segment. If threshold is reached or exceeded the axon 'fires'; if it is not reached it remains quiescent**.

16.4 OTHER EFFECTS OF SECOND-MESSENGERS

So far we have been considering only the effects which second-messenger systems may have on the magnitude and duration of EPSPs and IPSPs and on the initiation and adaptation of action potentials. This, of course, is at the very core of neurophysiology. But we have been emphasising in this book that the subject of molecular neurobiology brings together the strands of biophysics and biochemistry into a new, very powerful, synthesis. This synthesis is nowhere more apparent than in the operation of second messenger systems for, in addition to their wide-ranging affects on ion channels, they also **diffuse into the cytosol** of a neuron to influence many crucial links in its biochemistry.

One of the most intensively researched cases of the cytosolic activity of second messenger systems has been the melatonin-secreting **pinealocyte** of the pineal gland.

Our understanding of the pineal has come a long way since René Descartes apostrophised it as 'the seat of the soul'. Whilst in the lower vertebrates (the fish, amphibia and reptiles) it often functions as a 'third eye', in the birds and mammals it has lost all direct contact with light. Instead it elaborates a hormone, **melatonin**, which has been shown to be of importance in regulating reproductive cycles. Indeed Descartes may not have been so far off the mark when he speculated on the centrality of the pineal in human existence. For it has been argued that a mutation in the gene controlling the pineal's development is responsible for the delayed onset of reproductive maturity in *Homo sapiens*. The melatonin which the gland secretes inhibits the maturation of the gonads. In humans, unlike other primates, the pineal remains continuously active for the first 14 or 15 years of life, after which time it deteriorates, indeed calcifies. The prolonged childhood which this ensures is undoubtedly one of the most significant developments in the evolutionary path to mankind.

Returning, however, from these broad evolutionary perspectives to the neurochemical detail, we find that pinealocytes in the pineal have an adrenergic innervation which ultimately originates in the retina. This pathway is inhibited by light. Activation of the pathway only occurs in **low light intensities** or **short photoperiods**. The noradrenalin released operates in the way discussed in Chapter 7 to cause the synthesis of cAMP. cAMP diffuses into the interior of the pinealocyte where it causes a number of subsequent biochemical events. Let us concentrate on just one sequence of reactions. The cAMP first activates a protein kinase. The kinase, in turn, appears to phosphorylate a nuclear histone. Histones are closely associated with DNA in eukaryotic chromosomes. Phosphorylation of the histone throws a switch which allows a particular gene to be transcribed. Fresh mRNA from this gene can soon be detected in the cytosol. This mRNA programmes the synthesis of an important enzyme—**serotonin-n-acetyltransferase (SNAT)**. The cAMP may also be involved in the translation step of this synthesis. Finally SNAT catalyses the synthesis of melatonin from serotonin. The melatonin is secreted into the vascular system and on reaching the gonads exerts the effects mentioned above. The upshot of this complex sequence of events is thus to ensure that in many birds and infra-human mammals the gonads only become active when photoperiod increases.

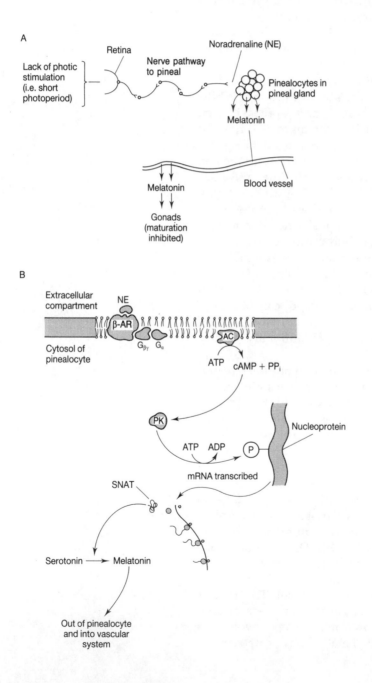

Figure 16.10   Second messenger activity in pinealocytes. (A) A multisynaptic pathway leads from the retina to the pineal. The final neuron in the chain releases noradrenalin (NE) on to the pinealocytes. This leads to the release of melatonin into the vascular system, which in turn inhibits the maturation of the gonads. (B) A collision-coupling mechanism in the pinealocyte membrane leads to the generation of cAMP. Protein kinase is activated which phosphorylates a nuclear histone. This switches on the transcription of mRNA for SNAT. Translation occurs at the ribosomes and the newly synthesised SNAT catalyses the production of melatonin from serotonin. Melatonin is released into the vascular system and circulates to the gonads. Note that this mechanism is not important in *Homo sapiens* as the pineal is largely inactive in adults of this species. Further explanation in text. SNAT = serotonin-*n*-acetyl transferase

We noted in Chapter 15 that mammalian neurons synthesise over 50 different **neuroactive peptides**. It is not difficult to see that these syntheses may be switched on and off in an analogous way by transmitter-activated second-messenger systems.

Cyclic AMP and cGMP are far from being the only second-messengers at work in the nervous system. We have, in fact, already met another second-messenger. This is the **calcium ion**. We have seen how this diffuses into a cell to bring about such vitally important phenomena as synaptic exocytosis. But Ca^{2+}

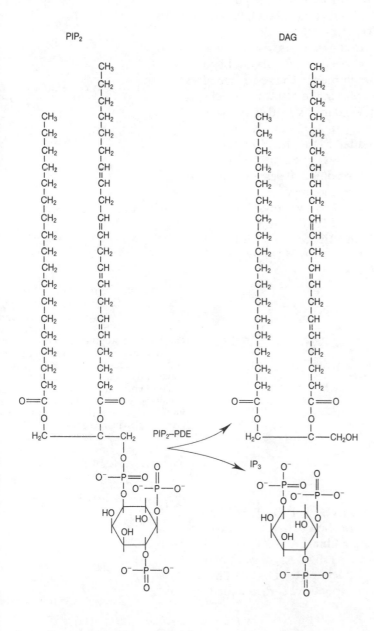

Figure 16.11 Origin of IP_3 and DAG from PIP_2. Phosphatidylinositol-4,5-biphosphate (PIP_2) is converted to diacylglycerol (DAG) and inositol triphosphate (IP_3) by the enzyme PIP_2-phosphodiesterase (PIP_2-PDE)

ions have many other control functions in the cell, from cell growth to cell movement. In addition to Ca^{2+} ions there are two other important second-messengers which so far we have not discussed. Both these second-messengers are derived from the phospholipid **phosphatidyl inositol (PI)** which, as we saw in Chapter 6, is predominantly located in the inner leaflet of the plasmalemma. First phosphatidyl inositol is converted to **phosphatidylinositol-4,5-biphosphate (PIP_2)** by the sequential addition of two phosphate groups from ATP. Next a **PIP_2-phosphodiesterase enzyme (PIP_2-PDE)** located in the membrane cleaves the PIP_2 into two moieties, **diacylglycerol (DAG)** and **inositol triphosphate (IP_3)**.

The production of the two second-messengers from phosphatidylinositol is again believed to be brought about by a collision-coupling mechanism in the membrane. The sequence of events is shown in Figure 16.12. A receptor in the membrane picks up a signal from a transmitter. Once again, as in the systems discussed in Chapter 7, a G-protein transmission mechanism is used to activate the membrane-embedded PDE. This then reacts with PIP_2 to produce IP_3 and DAG, as shown in Figure 16.11. IP_3 is a water-soluble molecule and hence it readily diffuses away into the cytoplasm. Here it may interact with the membranes of the ER, leading to a release of Ca^{2+}. These ions, as we noted above, are known to have many and varied effects on cellular biochemistry. Ultimately IP_3 is inactivated by inositol triphosphatase. DAG, on the other hand, is hydrophobic and hence remains behind in the membrane.

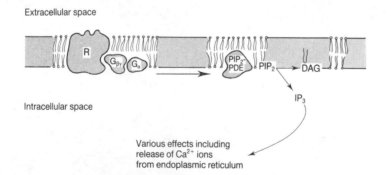

Figure 16.12 IP_3 as a second messenger. When the membrane receptor (R) is occupied by a transmitter a G-protein collision-coupling mechanism activates PIP_2-PDE, which cleaves PIP_2 into DAG and IP_3. DAG remains in the inner leaflet of the plasma membrane while IP_3 diffuses into the cytosol as a second-messenger. For further explanation see text. PIP_2-PDE = PIP_2-phosphodiesterase; DAG = diacylglycerol; IP_3 = inositol triphosphate

We haven't finished with the system yet. For the DAG left behind also has a job to do. Figure 16.13 shows that it interacts with a lipid-bound protein kinase, **protein kinase C (PKC)**. When the Ca^{2+} concentration of the cytosol rises (an effect, as we have just seen, of IP_3) PKC becomes attached to DAG. This interaction requires the presence of phosphatidyl serine which,

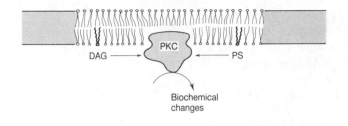

Figure 16.13 DAG as a second-messenger. Diacyglycerol (DAG) remains in the membrane and random movement brings it into contact with PKC, which is also in the inner leaflet of the membrane. Activation of PKC also requires the presence of phosphatidyl serine (PS), which is also normally present in the inner leaflet. For further explanation see text

as we saw in Chapter 6, is also concentrated in the membrane's inner leaflet. The aroused PKC can now activate proteins which elicit specific biochemical responses. In the case of blood platelets, for instance, PKC activates a hydrogen-ion exchange mechanism in the membrane. The consequent alteration in the pH of the cytosol can have profound consequences—not least on the synthesis of RNA. In neurons a number of effects have been demonstrated, including synthesis and secretion of neurotransmitters, alterations to the sensitivity of receptors and to the functioning of the cytoskeleton. Some recent studies have also suggested that PKC plays a role in determining synaptic plasticity. We shall return to this in Chapter 18, where we consider the molecular basis of memory.

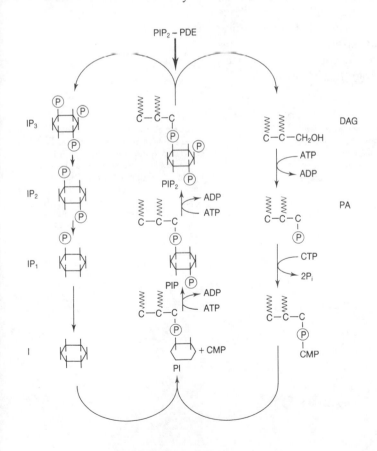

Figure 16.14 Resynthesis of PIP_2 from IP_3 and DAG. The enzyme PIP_2-PDE cleaves PIP_2 into IP_3 and DAG (see text). On the right hand side of the flow diagram DAG is phosphorylated first to phosphatidic acid (PA) and then interacts with cytosine triphosphate (CTP) to add cytosine monophosphate (CMP). On the left-hand side of the diagram IP_3 is dephosphorylated to inositol diphosphate (IP_2), inositol monophosphate (IP_1) and then to inositol itself (I). The two halves of the flow then come together to yield first phosphatidyl inositol (PI) (regenerating CMP), then phosphatidylinositol-4-phosphate (PIP) and lastly back to PIP_2. (After Berridge, 1985, *Scientific American*, **253**, 124–136.)

Finally—how is the phosphatidyl inositol replaced? Evidently the membrane cannot just lose this important constituent each time the second-messenger system operates. The resynthesis of PIP_2 is shown in Figure 16.14. The cycle requires the presence of ATP and CTP, which provide both energy and phosphate bonds. It is interesting to note that lithium ions block one of the steps in this resynthesis pathway: the step from inositol monophosphate to inositol. Whether the well-known effects of lithium in lifting depression can be connected to its action in this biochemical pathway is an interesting speculation—but as yet no more than a speculation.

16.5 THE SUBSYNAPTIC DENSITY

We noted at the beginning of this chapter that synaptosomes usually retain a portion of adherent subsynaptic membrane with a characteristic subsynaptic density or thickening. If a synaptosome is exposed to the strong detergent Triton X-100 the pre- and postsynaptic membranes are released from the rest of the complex. This, the so-called synaptic plasma membrane (SPM), may then be isolated from the other elements of the synaptosome by density gradient centrifugation. As indicated at the beginning of this chapter, the fact that the pre- and postsynaptic membranes stay together when the rest of the synaptosome has been liquidated suggests that they are held together by some electron-

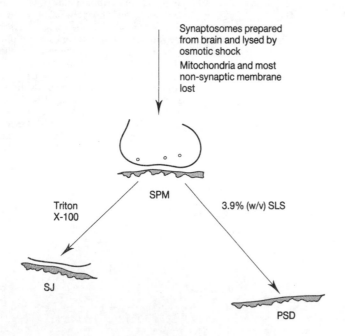

Synaptosomes prepared from brain and lysed by osmotic shock

Mitochondria and most non-synaptic membrane lost

SPM

Triton X-100

3.9% (w/v) SLS

SJ

PSD

Figure 16.15 Preparation of SPMs, SJs and PSDs from synaptosomes. Treatment of lysed synaptosomes (synaptic plasma membranes: SPMs) with Triton X-100 yields synaptic junctions (SJs); treatment of SPMs with sodium lauryl sarcosinate (SLS) yields postsynaptic densities (PSDs). (After Kelly and Cotman, 1977, *Journal of Biological Chemistry*, **252**, 786–793.)

translucent matrix. The analysis of this region can be carried a step further by subjecting the SPMs to 3.9% w/v sodium lauryl sarcosinate. This dissolves away all but the subsynaptic or postsynaptic density (PSD).

The proteins and polypeptides of the SPM and PSD can be analysed by polyacrylamide gel electrophoresis. In both cases the gel shows a large number of different bands, indicating a variety of molecules. The major molecule within the synaptic cleft seems to have a molecular weight of more than 95 kDa and to be a glycoprotein. The major proteins in the subsynaptic density appear to be smaller, having molecular weights of 52 kDa and 55 kDa, although there is evidence for at least five minor representatives with higher masses. Carrying the analysis a little further it can be deduced that the proteins in the subsynaptic density are extensively cross-linked, perhaps forming a network. There is also evidence that fibrous proteins, perhaps actin, tubulin and (possibly) neurofilaments, are constituents of the network. It is easy to speculate that this intricate network anchors receptor molecules in the subsynaptic membrane.

Evidence to support this speculation has come from studies of the neuromuscular junction (Section 9.1.3). Electron microscopy shows that the subsynaptic membrane of the junction is folded into a large number of invaginations and that there is a filamentous meshwork beneath it. It can be shown, furthermore, that the acetylcholine receptors are clustered on the crests of the folds. The density of AChRs on the crests may reach 10 000 μm^{-2}, compared with about 20 μm^{-2} on the rest of the sarcolemma.

We noted in Chapter 9 that the electric organs of electric fish provide a spectacular source of cholinergic neuromuscular junctions. The electrocytes of the electric ray, *Torpedo*, have thus been used in investigations of the structure and function of the neuromuscular subsynaptic meshwork. It has been found that the subsynaptic material can be removed by alkaline solutions or low concentrations of lithium diiodosalicylate. Analysis of the extract by gel electrophoresis reveals a number of proteins and in particular a group with a molecular weight of about 43 kDa. If antibodies are raised against this protein, tagged with colloidal gold particles and then reacted with the *Torpedo* electrocyte, the **cytoplasmic faces** of the *crests* of the subsynaptic membrane are labelled. This suggests that it is indeed part of the subsynaptic apparatus.

There is suggestive evidence that the 43 kDa protein plays a role in anchoring nAChRs into the subsynaptic membrane. A number of techniques for determining the mobility of large proteins such as the nAChR in biomembranes is available. For instance, electrocyte membranes may be fused with liposomes.

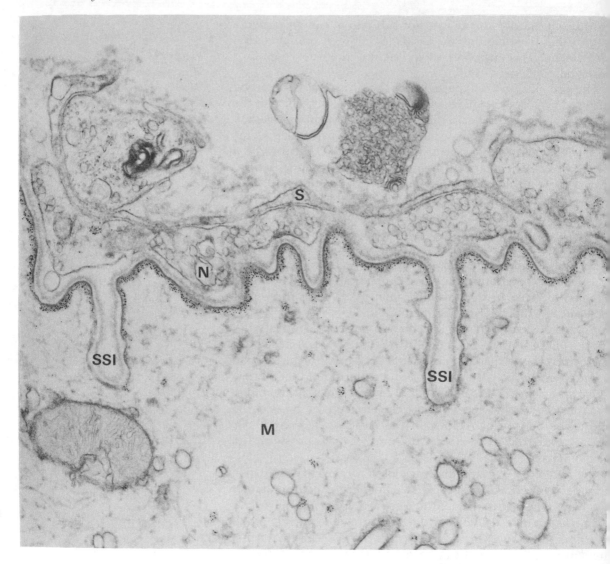

Figure 16.16 *Torpedo* electrocyte membrane labelled with anti-43 kDa protein antibody. The black dots are 5 nm gold particles attached to the anti-43 kDa protein antibody. It can be seen that these particles are concentrated on the cytoplasmic side of the crests of the subsynaptic folds and do not extend deep into the invaginations. For further explanation see text. N = nerve terminal; S = Schwann cytoplasm; M = sarcoplasm of muscle; SSI = subsynaptic invagination; ×38 000. (Reproduced from Sealock, Wray and Froehner, 1984, *J. Cell Biol.*, **98**, 2239–2244 by copyright permission of the Rockefeller University Press.)

If this is done it is found that nAChRs do not diffuse freely throughout the hybrid membrane. If, however, the electrocyte membranes have their subsynaptic network removed by alkali extraction the lateral diffusion is much enhanced.

Evidence is thus accumulating from various different sources to support the view that subsynaptic densities represent anchorages for neurotransmitter receptors. These anchorages are associated with elements of the cytoskeleton, especially actin and fodrin (Chapter 6). It is likely that the rather amorphous densifications seen by the electron microscopist (Chapter 1) will turn out to have an intricate multimolecular architecture.

16.6 CONCLUSION

This chapter has emphasised the developing recognition that the subsynaptic membrane is of equal importance to the presynaptic terminal in the functioning of synapses. But the connections between neurons are not only of importance in the neurophysiology of information processing in the adult brain. They are also of profound importance in the morphogenesis of the brain, in memory and, when they are in some way disabled, in causing numerous distressing neuro- and psychopathologies. It is to these matters that we turn in our final group of chapters. We shall see, once, again that subtle variations in molecular structure are multiplied up through the intricacies of neuroanatomy to end in massive effects on brain, behaviour and human well-being.

Chapter 17
Epigenetics of the brain

Human brains consist of at least 10^{11} cells and upwards of 10^{14} synapses. We have noted the heterogeneity of neuronal membranes and in Chapter 15 we reviewed the ever increasing number of different synaptically active substances. Yet it is a truism that this vast number of units, this immense heterogeneity, is organised into a harmonious functioning unity. How? The brain is perhaps the ultimate challenge for the developmental biologist! In this chapter we shall look at a few promising molecular approaches.

First of all let us clear out of the way any idea that the structure of the brain (and thus its functioning) might be completely **preformed**—directly specified in the 'blueprint' of the genes. It is easy to eliminate this notion. We only have to look at the numbers. It has been calculated that the human genome stores no more than about 10^{10} bits of information: yet we have just seen that there are at least 10^{11} neurons and 10^{14} synapses! Clearly the numbers don't add up: the genome is just not large enough to specify the co-ordinates of each and every neuron, let alone each and every synapse. Preformationism is not an option. Instead we have to consider some mechanism of **epigenesis**— some mechanism of gradual differentiation and elaboration.

The brain is very different from other tissues in its immense interconnectivity. It is not enough that its unit cells should differentiate. They must also form appropriate connections with each other. This compounds the problem set out in the previous paragraph. To use the computer analogy—it is not only that transistors must differentiate from resistors and resistors from capacitors but also that they must all somehow come to be interconnected in the proper way. The genome not only has to specify the position and nature of each cell but also its interconnections. Preformationism seems even more a huge impossibility. It seems that the genes could only specify a broad outline plan. Perhaps they direct the laying down of some crisscrossing of chemical gradients through which the growing neurons have to find their way. This criss-cross has sometimes been called a **morphopoietic field** or, alternatively, an **epigenetic 'landscape'**. The intersection of comparatively few morphopoietic gradients could lead to an immensely varied epigenetic landscape—see Figure 17.1.

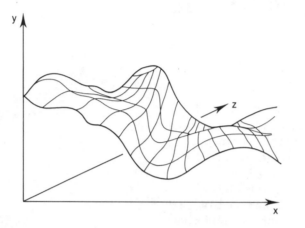

Figure 17.1   An epigenetic 'landscape'. Three chemical gradients laid down along the x,y and z axes of the diagram would create a complex chemical 'landscape' through which a developing neuron would have to find its way. (After Waddington, 1957, *The Strategy of the Genes*, London: Allen & Unwin.)

Before considering the neurochemical possibilities in this concept more closely let us look at the more general nature of neurogenesis: the building of a nervous system. We shall, as usual, confine ourselves principally to the vertebrate central nervous system.

17.1 THE ORIGINS OF NEURONS AND GLIA

We noted in Chapter 1 that the vertebrate central nervous system originates as a longitudinal strip of cells on the dorsal surface of the early embryo. We saw that this strip of cells soon sinks inwards and rolls up to form the neural tube. This process is termed **neurulation** and is shown in Figure 17.2.

Figure 17.2 shows that a strip of ectoderm left outside when neurulation is complete is called the **neural crest**. This strip of tissue is the precursor of all the sensory nerve fibres, the peripheral autonomic nervous fibres and the Schwann cells. All the other cells of the nervous system originate in the neural tube.

Initially the number of cells in the neural tube is quite small. In amphibian embryos it is believed to be about 125 000. Once the neural tube is complete, however, a rapid **proliferative** stage begins. The single layer of cells which originally formed the neural

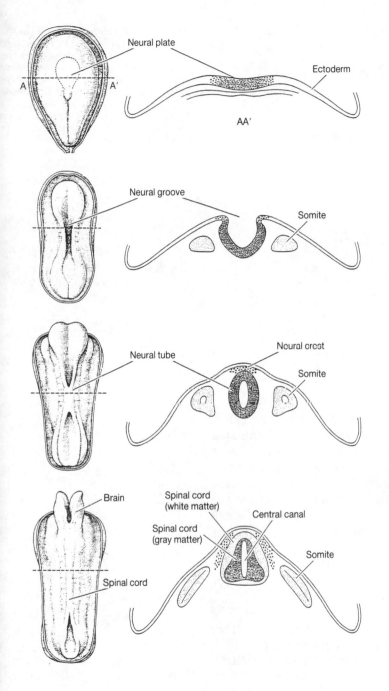

Neural plate

Ectoderm

A   A'

AA'

Neural groove

Somite

Neural tube

Neural crest

Somite

Brain

Spinal cord
(white matter)

Central canal

Spinal cord
(gray matter)

Somite

Spinal cord

Figure 17.2 Neurulation. The left-hand column of drawings shows the development of the human embryo (third to fourth week after conception) from above and the right-hand column shows transverse sections through these embryonic stages at the position marked by the broken line. (Reprinted with permission from Cowan, 1979, *Scientific American*, **241**, 107–117. Copyright © 1979 by Scientific American Inc. All rights reserved.)

plate quickly becomes transformed into a multilayered wall. This proliferative stage is, however, interestingly complex. Figure 17.3 shows that the stages of mitotic division are co-ordinated with movement up and down through the cell layers.

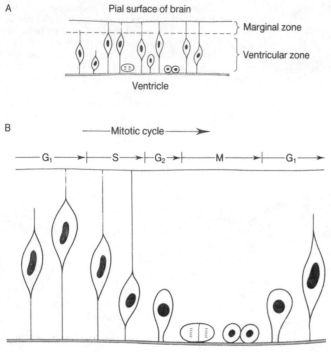

A

Pial surface of brain

} Marginal zone

} Ventricular zone

Ventricle

B

——Mitotic cycle——→

G_1 → | S → | G_2 → | M → | G_1 →

Ventricle

Figure 17.3 Proliferation of cells in the wall of the neural tube. (A) The wall of the neural tube at an early stage consists of two layers: a marginal zone consisting of processes and a ventricular zone where the cell bodies are located. (B) The mitotic cycle of the proliferating neurons is associated with movements up and down through the ventricular zone. For further explanation see text

During the G_1-**phase** of the mitotic cycle (where the cell is actively metabolising but otherwise quiescent) the cell is situated in the middle of the neuroepithelium. At the onset of DNA synthesis (the **S-phase**) the cell nucleus begins to move down toward the ventricular surface. During the G_2-**phase** the nucleus is close to the ventricular surface of the neuroepithelium and the lengthy cytoplasmic processes are withdrawn so that the cell rounds up ready for mitotic division. Mitotic division then occurs (**M-phase**), so that the cell is duplicated. The two daughter cells then enter the G_1-**phase** once more, their cytoplasmic processes re-form and the nuclei return to their original position in the centre of the epithelium.

This sequence of events may be repeated many times. The **number of repetitions** varies from one brain region to another and appears to be highly characteristic of a given region. What determines this number is as yet unknown. But it is crucially important. For once the cell's DNA synthesis has been switched off the cell migrates out of the ventricular, proliferative, zone into an **intermediate zone**. Not only this but the cell's 'fate' is also to an extent **determined**. In other words if its 'date of birth' is known (i.e. the time when it loses its capacity for DNA synthesis) then its final position in the brain, its type and to a large extent its interconnections can be predicted.

It is found that both neurons and neuroglia originate at much the same time. However, the reproductive rate of neurons is at first far greater than that of glia. In the human fetus the proliferation of neurons occurs during the first 18 weeks after conception. After this period neurons cease proliferating (though there are exceptions in some parts of the brain, e.g. the olfactory epithelium). Glial cells, on the other hand, although slow starters, continue dividing for a much longer period—indeed well into post-natal life.

Another feature of the proliferative phase which is worth noting is that the **larger** ('principal' or 'projection' (see Chapter 1)) neurons are the first to develop; the **smaller** ('local circuit' or 'inter-') neurons appear later.

The next stage in the development of the brain (though not of the spinal cord, where neurons remain central) is the migration of neurons from around the ventricle to the outer surface. This surface, because it abuts the innermost of the meninges, the pia mater, is called the **pial** surface. Neurons appear to migrate 'upwards' towards the pial surface along the lengthy processes of **radial glia** (see Chapter 1). The cell bodies of these glia line the **ventricular surface** of the neural tube and a lengthy process stretches right across the wall of the tube to terminate against the endothelial wall of one of the blood vessels in the pia mater.

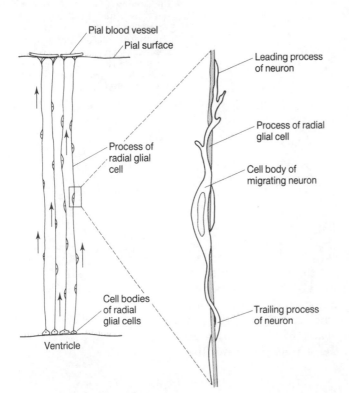

Figure 17.4   Migration of neurons along processes of radial glia. The processes of the radial glial cells extend from the ventricular to the pial surface of the developing cerebrum. On the right of the diagram is an enlargement to show a neuron migrating up a glial process towards the pial surface. (After Racik, 1979, in *The Neurosciences, Fourth Study Program*, eds F. O. Schmitt and F. G. Worden, Cambridge, Mass: MIT Press, pp. 109–127.)

Pial blood vessel
Pial surface
Leading process of neuron
Process of radial glial cell
Process of radial glial cell
Cell body of migrating neuron
Cell bodies of radial glial cells
Trailing process of neuron
Ventricle

The movement of neurons along glial processes seems to be a type of amoeboid locomotion. A leading process entwines itself around the glial fibre and the nucleus is drawn up behind it. In some cases the the trailing process behind the neuron merely elongates as the nucleus moves up towards the pial surface. This process may then form the axon. In other cases the trailing process is drawn up behind the nucleus as it makes its slow journey, in yet other cases it becomes detached and is broken down and removed by neighbouring (non-radial) glial cells.

There is evidence for a strong **symbiotic relationship between radial glia and migrating neurons**. Not only do radial glia act as guidelines for postmitotic neurons but vice-versa postmitotic neurons appear to be essential to prevent embryonic astroglia continuing their proliferative phase. Without such an association astroglia fail to assume their characteristic fibrous form. This is a first example of the great importance of cell–cell contact in the development of the nervous system.

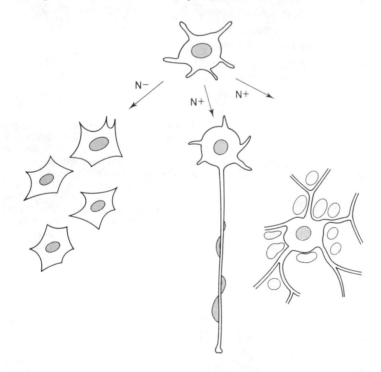

Figure 17.5 Effects of neurons on embryonic astroglia. Neurons and astroglia were rapidly separated from mouse cerebella and either mixed or kept separate. When neurons and glia were mixed (+N) the glia assumed their characteristic morphology: either developing a long process along which neurons could be seen to 'crawl' or developing radial arms which seemed to 'compartmentalise' the neurons. In the absence of neurons (-N) the glia remained undifferentiated and continued to proliferate. (After Hatten and Mason, 1986, *Trends in Neurosciences*, **9** 168–174.)

The significant role which the fibres of the radial glia play in guiding neurons to their final destination has been examined in mice homozygous for the **weaver** mutation (wv/wv). This mutation results in the granule cells of the cerebellum failing to reach their correct position, which leads to the disastrous behavioural upset summed up in the name given to the mutation—weaver.

The weaver mutation expresses itself in the granule cells. They appear to lack some membrane component which is essential for the proper differentiation of radial glia. The granule cells thus have no means of climbing to their proper position in the cerebellum. The structure and functioning of the cerebellum is consequently severely disrupted.

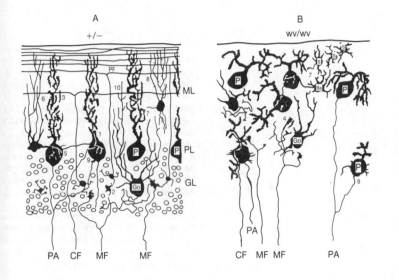

Figure 17.6 The structure of normal $(+/-)$ and weaver (wv/wv) cerebella. (A) Normal mouse cerebellum. (B) Cerebellum of mouse homozygous for the weaver mutation. Both cerebella are taken from 3-week-old mice and stained by the Golgi technique. The granule cell layer is completely missing from the weaver cerebellum and the other cells and cell processes are highly disorganised. P = Purkinje cell; Go = Golgi cell; Ba = basket cell; S = stellate cell; PA = Purkinje axon; CF = climbing fibre; MF = mossy fibre; GL = granule cell layer; PL = Purkinje cell layer; ML = molecular layer; PF = parallel fibre; the numbers refer to specific types of synapse. (From Rakic, 1979, in *The Neurosciences, Fourth Study Program*, eds F. O. Schmitt and F. G. Worden, Cambridge, Mass: MIT Press, pp. 109–127; with permission.)

Finally, let us consider the migration of neurons from ventricular to pial surface in a little more detail. This migration is shown in Figure 17.7. It brings about a progressive thickening of the neural tube. The original proliferative wall is shown at (A). Two layers are recognisable. A **ventricular zone (VZ)** in which proliferation is proceeding and a **marginal zone (MZ)** in which only the outermost proceeses of the embryonic neurons are ever present. The first cells to lose their DNA-replicative ability (i.e. to stop proliferating) move up from the ventricular zone to form an **intermediate zone (IZ)**. In the forebrain we find that further migrating cells pass through the IZ to form a **cortical plate (CP)**. The CP later differentiates to give the typical six- or three-layered structure of the neo- or allo-cortex.

Ultimately the cerebral cortex is formed from the original marginal zone (MZ) plus the cortical plate (CP). The intermediate zone (IZ) beneath the CP becomes the subcortical white matter whilst the original VZ is transformed into the ependymal lining of the ventricle. Above the ependyma a thin layer—the subventricular zone (SZ)—remains as a proliferative region where glia cells continue to multiply.

The migration of neurons along the guidance fibres of radial glia goes far to ensure that neurons originating in the same region of the neural tube remain together in the adult cortex. It is likely that this developmental process underlies the **columnar organisation** of the cerebral cortex. It appears, in other words, that the cortical modules which we discussed in Chapter 1 (see Figure 1.23) consist of cells which have been together since their birth. Perhaps they all share similar membrane characteristics (see Section 17.4) which ensure that they stick together in a more than figurative fashion.

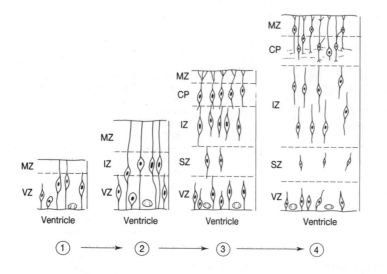

Figure 17.7 Maturation of the neural tube. (1) At an early stage the neural tube consists of two layers: the marginal zone (MZ) consisting of processes and the ventricular zone (VZ) consisting of proliferating cells. (2) Cells which have finished proliferating migrate upwards to form the intermediate zone (IZ). (3) In regions of the brain which are to develop a cortex the cells continue migrating upwards to form a cortical plate (CP). (4) Finally the cortex differentiates from the MZ and the CP; the IZ forms subcortical white matter; glial cells continue proliferating in the SZ; the VZ becomes the ependymal lining of the ventricle. For further explanation see text. (After Jacobson, 1978, *Developmental Neurobiology*, New York: Plenum.)

The **differential stickiness** of neurons has indeed been shown in numerous experiments. Disaggregated neocortical and hippocampal neurons cultured in appropriate conditions reaggregate into distinct clumps consisting of either cortical or hippocampal cells. Such clumps even show the beginnings of lamination. This indicates that some sorting of the dissociated cells into their definitive positions occurs. Similar experiments have been carried out on the retina. Disaggregated retinal cells tend to re-establish their original organisation. Furthermore it can be demonstrated that disaggregated chick retinal cells adhere preferentially to those parts of the optic tectum to which they would normally project. We shall return to the topic of 'differential stickiness' in later parts of this chapter—especially in Section 17.5, where we review some of the features of **cell adhesion molecules (CAMs)**.

17.2 MORPHOGENESIS OF NEURONS

It is a truism that neurons have intricate shapes. Yet we left them as simple bipolar forms clambering along the guidance fibres of the radial glia. How do they achieve their adult morphology?

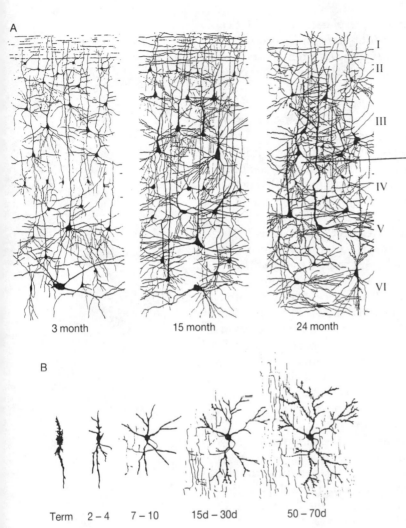

A

I
II
III
IV
V
VI

3 month   15 month   24 month

B

Term   2 – 4   7 – 10   15d – 30d   50 – 70d

Figure 17.8 Morphogenesis of cortical neurons. (A) Tracings from Golgi-stained sections of the temporal cortex of 3-month, 15-month and 24-month human brains. The increased dendritic arborisation and in the 24-month preparation the strong development of dendritic spines are clearly visible (*see enlarged area*). (B) Tracings from Golgi-stained sections of the cerebellar cortex of kittens at various ages. The dendritic processes of the granule cells show great development during the first 70 days of life, and in the 50–70 day section dendritic spines are again clearly visible. (From Altman, 1967, in *The Neurosciences*, eds G. C. Quarton, T. Melnechuk and F. O., Schmitt, New York: Rockefeller Press; with permission.)

Figure 17.8 shows the progressive development of neurons in the cerebral cortex of the human brain. It is clear that at birth the neurons are in a very immature state. They may be in the right place but their dendritic trees are hardly formed and in many cases their axons have yet to find their correct destination.

Each class of neurons has its own distinctive morphology. Pyramidal cells are not to be mistaken for stellate cells; Purkinje cells are completely different from granule cells, etc. These differences persist even when the cells are cultured outside the nervous system. Such major morphologies are evidently genetically determined. The genetic determination, however, probably goes further. Physiologically identified neurons can be filled with dye and their dendritic arborisations carefully studied by serial sectioning. It turns out that similar neurons of genetically identical animals show remarkably similar dendritic branching patterns and the initial routes (at least) of their axons are also remarkably the same. Thus, at this level, **genetic determination** evidently plays a major role.

The fine detail of synaptic connectivity and dendritic and telodendritic 'twig' pattern is, however, under **epigenetic** control. Young neurons can be seen to undergo a period during which an extravagant growth of dendrites occurs. Many of these hopeful sprouts are withdrawn. This phase of exuberant arborisation is timed to coincide with the arrival of afferent fibres. It is likely that dendritic sprouts require stabilisation by the establishment of synaptic junctions if they are not to be resorbed. Afferentation can thus be seen as a process of **'negative sculpturing'**. The characteristic pattern of a dendritic tree is sculptured by incoming afferents from an originally somewhat inchoate dendrite thicket. We shall consider evidence for these long-range effects on dendritic form in Section 17.6. The concept of 'negative sculpturing', of chipping away unwanted material, to reveal an appropriate pattern is very important. We shall find it at work not only in our considerations of neural epigenesis but also in our considerations of the molecular basis of memory. It has also been used to explain the way in which the cerebellum moulds the pattern of impulses by which it co-ordinates muscular activity. 'Negative sculpturing', indeed, might almost be seen as the Darwinism of the nervous system.

In addition to global effects the 'local' environment also plays a part in determining neuronal morphology. There is good evidence, for instance, that the position of a neuron in the cerebellar cortex affects its pattern of branching and the position of a pyramidal cell in the cerebral cortex—in the comparatively thin cortex of a sulcus or the thicker cortex of a gyrus—again affects its morphology.

17.3 GROWTH CONES

Neural processes (neurites)—axons and dendrites—grow by means of **growth cones**. Growth cones, as Figure 17.9 shows, are rather like outspread hands, palms down, at the ends of neurites. They only form when the neurite is in contact with an appropriate substratum. The 'palm' of the growth cone is typically about 5 μm in diameter and the numerous fingers (**microspikes**) are long (up to 50 μm) and narrow (diameter: 0.1–0.2 μm). They are in constant movement—stretching out, waving to and fro, retracting back into the 'palm'. The 'palm' itself frequently divides, each half seemingly searching out the best route. The least successful

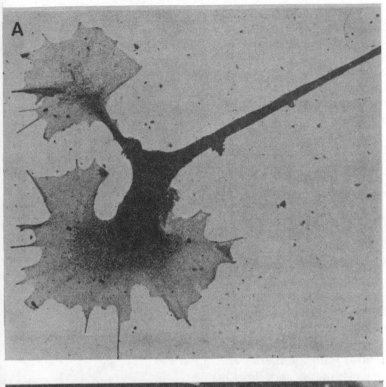

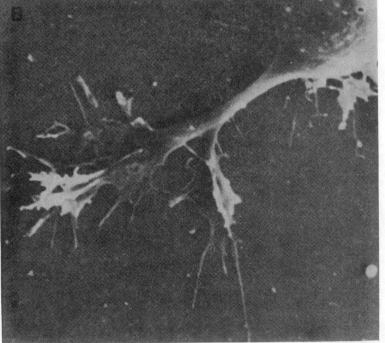

Figure 17.9 Growth cones of neurons in tissue culture. (A) Transmission electron micrograph of two growth cones at the end of the axon of a cultured rat sympathetic cell. (B) Scanning electron micrograph of cultured fetal rat hippocampal cell showing growth cones at the tip of a dendrite. ((A): courtesy of Dr M.J. Cochran and Dr M. Bartlett; (B): courtesy of Dr S.R. Rothman.)

half is usually resorbed although, especially in the case of dendrites, branch points may be established.

If the ultrastructure of a growth cone is carefully examined it can be seen to contain innumerable small vesicles, sometimes running together to give larger profiles resembling smooth endoplasmic reticulum. The cone also contains mitochondria and the characteristic filamentous elements of neurites: neurotubules, microfilaments (actin) and neurofilaments.

The growth of the neurite is probably accomplished by the synthesis of neurotubules and neurofilaments in the cell body and their continuous extrusion into the process. Labelling techniques have shown that these elements move out along an axon (and thus presumably also along dendrites) at 1 or 2 mm per day, i.e. a rate similar to slow axoplasmic transport (see Section 14.3). Whilst the neurite grows there is no disassembly of the tubules and filaments, just a gradual elongation. Superimposed upon this slow, steady elongation is a more rapid transport of membranous vesicles. These presumably carry new membrane to the cone, where it collects as the small vesicle population and smooth ER which, as we noted above, is characteristic of growth cone ultrastructure. The membranous material is ultimately added to the ever-growing plasmalemma of the growth cone by the process of exocytosis. The vesicle membrane fuses with the membrane of the growth cone and its lipoprotein constituents very quickly diffuse into the bilayer.

The restless probing activity of the growth cone depends on the actin microfilaments. If cytochalasin B, which inhibits actin polymerisation, is added to the culture medium, the ceaseless exploratory movements of the growth cone cease. It no longer puts out its microspike fingers and remains quiescent, fixed to the substratum.

17.4 PATHFINDING

Elongation of a neurite is not, of course, enough. It must find its way to its destination. The way in which this vital pathfinding job is accomplished is as yet still poorly understood. Two mechanisms are believed to be at work: growth along a chemical gradient and contact guidance. One or other, and probably a combination of both, mechanisms probably underlie neurite pathfinding.

By far the best known **neurotropic** substance is **nerve growth factor (NGF)**. Although NGF was first extracted from mouse sarcoma cells, its richest source is (for some unknown reason) the salivary gland. NGF exists in several different forms with various different molecular weights. Its most active form (**β-NGF**), however, has a molecular weight of 26.5 kDa and consists of a non-covalently bound dimer of two 118 amino acid units (Figure 17.10). The other forms of NGF are weakly bound associations of this fundamental structure.

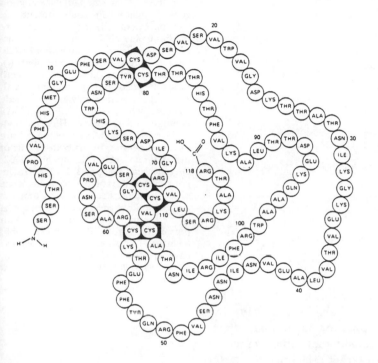

Figure 17.10 Molecular structure of a single unit of the major β-NGF dimer. There are 118 amino acids in the polypeptide chain and three disulphide linkages between cysteine residues (black rectangles) link different parts of the polpeptide together. (From Angeletti and Bradshaw, 1971, *Proceedings of National Academy of Sciences, USA,* **68**, 2417–2420; with permission.)

The major effect of NGF is on nerve cells derived from the neural crest. These, it will be recalled from Section 17.1, are autonomic and sensory neurons. Neurons belonging to the **sympathetic nervous system** (but not the parasympathetic system) are particularly dependent on NGF. If anti-NGF antibodies are injected into newborn mice the sympathetic nerve fibres are selectively destroyed. Vice versa, immunological techniques show that NGF is present on the target cells of sympathetic fibres.

The **neurotropic** effects of NGF are readily demonstrated in tissue culture. Figure 17.11 shows an experiment in which sympathetic neurons are plated on the central division of a culture dish. Scratches in the substratum ensure that neurites grow only to left or right. A silicon grease barrier divides the central plateau from the plateaux on either side. Silicon grease prevents the diffusion of NGF which is introduced into the medium of one of the side plateaux but not the other. The figure shows that the sympathetic neurites only grow into the NGF-containing compartment. Other experiments have shown that cultured sympathetic neurons will 'follow' a micropipette filled with NGF through a 180° turn.

A

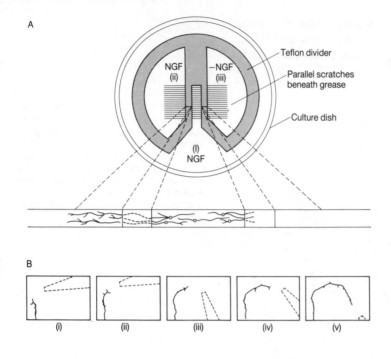

B

Figure 17.11 Neurotropic effect of NGF. (A) The culture dish has three compartments ((i), (ii) and (iii)) separated from each other by a Teflon wall which is sealed to the dish by a layer of grease. A culture of rat sympathetic ganglion cells is placed in compartment (i). Compartment (ii) contains culture medium plus NGF, whereas compartment (iii) contains medium without NGF. NGF is present in compartment (i). Parallel scratches (lined with collagen) under the grease prevent random growth of neurites. Neurites only grow into side chambers which contain NGF and if NGF is removed they regress. This is shown in the cross-sectional view of the culture dish and neurites in the bottom part of the diagram. (After Campenot, 1982, *Developmental Biology*, **83**, 1–21). (B) The growing neurite is on the left in this series of illustrations. It can be seen that the growth follows the nozzle of a pipette (dotted outline) containing NGF. (With permission from Ribchester, 1986, *Molecule, Nerve and Muscle*, Glasgow: Blackie; after Gundersen and Barrett, 1979, *Science*, **206**, 1079–1080, Copyright 1979 by the AAAS.)

We shall return to NGF in Section 17.6 for, in addition to the neurotropic (guidance) effect which we have been considering in this section, it also has a **neurotrophic** (or nutritional) effect. This, as we shall, see is of very considerable importance in stabilising synaptic connections with target cells once the latter have been 'found'.

The second major means by which neurites find their target cells is by **contact guidance**. Growth cones show a preference for substrata to which they can adhere strongly. Indeed no growth occurs at all if a suitable surface is not supplied. One surface to which growth cones adhere, both *in vivo* and *in vitro*, is that provided by other neurons. Thus when one pathfinder neuron has found its target others can 'feel' their way along it to the same or neighbouring targets. This helps to explain the neuroanatomical fact that nerve fibres frequently run in bundles, or **fasciculi**.

In tissue culture nerve fibres can be induced to grow along tracks of poly-*l*-lysine and polyornithine. These polypeptides have positively charged side chains (Table 2.1) which probably interact with negative charges on the cell membranes of the growing neurites. Indeed so 'sticky' is the substratum that in these cases not only the growth cone but also the rest of the neurite remains attached and thus records the track which the neurite has taken.

Other experiments have indicated that type 1 and type 4 collagens, fibronectin and especially the protein constituent of

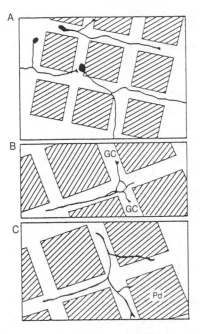

Figure 17.12 Track of cultured neurons on polyornithine. A dish has first been coated with polyornithine and then had patches of palladium deposited on top (hatched). Sensory neurons from chick embryos grow along the polyornithine lanes and only very rarely cross the palladium. Pd = palladium; GC = growth cone. (From Ribchester, 1986, *Molecule, Nerve and Muscle*, Glasgow: Blackie; after Letourneau, 1975, *Developmental Biology*, **44**, 77–91; with permission.)

basal laminae—laminin—when bound to a polyornithine substratum are extremely potent neurotropic substances. Yet other work has shown that the plant lectin, **concanavalin A (Con A)**, also acts as a powerful contact guide, at least for leech neurons. These tissue culture experiments hold great promise of determining the nature of the molecules which growth cones (indeed the growth cones of different types of neuron) recognise.

Having arrived at its target a growth cone must, of course, stop. This is another puzzle. It is not known what switches off the elongation process. One can only speculate that, once again, some chemical in the target cell membrane switches on a neurotubule/ neurofilament **disassembly** process in the growth cone. If and

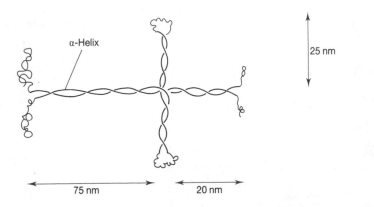

Figure 17.13 Molecular structure of laminin. Laminin is a cross-shaped molecule with a molecular weight of some 900 kDa. The arms and stem of the cross are formed of twin α-helices wound around each other to form a two-stranded rope. At each end of the cross the polypeptide chain forms a more disordered globular-type region which is believed to possess cell adhesion and/or neurite growth-promoting characteristics. (Partly after Davis *et al.*, 1985, *Trends in Neurosciences*, **8**, 528–532.)

when this happens the neurite will assume its adult condition. Neurotubules and neurofilaments will be assembled at the perikaryal end of the process and disassembled at the synaptic end. Axoplasmic flow will continue (as we noted in Chapter 14) but no elongation of the process will occur.

We have seen in the preceding paragraphs that the elongation and direction-finding of neurites depends on **contact adhesion** and the following of chemical pathways and 'signposts'. We can see, in a general sort of way, that the ceaseless probing of the microspike 'fingers' could very well be a searching out of such chemical route markers. We have already considered the evidence that gradients of NGF may form beacons for sympathetic neurons. Let us turn next, however, to a consideration of what form the **contact signals** might take.

17.5 CELL ADHESION MOLECULES (CAMs)

Three classes of **cell adhesion molecule (CAM)** are presently known: liver cell adhesion molecule (**L-CAM**), neural cell adhesion molecule (**N-CAM**) and neuron-glia cell adhesion molecule (**Ng-CAM**). We shall only concern ourselves with the last two. Both N-CAMs are membrane-embedded glycoproteins. N-CAM itself is found in the membranes of all neurons; Ng-CAM appears to be a 'secondary' CAM as it is not found in the membranes of neurons during the proliferative stage and only appears after mitosis has ceased. The great importance of neuron–glia interactions was emphasised in Section 17.1.

The two neural adhesion molecules also have somewhat different binding properties. N-CAM shows '**homotypic**' binding, i.e. N-CAM in one neural membrane binds to N-CAM in a neighbouring neural membrane. Ng-CAM, in contrast, shows

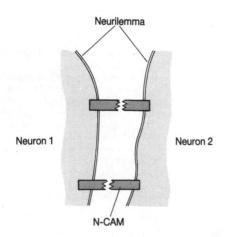

Neurilemma

Neuron 1

Neuron 2

N-CAM

Figure 17.14 Homotypic binding between N-CAMs. The schematic shows the principle of homotypic binding between N-CAMs of two neighbouring neurons

'**heterotypic**' binding. Ng-CAM in a neural membrane binds to a different (so far undiscovered) CAM, or some other receptor, in a glial cell's membrane.

The detailed structure of CAMs has yet to be established. A 100 kbp segment of genomic DNA containing the entire N-CAM sequence has, however, been successfully cloned using the cosmid technique (Chapter 5). This should soon clarify the structure of the molecule. At present all that can be said is that N-CAM appears to consist of two polypeptide chains of approximately 160 kDa and 130 kDa, whilst Ng-CAM, of which even less is presently known, seems to consist of three polypeptides of 200 kDa, 135 kDa and 80kDa, respectively. N-CAM also differs from Ng-CAM in showing a radical change in its carbohydrate composition during embryology. This change, which is termed the **E to A conversion** (i.e. embryonic to adult conversion), consists of a reduction by at least a third in the sialic acid content of the molecule. This greatly increases the mutual adhesion between adposed N-CAMs. Ng-CAM does not show an E to A conversion. Our present understanding of the major structural features of N-CAMs is shown in Figure 17.15.

Figure 17.15   Major features of E-type N-CAMs. (A) Both the 160 kDa and the 130 kDa N-CAMs appear to consist of three domains: a cell attachment domain which contains the C-terminal end of the molecule; a sialic acid domain which has three attachment sites for large amounts of the negatively charged carbohydrate; and a binding domain which terminates in val, glu and leu. (B) Schematic to show one possible mode of binding between adjacent N-CAMs. The negatively charged sialic residues are brought into the near neighbourhood of each other and may tend to destabilise the union by deformation of the polypeptide or simple charge repulsion. The strength of the binding between N-CAMs is found to undergo up to a fourfold increase if the sialic acid residues are removed. Sialic acid residues are shed when the E to A conversion occurs. (After Edelman, 1986, *Annual Review of Physiology*, **48**, 417–430.)

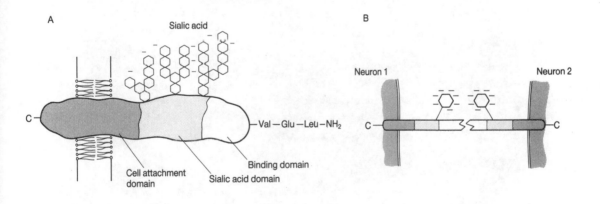

Figure 17.15 shows that N-CAMs are large membrane-bound glycoproteins. When isolated and viewed in the electron microscope they show a striking resemblance to clathrin triskelions (Figure 17.16). The different polypeptide domains are all believed to be derived from a single gene. The fact that at least four different sized N-CAM mRNAs can be detected in the young postnatal mouse brain (7.4, 6.7, 4.3 and 2.9 kbp) suggests that this single gene consists of a number of exons. Differential splicing of the primary transcript can then provide different N-CAMs at different developmental stages and in different brain regions. It can, indeed, be shown that there are great variations in the quantity of N-CAM mRNA present in the brain during

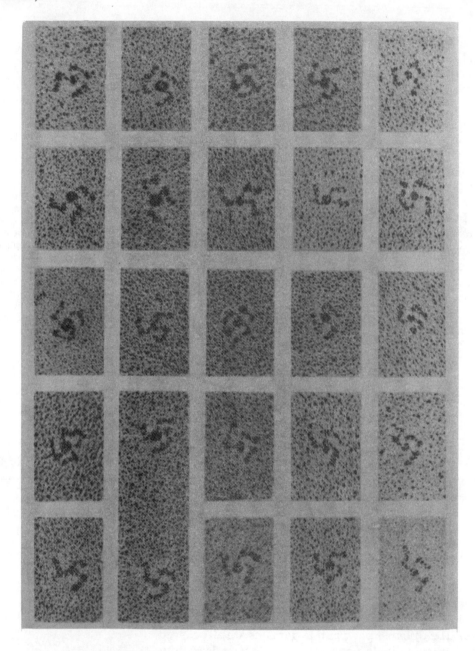

development. In the mouse the quantity of N-CAM messenger peaks near birth and falls by about 80% during development.

It is believed that about 100 000 N-CAM molecules are developed in the neurilemma of an average neuron. There is thus much opportunity for homophilic binding between neurons. But, it might reasonably be asked, how does this help us with understanding the contact adhesion theory of pathfinding? Would

Figure 17.16 N-CAM triskelions. Electron micrographs of N-CAM triskelions from embryonic chicken. The triskelions were rotary-shadowed and viewed at a magnification of x 200 000. Each arm measures about 40 nm. (Reproduced with permission from Edelman, 1984, *Annual Review of Neuroscience*, **7**, 339–377; © by Annual Reviews Inc.)

not all paths look the same to the probing microspikes of a growth cone? The answer to this question seems to be that different neurons have different spatial and temporal patterns for N-CAM expression. We have already noticed the possibilities inherent in differential splicing of N-CAM mRNAs. Moreover different timings and degrees of E to A conversion in different regions of the brain ensure that different adhesions are expressed in different brain areas.

17.6 DIFFERENTIAL SURVIVAL

The phenomenon of neurogenesis is far from over when neurons and their processes reach their definitive positions. There is good evidence that there is very considerable over-production of neurons followed, once again, by a process of 'negative sculpturing'.

In those systems which have been carefully studied (spinal cord of *Xenopus*, various parts of chick CNS, etc.) the over-production ranges from 40 to well over 100%. The cell loss, moreover, does not occur at random, spread over a lengthy period of time. It occurs at a definite period in development which can be predicted with some certainty. In the lateral motor column of the chick's spinal cord, for instance, a population of over 20 000 neurons is reduced to just over 12 000 in 72 hours (Figure 17.17(A)); in *Xenopus* spinal cord a reduction from 4000 to 2000 cells occurs in about the same period of time.

It can be shown that the degenerating perikarya are **not** merely the last to arrive, denied their 'place in the sun'. Rather the evidence points to the causal agent being at the far end of the axons, at the growth cones. If, for instance, the target field is partially or completely **extirpated** the loss of cell bodies is proportionately **greater**, and this loss, moreover, occurs at the same time as naturally occurring cell loss. Vice versa, if the target field is **increased** in area (by, for instance, implanting a supernumerary limb bud into the limb field of a chick embryo) then the cell loss in the appropriate motor area of the spinal cord is much **reduced**.

There is evidence that this initial over-production and subsequent selective pruning is a feature of all neural systems. How are the 'successful' neurons selected? What is the 'causal agent' at the growth cone's destination? Is it some 'trophic factor' necessary for the continuing life of the neuron? Is this 'trophic factor' rationed in such a way that only a fraction of the questing growth cones can be satisfied?

We have already met one such factor in the guise of nerve growth factor (NGF). As we saw in Section 17.4 this factor, in

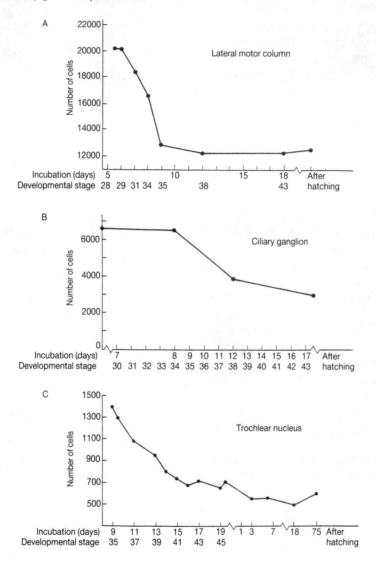

A — Lateral motor column

B — Ciliary ganglion

C — Trochlear nucleus

Figure 17.17 Cell death in embryonic chick central nervous system. In each region a great loss of neurons occurs at particular developmental stages and particular times of incubation and after hatching. ((A): from Hamburger, 1975, *J. Comp. Neurol.*, **160**, 535–546: with permission; (B): from Landmesser and Pilar, 1974, *J. Physiol.*, **241**, 737–749: reproduced by permission of The Physiological Society; (C): from Cowan and Wengler, 1967, *J. Exp. Zool.*, **164**, 267–280: with permission. After Purves and Lichtman, 1985, *Principles of Neural Development*, Sunderland, Mass: Sinauer.)

addition to being a **tropic** factor, is also a **trophic** factor. Not only does it guide sympathetic neurites to their destination, but it is also taken up by synaptic terminals and transported in a retrograde direction towards the perikaryon. If this take-up is prevented by axotomy or by injection of anti-NGF antibodies, sympathetic neurons undergo a series of metabolic and structural changes and ultimately die. These consequences can be reversed and/or prevented if NGF is presented to the cut end of the axon.

It can be shown that sympathetic terminals have specific **NGF receptors** in their membranes. When a receptor–NGF complex is formed endocytosis occurs at the terminal and the endocytotic vesicle so formed is transported in the retrograde stream along

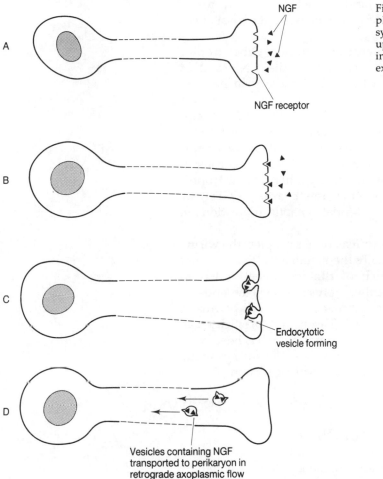

A

NGF

NGF receptor

B

C

Endocytotic
vesicle forming

D

Vesicles containing NGF
transported to perikaryon in
retrograde axoplasmic flow

Figure 17.18 Endocytosis and axo-plasmic transport of NGF in a sympathetic fibre. Schematic to show the uptake and retrograde transport of NGF in sympathetic axons. For further explanation see text

the axon to the perikaryon. Once in the perikaryon the NGF is released and can there exert its various metabolic effects. One such effect is to induce the manufacture of **tyrosine hydroxylase (TH)**. It will be recalled from Chapter 15 that this is the rate-limiting enzyme in the synthesis of noradrenaline in adrenergic neurons.

Although, as mentioned in Section 17.4, NGF's major activity is on sympathetic neurons it has also, more recently, been shown to have an effect in the CNS. Somewhat surprisingly it does not affect central catecholaminergic neurons. Instead it has been shown that if NGF is injected into the brains of adult rodents it is taken up and transported in a retrograde direction by **cholinergic** neurons. It causes an increased synthesis of choline acetyltransferase (CAT) and thus a general activation of cholinergic pathways. Endogenous NGF can be detected in rat

hippocampus and **neocortex** and it can be shown to be transported from there to cholinergic cell bodies in the basal nuclei of the forebrain.

NGF is by far the best-known trophic factor. Other trophic factors have, however, been detected in the CNS and at cholinergic neuromuscular junctions. The pig's brain has, for instance, yielded a 12.3 kDa factor which maintains the growth of sensory neurons in tissue culture. This factor is called **brain-derived growth factor (BDGF)**. The neuromuscular junctions of vertebrate skeletal muscles synthesise a factor (**cholinergic nerve growth factor (CNGF)**) which supports cholinergic neurons. It is not unreasonable to suppose that many other specific trophic factors (sometimes called **polypeptide growth factors (PGFs)**) are present in minute amounts at potential synaptic appositions in the developing brain.

However, as we noted at the outset of this chapter, the wiring of the vertebrate brain—especially the mammalian brain—is not completely pre-ordained. Much of the fine detail is left to environmental 'moulding'. In other words the detail depends on the brain's activity. It depends, ultimately, on which pathways and synapses are most heavily used. This neural 'plasticity' can be studied in various of the brain's systems but it has been most extensively examined in the visual pathways. We shall examine the plasticity of these systems in the next two sections of this chapter.

17.7 MORPHOPOIETIC FIELDS

The best-known example of a morphopoietic field is provided by the **retino-tectal** visual system in the lower vertebrates. In infra-mammalian vertebrates the retina does not project to a visual cortex developed from the telencephalon but to an optic **tectum** which develops in the roof of the midbrain (Figure 17.19). In fish and amphibia, moreover, regeneration of the optic nerve fibres occurs if they are sectioned. Because the optic nerve fibres have their cell bodies (the ganglion cells) in the retina this regeneration occurs **from** the retina **to** the tectum.

The original experiments on this system were performed by Roger Sperry in the 1940s and 1950s. He showed that if the optic nerve of a frog was sectioned regrowth would occur in such a way that within a few weeks normal vision (judged by appropriate visual reflexes) was restored. Electrophysiological recording also showed that photic stimulation of a patch of retina elicited activity in the correct part of the tectum. Now this accurate regrowth might well be explained by the pathfinding mechanisms we have already discussed. Indeed Sperry's interpretation—called the

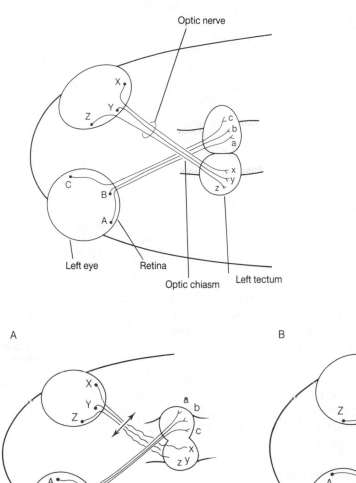

Optic nerve

X
Y
Z

c
b
a

C
B
A

x
y
z

Left eye   Retina

Optic chiasm   Left tectum

Figure 17.19 Visual pathway in fish and amphibia. In fish and amphibia the optic nerve fibres cross completely at the chiasm to innervate the contralateral tectum. The figure shows (diagrammatically) that a 'map' of the contralateral retina is formed in each tectum. Stimulation at A gives tectal activity at a, stimulation at Y gives activity at y, etc

Figure 17.20 Schematic to show the principle of optic nerve section experiment. (A) The optic nerve from the right eye is sectioned (double-headed arrow). The optic nerve fibres degenerate between the section and the tectum. (B) Regrowth occurs from the cut ends of the optic nerve fibres. Electrophysiological testing shows that the fibres have reformed the tectal map as it was before the nerve was sectioned

A

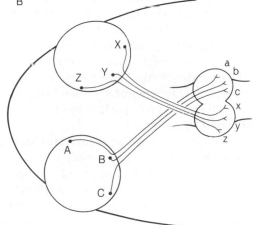

X
Y
Z

a
b
c

x
z y

A
B
C

B

X
Y
Z

a
b
c
x
y
z

A
B
C

chemoaffinity hypothesis—suggested just this. Figure 17.20 schematises the experiment.

Sperry followed up his original experiments by showing that if, after sectioning the optic nerve, he cut the extrinsic eye muscles and rotated the eyeball the optic fibres regrew in an anatomically 'correct' but behaviourally 'incorrect' way. As Figure 17.21 shows the tectal map is 180° out of phase with the retina; motor outflow from this map thus leads to behaviourally absurd responses. A frog, always striking 180° out of true, can never catch a nutritious fly and hence is apt to starve to death in the midst of plenty. Once again the chemoaffinity hypothesis seems adequate to explain this finding.

A   B   C

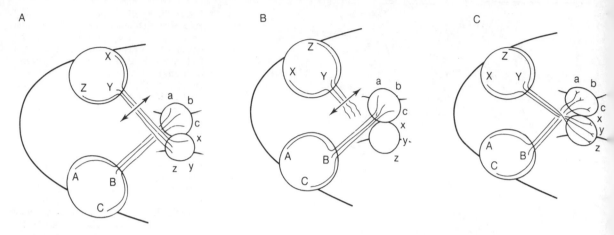

Figure 17.21 Rotation of the frog eye through 180°. (A) The optic nerve from the right eye is sectioned (double-headed arrow). (B) The eye is rotated through 180°. (C) The optic nerve is allowed to grow back to the tectum. Electrophysiological testing shows that the original map has been regenerated. Behaviour is now 180° out of line. For further explanation see text

To make sure that the nerve fibres were not merely growing back along the old myelin sheaths left behind after degeneration Sperry introduced a barrier into the path of the regenerating fibres. The fibres had to find their way around this barrier before they could make their way to the tectum. In spite of this scrambling Sperry was able to show that the fibres found their way back to their anatomically correct place in the tectum. It seemed, therefore, that retinal ganglion cell and optic tectal cell were in some way chemically matched. The axon from the ganglion cell would grow back to the tectum and search around until it met its complement.

However, more recent work has shown that things are not quite as simple as this. First of all it can be shown that the apparently rigid point for point relation between retina and tectum is not established until a certain **critical** or **sensitive** period in the amphibian's development has been passed. If the rotation experiments are done before this period has passed the retino-tectal projection regenerates in a **behaviourally** appropriate manner. If a chemical complementarity between individual ganglion and tectal cells exists it must develop after this period has elapsed. Critical or sensitive periods are found in the development of all vertebrate nervous systems. We shall note the existence of similar periods in the development of the mammalian nervous system in the next section.

Secondly, Sperry's original interpretation has been subverted by experiments in which either the retina or the tectum have been halved. If the optic nerve is sectioned and the tectum is halved we may legitimately wonder what the regrowing optic fibres will do. The chemoaffinity hypothesis in its simplest (perhaps 'simplistic') form would suggest that half the regrowing axons, finding their tectal destinations eliminated, would despair and die. This, however, is not what is found to happen. The regenerating axons in fact all tend to cram into the remaining half tectum. They cram in, moreover, in a regular manner. It is as if the half tectum holds the original sensory map but at twice the density.

Vice versa, if the optic nerve is sectioned and half the retina removed then the remaining optic nerve fibres grow back and initially innervate half the tectum. Slowly, however, the map from the half retina expands until (in a few months) the whole tectum is innervated. Once more the hypothesis of a precise point for point 'targeting' cannot be sustained. The notion of a '**morphopoietic**' field begins to seem more appropriate.

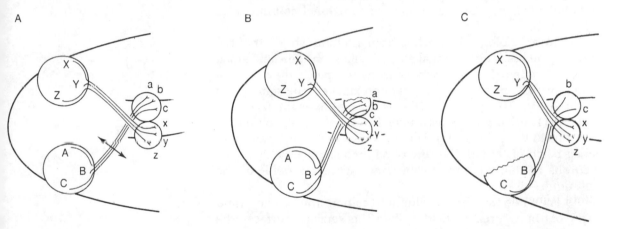

A   B   C

Much recent work in general embryology indicates that field effects are fundamental to development. The nervous system is thus in no way unusual in displaying this feature during its development. Indeed it has been possible to transplant an embryonic eye into the flank of a developing tadpole and show that the polarity characteristic of the flank is imposed on the retina. When the eye is replaced in the orbit its ganglion cells form connections with the tectum which reflect this imposed polarity rather than the polarity appropriate to its position in the orbit.

Unfortunately it is still too early to give a molecular explanation of embryonic morphopoietic fields. We must thus leave this topic at the phenomenological level and pass on to the penultimate section of this chapter. In doing so, however, we shall not leave behind our consideration of the visual system. For we shall find that this system also provides intriguing examples of functional sculpturing.

Figure 17.22 Expansion and compression of tectal maps of the retina. (A) The left optic nerve is sectioned (double-headed arrow). (B) Following section of the optic nerve half the right tectum is removed. The optic nerve fibres grow back to the remaining part of the tectum to create a miniaturised map. (C) Following section of the optic nerve half the left retina is removed. The optic nerve fibres grow back eventually to fill the whole right tectum with a map of the remaining part of the retina. For further explanation see text

17.8 FUNCTIONAL SCULPTURING

We noted in Section 17.6 that although many neurons are formed rather few are ultimately chosen. In this section we shall see that even those which are chosen depend on **use** for the persistence of their synaptic connections. Although the overall plan of neuronal connectivity is determined by 'nature' the relative strength of the connections is controlled by 'nurture'. Some of the best studied examples of this activity-dependent sculpturing are found in mammalian visual systems.

As a first example let us consider the mammalian **primary visual cortex** (cortical area 17). A great deal is now known about the anatomy and physiology of this region of the brain. Following the pioneering studies of Hubel and Wiesel in the 1960s it has become clear that this cortex, like other parts of the neocortex, is subdivided into a large number of **functional columns** (see Chapter 1).

Electrophysiological recording from a column shows that the neurons all respond to visual stimuli falling on the same small patch of retina. For different neurons the patch may be of a different size—but it is always in approximately the same place in the retina. This patch of retina is referred to as the **receptive field (RF)** of the nerve cell under investigation. A column of neurons in the primary visual cortex thus 'looks' at a particular small patch of retina. The sum of all the receptive fields of the neurons in that column is called the '**aggregate field**' of the column.

As one progresses from column to column the position (and size) of the aggregate field shifts. The sensory surface—the retina—is thus mapped on to the primary visual cortex. The map is not isomorphous. Those regions of the retina which are of greatest biological importance—the fovea, for example—have many more columns devoted to them than do areas of lesser importance at the retina's periphery.

Now one of the first things to be found when the electrophysiology of the neurons in the visual cortical columns was investigated was that many of them responded best to **bar stimuli** flashed—about 1 second exposure—to the retina. The stimuli could be strips of light or dark bars. Circular spots of light presented to the retina provoked no response from these cortical cells (except in layer lVc). Furthermore the orientation of these bar stimuli was crucially important. All the cells in a given column respond to bar stimuli of a particular **orientation**. Cells in neighbouring columns will respond to bars of different orientation.

A great deal more fascinating neurophysiology has been done on the visual systems of mammals. Interested readers should once again consult references listed in the bibliography. For our

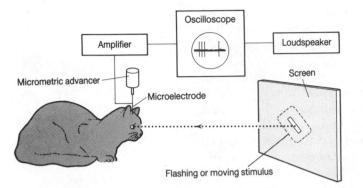

Figure 17.23   Technique for investigating the response of cells in the cat's primary visual cortex. A spectacle lens keeps the eye of the anaesthetised cat open. A flashing or moving stimulus is displayed on the oscilloscope screen. A micro-electrode stereotactically inserted into the visual cortex records the response of cortical neurons. (From C. Blakemore in R.L. Gregory and E.H. Gombrich, 1973, *Illusion in Art and Nature*, London, Duckworth, by permission of Duckworth.)

purposes it is sufficient to understand that in the normal cortex cells responding to all possible orientations of a bar stimuli will be present—in approximately equal quantities.

Let us now return to our epigenetic concerns. How much of the organisation underlying this visual physiology is inborn, and how much due to visual experience?

Kittens are born with their eyes closed. They do not open for about 10 days. They remain cloudy for another couple of weeks and there is little sign of accurate visuo-motor co-ordination at this early period. Electrophysiological recording does not reveal responses to specifically orientated bar stimuli. Soon after the ocular cloudiness clears up, however, the receptive fields become tuned to bar stimuli in the way described above. This immediately suggests that visual **experience** plays a significant role in moulding the neural pathways underlying vision.

It is not difficult to design experiments to test the significance of visual experience. Kittens can be reared in the dark or in environments of fixed (or moving) stripes of a particular orientation. The results confirm the importance of sensory experience. Kittens reared in the dark show little sign of possessing orientation-selective cells in the primary visual cortex. Kittens reared in visual environments of, say, vertical stripes develop cortices in which the majority of cells respond to vertical bar stimuli.

It should be noted that these experiments are only effective on kittens during the **sensitive** or **critical** period (see above) of their development. They are ineffective with adult cats. There is no doubt, however, that during this period the neural circuitry responsible for the orientation detector cells in the primary visual cortex is in a 'plastic' state: open to environmental moulding; responsive to use and/or disuse.

The kitten's visual system can be used for another interesting investigation of the nature/nurture issue. It can be shown, firstly, that the neurons in an adult cat's primary visual cortex (except those in layer lVc) can be 'driven' from both eyes. This so-called **'binocular drive'** plays a central role in stereoscopic vision. It is thus particularly well developed in highly 'visual' animals such as felines and primates.

Now just as the primary visual cortex is built of a series of 'orientation' columns so it is also subdivided into a series of **'ocular dominance'** columns. The neural pathway from the retina is arranged in such a way that fibres originating in the left eye are directed to layer lVc of one column and from the right eye to layer lVc of the adjacent column. Above and below lVc transverse connections ensure that activity from **both** eyes is delivered to a cortical cell. This arrangement is shown in Figure 17.24.

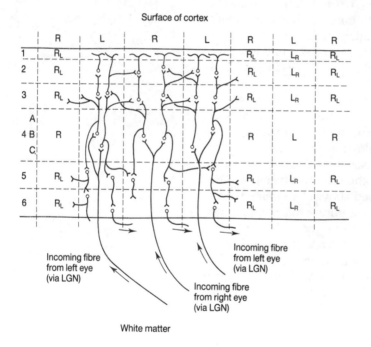

Figure 17.24 Schematic to show ocular dominance columns in cat primary visual cortex. This schematised diagram shows that fibres from the lateral geniculate nucleus (LGN) of each eye terminate in alternate columns of layer 4c. The fibres from each eye are kept separate in the LGN, which is a relay station on the route from the retina to the primary visual cortex. The diagram shows that above and below 4c transverse connections ensure that the sub-dominant eye has some influence on the activity of the cortical neurons

Once again this system lends itself to experimental manipulation. If one eye is patched during the kitten's sensitive period it is found that binocular drive is lost. It seems that the neural pathway from the patched eye weakens. If, however, both eyes are patched no great harm is done. After removal of the patches binocular drive is present almost as normal. It seems, therefore, that there is some form of **competition** between pathways. It seems that if one is active and the other inactive the synapses of the latter atrophy or detach.

The experimental analysis of this system can be taken further. It can be shown that if the patched eye is opened during the third

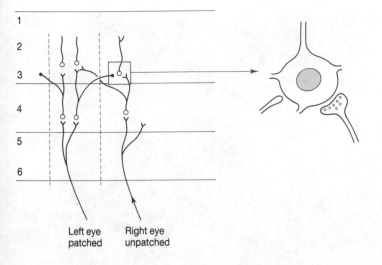

Figure 17.25 Effect of eye patches on ocular dominance in the visual cortex. The schematic diagram shows that if the left eye is patched its ability to control cells in the right eye column (i.e. to induce binocular drive of cells in layer 3) is eliminated or greatly reduced

Left eye patched   Right eye unpatched

or fourth week after birth and the previously open eye patched then reversal of the pathways occurs. The previously inactive pathway is **reconstructed** and the previously active pathway fades. Clearly during this early period of the kitten's life the visual pathways are very open to environmental sculpting.

But how often can the patches be reversed? What happens if both eyes are allowed visual experience but never at the same time? Does binocular drive develop in these circumstances?

It can be shown that if the patches are reversed every 24 hours binocular drive does not develop. Only when pathways from both eyes are operational at (approximately) the same time does binocular drive become established. Indeed it can be shown that if input from the two eyes is separated by **10 seconds** or more binocular drive tends to be lost. It looks as though, in the visual system at least, two synapses have to fire at nearly the same instant if they are to stabilise each other. Any substantial length of time between firing enables one synapse to establish itself at the expense of the other. We shall return to this observation in the next chapter for it suggests a possible mechanism for associative memory.

A further interesting experimental manipulation of the binocular drive system has used the macaque visual system rather than that of the cat. It has proved possible to visualise ocular dominance columns by injecting a radio-labelled amino acid into one eye. This is taken up by the ganglion cells of the retina and passed back to the visual cortex. After allowing an appropriate length of time for this transport to occur the animal is sacrificed and autoradiographs prepared of tangential sections of its visual cortex. As expected the ocular dominance columns show up as a complex pattern of stripes. The light stripes represent the radio-

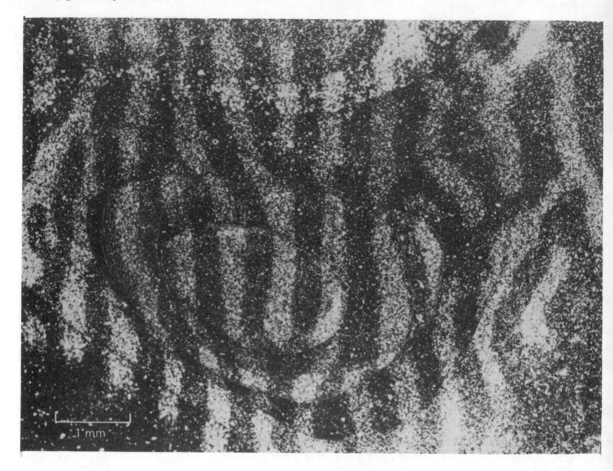

.1`mm

labelled amino acid from the injected eye. The dark stripes represent the input from the unlabelled eye.

If this experimental procedure is combined with the patch procedures described above the electrophysiological analysis is confirmed. Figure 17.27 shows the result of rearing a macaque through its sensitive period with one eye patched and then injecting the **unpatched** eye with the radio-labelled amino acid. The figure shows that the columns innervated from the unpatched eye (white) have expanded greatly at the expense of the columns innervated by the patched eye (dark).

Let us consider what the result of this experiment means. The size of the visual cortex has not diminished, nor have the number of cells. What has happened is that the synaptic terminals from the unpatched eye have invaded territory normally occupied by the terminals of fibres from the patched eye. Once again the conclusion seems to be clear. Synaptic **activity** is required for synaptic stability. Inactive synapses lose the struggle for survival.

Figure 17.26 Tangential section through radiolabelled ocular dominance columns. Radiolabelled proline is injected into one of the macaque's eyes and after 10 days the animal is sacrificed and autoradiographs prepared of tangential sections of the visual cortex. The light stripes show where the radiolabelled proline has accumulated. It can be seen that the light stripes (representing input from the labelled eye) and the dark stripes (input from the unaffected eye) are approximately equal in width. (From Hubel, Wiesel and LeVay, 1977, *Philosophical Transactions of the Royal Society (B)*, **278**, 377–409; with permission.)

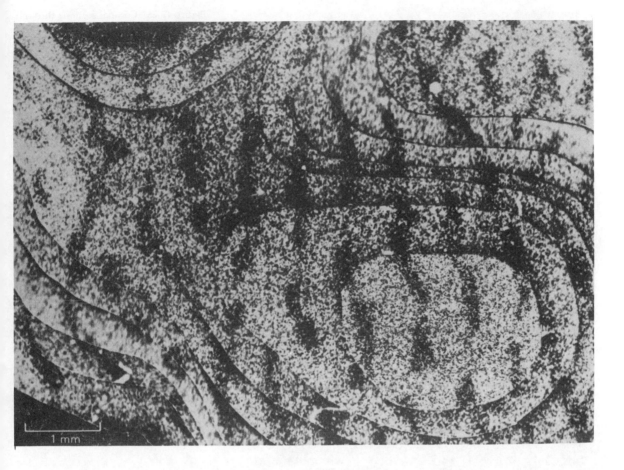

Let us conclude this section by turning from mammalian visual systems back to the amphibian systems we discussed in Section 17.7. For we can find a striking analogy in an experimentally manipulated frog to the ocular dominance columns we have just discussed.

It has proved possible to transplant an embryonic frog eye to an anterior position on another embryonic frog. This frog thus has three eyes: two of its own and a transplant. But a frog only has two optic tecta. The optic nerve from the third eye grows back to innervate one of these tecta. In other words one of the frog's optic tecta is innervated by two eyes. Both sets of optic nerve fibres attempt to expand to fill the whole of the tectum. But they find themselves in unexpected competition with the second set of fibres. It turns out that they sort themselves out into stripe-like territories which are highly reminiscent of mammalian ocular dominance columns.

The explanation of this striking finding is identical to that which

Figure 17.27 Tangential section through radiolabelled ocular dominance columns after patching one eye during the sensitive period. One of the macaque's eyes is patched during the sensitive period of the monkey's development. Radiolabelled proline is then injected into the **unpatched** eye and autoradiographs of the visual cortex prepared. It can be seen that the ocular dominance columns connected to the unpatched eye (light stripes) are much more extensive than those driven from the patched eye (dark stripes). (From Hubel, Wiesel and LeVay, 1977, *Philosophical Transactions of the Royal Society (B)*, **278**, 377–409; with permission.)

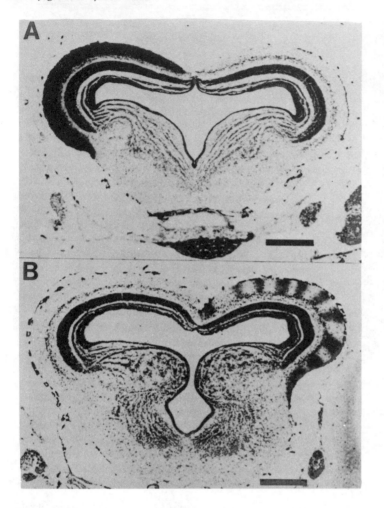

Figure 17.28   Coronal sections through optic tecta of normal and three-eyed frogs. (A) Normal otpic tecta. The frog's left eye was injected with radiolabelled proline 3 days before sacrifice. The autoradiograph shows that the entire superficial layer of the right tectum is filled with developed silver grains, indicating the space occupied by the terminals of optic fibres from the left eye (B) Optic tecta of three-eyed frog. The frog's left eye was once again injected with radiolabelled proline. The supernumerary eye also projects to the right tectum. It is clear that the synaptic territories in the tectum have sorted themselves into regularly spaced columns. Scale bar = 400 μm. For further explanation see text. (From Constantine-Paton, 1981, in *The Organisation of the Cerebral Cortex*, eds F. O. Schmitt *et al.*, Cambridge, Mass.: MIT Press, pp. 47–67; with permission.)

we have discussed above. Synapses with simultaneous (or near simultaneous) activity stabilise. Hence all synapses developed on the terminals of fibres from one eye, being simultaneously activated, stabilise each other. Gradually, by competition, the territories shown in Figure 17.28 become established.

The molecular mechanism(s) underlying this selective stabilisation are as yet unknown. One attractive speculation suggests that postsynaptic cells are induced by active presynaptic terminals to secrete an antagonist which inhibits the formation of other synapses. Only active terminals are protected from the effects of this antagonist. What this antagonist might be there is as yet no knowledge. It is, however, of some interest to note that NMDA receptors (Section 9.4) may be involved. It has been shown that agents which block the NMDA receptor (e.g. D-AP5) also prevent the clear demarcation of optic fibre territories in the tectum of three-eyed frogs. A similar effect can be demonstrated in the monocular kitten. If an antagonist is being induced by synaptic activation could it be that it is inhibited by activation of the NMDA receptor? Could it be that the second-messenger activity of the Ca^{2+} ions which flow through the NMDA receptor channel switch off the synthesis of the putative synapse-forming antagonist? It will be recalled from Chapter 9 that only when a subsynaptic membrane has been depolarised by some 30 mV is the Mg^{2+} blockade of the NMDA channel lifted. This might well require two or more closely set excitatory (non-NMDA) synapses to be (nearly) simultaneously active. It is clear that the NMDA channel provides a possible mechanism. We shall return to a similar speculation in Chapter 18, where we shall see that the NMDA receptor has also been implicated in the plastic change responsible for memory.

These speculations provide a suitable end-point for this chapter. They show how molecular neurobiology is beginning to provide a theory of the brain. They show, in other words, how molecular investigations in one part of the subject (neuro-pharmacology) are beginning to impinge on and illuminate quite a different part (neuroembryology). It must be borne in mind, however, that these ideas are as yet only speculations Like all speculations they have many competitors which might also account for the facts. Like the synapses themselves only use (i.e. further research) will winnow out the false and reveal the truth.

17.9 CONCLUSION

We observed at the outset of this chapter that the brain is perhaps the ultimate challenge for the developmental biologist. It is clear from the remainder of the chapter that we still have far to go. Yet the molecular approach here, as elsewhere, is beginning to yield dividends. It begins to seem feasible that increasing knowledge of the selective stickinesses of membranes, of the subtleties of a cell's control of N-CAMs, of the distribution, uptake and effect of tropic and trophic factors and their distribution in morphopoietic fields, and of the fine tuning resulting from use and disuse, will begin to provide a framework for an under-standing. Neuroembryology, furthermore, does not stand apart from the rest of neuroscience. Its growth depends on the development of our knowledge of synapses and their pharma-cology, on the biophysics and molecular biology of channel proteins, as well as on behavioural biology and neuropathology. The prize is a great one. If we can begin to understand how the nervous system develops its harmonious and intricate structure we shall be in a better position to repair it when it is disrupted by injury or disease.

Chapter 18
Memory

Fifty years ago a great neuroscientist, E. R. Hilgard, wrote that 'It is a blot upon our scientific ingenuity that after so many years of search we know as little as we do about the physiological accompaniments of learning.' Half a century has passed since those words were written. Half a century in which a vast amount of research has been directed to discovering 'the physiological accompaniments of learning'. Yet, by and large, the blot remains. We still know surprisingly little about what happens in the brain when learning occurs and memories are 'laid down'. In quite recent years, however, a number of openings have appeared. The horizon, to change the metaphor, begins to seem a little brighter. Perhaps in the late eighties and early nineties of the twentieth century we are really beginning to see a glimmer of a solution to the perplexity. This glimmer, moreover, comes from studies at the molecular and biophysical levels. It comes, in addition, from studies on invertebrate organisms which might not have immediately commended themselves to the neuroscientists of the 1930s.

The solution to the problem of memory requires one of the great syntheses of neurobiology. This is why we have left it to the eighteenth of our nineteen chapters. It involves ion flows, second messengers, gene derepressions, channel proteins, membrane structure. It also involves levels above the molecular and ultrastructural. In mammals, and after all it is human memory which ultimately concerns us, the intricate anatomy of the brain is crucially involved. The study of memory concerns psychologists and ethologists, cognitive and computer scientists, as well as neurobiologists.

Yet the effort is well worthwhile. Memory is very central to our life. To an extent we are bundles of memories. If we suffer total amnesia we lose touch with who we are. There can be few greater personal tragedies or sufferings. Consciousness itself loses its depth. All that is left is the thin patina of the existential present.

Yet to a degree we all face at least the beginnings of this tragedy. Old age customarily brings with it loss of memory. The worst scourge of old age—dementia of the Alzheimer type—is characterised by ever deepening amnesia.

To a degree, also, we could all benefit by an improvement in the memory we have. Certainly the multibillion-pound world-wide educational profession could hardly help benefiting from a deeper knowledge of the mechanisms at work when learning is occurring and memories are being established.

Finally the world of computer science undoubtedly has much to learn from a system which can store as much information as a Shakespeare, a Darwin or an Einstein and retrieve it so effortlessly and so rapidly. Human brains have taken a thousand million years to evolve: it is likely that they have a few lessons to teach the parvenu advocates of artificial intelligence.

18.1 SOME DEFINITIONS

The terms 'learning' and 'memory' are closely allied. Perhaps in the common usage both have a connection with consciousness. Yet this need not be so. We are nowadays quite accustomed to the idea of 'unconscious' memories and we are quite prepared to say of someone that he learnt no end of a lesson without supposing that he was aware at the time that he was doing so. Thus even in the common usage 'learning' and 'memory' tend to become generalised. In the world of biology they are generalised yet further. Certainly the notion of conscious awareness plays no essential role in the concepts.

In its most general form we can define learning and memory in behavioural terms as a **changed response to a repeated stimulus**. This very broad definition allows us to attach the terms 'learning' and 'memory' to many non-neurological systems. For instance both bacteria and protozoa show behaviour which falls under this definition. Behavioural adaptation to repeated stimuli is a very general feature of all living forms. The immune system is another instance where, according to our definition, learning and memory occur. Everyone knows that the immunological response is very different the second time the system is challenged.

In this book, however, we are restricting ourselves to neurobiological instances. Even so our definition will include phenomena which may not immediately commend themselves as instances of learning and memory. **Habituation** and **sensitisation** are two such instances. We all experience habituation to monotonous stimuli: we may, for example, become so accustomed (habituated) to the ticking of a clock that we only become aware of it when it stops. Vice versa the smallest intimation that a painful experience may be about to be repeated is likely to induce a vivid avoidance reaction: we are sensitised.

Both habituation and sensitisation are variations in the intensity of an already existing response to a stimulus. In this regard they show a resemblance to the immune response. In contrast to these phenomena, however, is **associative learning**. Here a response is developed to a previously 'neutral' stimulus. Some authorities insist that this type of learning is the only type worthy of the name.

Associative learning can also be classified into various subtypes: Pavlovian (= classical) conditioning, instrumental (= operant) conditioning, imprinting, insight, etc. In all cases a stimulus (or constellation of stimuli) which initially did not induce response A is brought to induce that response. Details of these different forms of associative learning and the 'training' procedures involved are to be found in texts of physiological psychology.

Here we shall very briefly describe the two fundamental subtypes—**classical** and **operant** conditioning—as they are both crucial to experimental approaches to the molecular basis of memory.

Classical conditioning. The paradigmatic examples of classical conditioning are those carried out at the beginning of this century by Ivan Pavlov. Pavlov's initial interests were in digestive physiology and from this interest grew his classical research into the response of his experimental animals—dogs—to the sight or other clue of dinner. One of the inborn alimentary reflexes to the presence of food in the mouth is salivation. By collecting the saliva produced it is easy to measure the strength of this reflex response. This reflex salivation would, of course, not normally occur in response to some **neutral** stimulus such as bell, a red light, or a gentle touch. However, Pavlov was able to show that if the neutral stimulus **preceded** the placing of food (or dilute acid) in the mouth sufficiently frequently then salivation would occur in response to the neutral stimulus alone.

The following terminology has been developed to describe this type of reflex. The 'neutral' stimulus is termed the **conditioned stimulus (CS)**, the food or dilute acid is called the **unconditioned stimulus (UCS)**, the inborn salivary response to the food or acid is called the **unconditioned reflex (UCR)** and the same response when elicited by the CS is called the **conditioned reflex (CR)**.

Because, as we saw above, Pavlov was able to quantify the CR he was able to work out some important properties of classical conditioning. One of the most important of these properties has to do with the time interval between the CS and the UCS. **The CS must precede the UCS**. In Pavlov's case the optimal interval

A

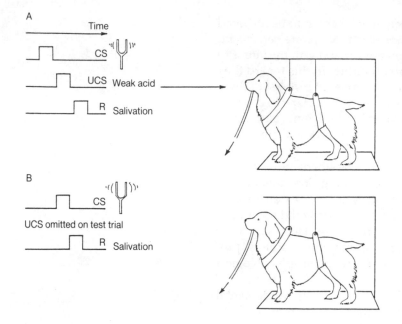

Time

CS ·((∪))·

UCS Weak acid

R Salivation

B

CS ·((∪))·

UCS omitted on test trial

R Salivation

Figure 18.1 Pavlovian (classical) conditioning. (A) Conditioning. The conditioned stimulus (CS) and the unconditioned stimulus (UCS) are paired and the response (R), salivation, measured. (B) Eliciting the conditioned response. The UCS is omitted and the reflex salivation is obtained to the CS alone. (After Racklin, 1976, *Introduction to Modern Behaviourism*, New York, W.H. Freeman, with permission.)

between the CS and the UCS (the **interstimulus interval (ISI)**) turned out to be about 0.5 seconds. This time period seems to obtain in many organisms, vertebrate and invertebrate. However, there are well known instances, for instance taste aversion, where the ISI may be a matter of hours. To establish the CR the CS–UCS pairing must be repeated a number of times. This is called **reinforcement**. If the sequencing of the stimuli is reversed, if in other words the UCS precedes the CS, then the CS weakens and ultimately disappears. This is known as **extinction**. Extinction will also occur if the CS is presented a number of times on its own.

Operant conditioning. We saw in the preceding section that Pavlovian CRs are in a sense 'elicited' from the animal. In Pavlov's case the dog is held in a harness, appropriate stimuli presented and the salivary response measured. In a sense the **dog** is not involved at all. This is not the case in operant conditioning. Here the whole animal **responds**. The initial investigations of this second type of CR were carried out by B.F.Skinner. The piece of apparatus he devised is now well known—the **Skinner box**—and operant conditioning itself is often known as **Skinnerian conditioning**.

The essence of Skinnerian conditioning is that the animal has to press a lever, or (if a bird) peck at a key, or perform some other **operant** once or a number of times to receive a reward—food or drink. The reward **reinforces** the operant behaviour. It is said to be **contingent** upon that behaviour. The strength of the operant behaviour can be measured in terms of the number of bar presses,

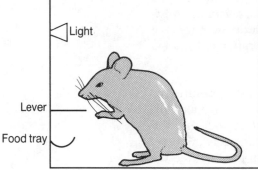

Figure 18.2 Skinner box. For further explanation see text

pecks, etc. The operant, moreover, is open to different types of reinforcement. **Negative reinforcement** occurs, for instance, when an animal emits the operant in order to **avoid** a painful stimulus. **Secondary reinforcement** is induced when, for example, every time a food pellet is to be delivered into a Skinner box a light switches on. Frequency and duration of bar pressing will then be increased when the light is switched on and reduced when it is off.

Skinnerian conditioning shares some characteristics with the Pavlovian type but differs in others. In particular operant conditioned reflexes are much more stable than Pavlovian reflexes, which require frequent reinforcement if they are not to fade to extinction.

It is not difficult to see that Skinnerian reflexes merge into trial and error learning (including that sort of trial and error learning 'done in the head' which is sometimes called 'insight learning') and into behaviours such as maze-learning and exploratory behaviour.

18.2 SHORT- AND LONG-TERM MEMORY

One of the ground rules of scientific theorising was summed up by William of Occam in the thirteenth century: 'Entia non sunt mutiplicanda praeter necessitatem'—entities are not to be multiplied beyond necessity—an aphorism which has come to be known as **Occam's razor**. This principle holds as strongly in the study of memory as elsewhere in science. Neurobiologists hope to find a single mechanism at work underlying the phenomenon. Yet the facts may be otherwise. It may be that memory is a multifaceted function of the brain. At the time of writing the issue is still unsettled. We, however, shall follow Occam's recommendation and assume that memory is the outcome of one underlying process.

One very common distinction made by students of the formation of memory is to divide the process into a 'labile', **short-term memory (STM)** and a more 'stable' **long-term memory**. We shall make use of this distinction in our consideration of putative molecular bases of memory in Section 18.5.

Short-term memory (STM) endures for seconds, minutes or hours. It is the type of memory which we use when we look up a telephone number and then dial it. It is just as well that the number does not remain in the memory more than a few minutes. If we stored all the numbers we had looked up in a lifetime we might well not be able to concentrate on more important matters. Indeed this is likely to be the biological significance of this type of memory. It enables an animal to **forget** the trivialities of its life. Its transience and lability suggests that it has a 'physiological' basis—perhaps a transient alteration in the synaptic 'resistance' of certain pathways in the brain.

Long-term memory (LTM) endures for days, years, decades. This holds the significant data of an animal's life—where to find food or a mate, where to avoid a predator or a poison. In the lives of most English men and women the date of the battle of Hastings is of sufficient significance to be in the LTM. 1066 AD may remain firmly embedded for 70 or 80 years. This permanence argues for a permanent alteration in a cerebral pathway (or pathways). Whenever William the Conqueror, Hastings, or the Bayeux Tapestry are voiced, read or otherwise understood, AD 1066 becomes available.

Relation between STM and LTM. It is generally believed that information to be memorised passes first into the STM and then into the LTM. This transfer is called **consolidation**. Now we have already noted that STM may be distinguished from LTM by its greater 'lability'. It is not too difficult to disrupt STM. LTMs, however, are very difficult to displace. It follows that we can prevent consolidation by disrupting the STM phase. This can be

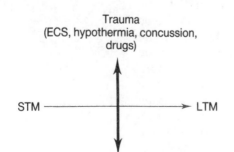

Figure 18.3   Trauma affects transfer of information from STM to LTM

done by exposing the brain to any one of a number of different 'insults': concussion, electroconvulsive shock (ECS), hypothermia, certain drugs, etc. Many of us may have had personal experience of this. It is quite common to find that after severe concussion the period immediately before the concussion cannot be remembered. This phenomenon is known as retrograde amnesia (RA).

The phenomenon of retrograde amnesia is amenable to experimental investigation in laboratory rodents. If the brain is insulted in one or other of the ways mentioned shortly after operant conditioning the chances of the operant behaviour becoming established is much reduced.

We should not finish this section without observing that not all investigators accept the STM–LTM scheme outlined above. Some workers suggest that it is not so much the differential laying down of memories which we are looking at but differential **retrieval** of memories. There is some evidence for this interpretation both from animal studies and from human experience. For it is well known that with time the period of retrograde amnesia shrinks. More and more of the events preceding the concussion become available though probably not all. However, it would take us too far from the subject of molecular neurobiology to pursue the pros and cons of this argument further.

We can conclude, therefore, by noting that the problem set to molecular neurobiologists by their behaviourist and psychological colleagues is to provide a molecular mechanism which can account for STM, LTM and the transfer (consolidation) between one and the other.

18.3 WHERE IS THE MEMORY TRACE LOCATED?

In Sections 18.1 and 18.2 we have been discussing memory in a very general sense. The experiments described have been behavioural and they have provided some parameters which any molecular mechanism must obey. But in order to investigate events at the molecular level we must know **where** in the brain they are occurring.

This is much easier said than done. Karl Lashley, one of the great pioneers in the neurobiology of memory, wrote at the end of his research career in the 1950s that 'I sometimes feel, reviewing the evidence on the localisation of the memory trace, that the necessary conclusion is that learning is just not possible!'.

The best-known outcome of Lashley's research is the so-called law of '**mass action**' or '**equipotentiality**'. Working with rats he was able to show that their ability to memorise a maze depended not so much on which fragment of the cerebral cortex was excised but on **how much** was removed. According to this interpretation memory of a maze was 'smeared' throughout the cortex, not located in one area more than another. Later, in the 1970s, electrophysiological recording from unrestrained rats undergoing operant training in a Skinner box provided similar results. It seemed that cells throughout the brain were activated during the learning procedure.

In spite of these results it is now beginning to seem more likely that 'memory circuits' are localisable within the brain. It may well be that the 'mass action' observations merely indicate a general arousal throughout the brain when learning is occurring (memories being laid down) but that the actual pathways or 'circuits' where the changes are occurring are quite discrete.

It is nowadays believed that the areas primarily involved in the laying down of memory traces are the **cerebellum**, **hippocampus**, **amygdala** and **cerebral cortex**.

There is good evidence that a number of adaptive conditioned reflexes to aversive stimuli involve the cerebellum. One of the favourite reflexes in these studies has been the eye-blink (UCR) in response to a puff of air (UCS). This can be coupled to a tone or other conditioned stimulus (CS). Pairing of CS and UCS ultimately elicits the eye-blink in response to the CS alone. This reflex has all the characteristics of a classical Pavlovian conditioned reflex.

Careful experiments involving lesioning, microinfusion of drugs, electrophysiological recording and electrical microstimulation show that certain regions of the cerebellum are crucial to the establishment and maintenance of this conditioned reflex. These regions include the ipsilateral **interpositus nucleus** (in the base of the cerebellum) and identifiable **Purkinje cells** in the cerebellar cortex. Figure 18.4 shows that inputs from both the UCS and the CS meet on Purkinje cell dendrites and on cells in the interpositus nucleus. We shall see (especially in section 18.6) that synaptic conjunctions of this type are believed to be an essential part of memory mechanisms.

There is overwhelming evidence that the cerebellum plays a crucial role in the performance of skilled movements. It is thus not surprising to find that it is also deeply involved in learning adaptive responses to aversive stimuli.

Another region of the brain which is deeply involved in memory is the **hippocampus**. It has been known for many years that injury to human hippocampi causes a profound upset of STM. If their attention is distracted, patients are unable to remember lists of words or names of objects which they have memorised just a few moments previously. They cannot remember what day it is or what they had for breakfast. Yet their

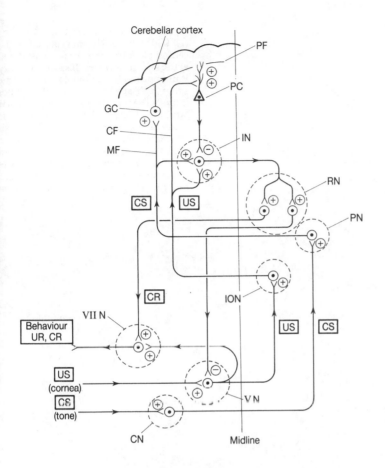

Cerebellar cortex

PF

PC

GC

CF

MF

IN

RN

CS

US

PN

CR

ION

VII N

RN

Behaviour
UR, CR

US

CS

US
(cornea)

CS
(tone)

V N

CN

Midline

Figure 18.4 Anatomy of the air-puff conditioned reflex. This complicated diagram shows the neuronal pathways underlying the eye-blink reflex. Impulses generated by an air puff to the cornea (unconditioned stimulus, US) make their way via the Vth cranial nerve to its nucleus in the midbrain (V N) and thence via the inferior olivary nucleus (ION) to the dendritic tree of a Purkinje cell (PC) in the cerebellar cortex. A branch from this pathway leads to the VIIth cranial nerve nucleus VII N) and thence to the muscles of the eyelid. Impulses generated by a tone (the conditioned stimulus, CS) make their way from the ear via the cochlear nucleus (CN) to the pontine nucleus (PN) and thence via a synapse with a granule cell (GC) to the dendritic tree of the Purkinje cell. The output from the Purkinje cell passes first to cells in the interpositus nucleus (IP), then to cells in the red nucleus (RN) and finally to the output to the eyelid muscles from the nucleus of the VIIth cranial nerve. It can be seen that inputs from both the US and the CS meet at the PC and the IN. It can also be seen that the output from the PC runs to both V N (inhibitory) and VII N (excitatory). CF = climbing fibre; CN = cochlear nucleus; CR = conditioned response; CS = conditioned stimulus, GC = granule cell; IN = interpositus nucleus; ION = inferior olivary nucleus; MF = mossy fibre; PC = Purkinje cell; PF = parallel fibre; PN = pontine nucleus; RN = red nucleus; UR = unconditioned response; US = uncondi-tioned stimulus; V N = nucleus of Vth cranial nerve; VII N = nucleus of VIIth cranial nerve; + = excitatory synapse; - = inhibitory synapse. (After Thompson, 1986, *Science*, **233**, 941–947.)

long term memories are comparatively intact. We shall see in Chapter 19 that Alzheimer's disease in which the hippocampi are particularly affected is characterised by a profound loss of short-term memory.

In rats it can be shown that the hippocampus is crucially involved in behaviours which involve spatial orientation. Means of testing such behaviour are shown in Figure 18.5. A rat may, for instance, be placed on the central platform of a radial maze. Each arm of the maze is baited with food. The optimal strategy is to visit each arm in turn thus ensuring that time and energy is not wasted in entering an empty arm. If rats can orientate themselves by observing visual cues above and around the maze they often do not visit each arm in turn but run to each apparently at random, remembering from the visual cues which arm they have visited and which they have not. Similarly if a rat is forced to find a platform concealed beneath cloudy water it can only do so by learning the visual cues in the room surrounding the tank. It is said that the animals carry a 'cognitive map' in their brains.

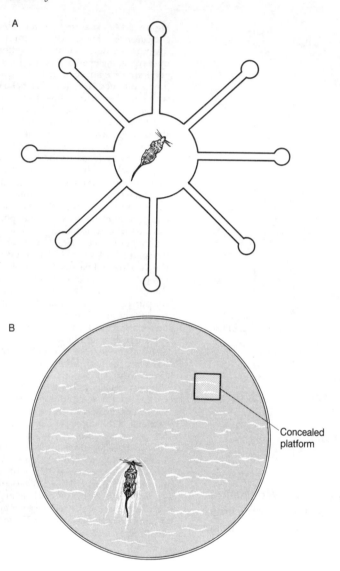

A

B

Concealed
platform

Figure 18.5 Radial and water 'mazes'. (A) Radial maze. The rat is placed on the central platform. Food or water is placed at the end of each arm. If spatial memory is unimpaired the rat should not enter the same passageway twice. (B) Water 'maze'. The rat is placed in a large circular tank filled with water. The water is commonly made cloudy by adding milk. At some point in the tank, just below the surface, is a platform. The rat is required to memorise its surroundings (the positions of lights, doors, tables etc.) in order to navigate rapidly to the platform

Rats with lesioned hippocampi perform significantly less well in these tasks. It is as if their ability to form and/or store a cognitive map has been damaged. Current evidence suggests, however, that although the hippocampus is massively involved in learning and STM, the LT memory traces are held elsewhere.

We shall return to the mammalian brain later. It is time now, however, to turn our attention to the nature of the memory trace. We have seen something of what it is required to do; we have looked briefly at where it may be laid down; but what form does it take?

The physical basis of memory, we have seen, must be some alteration in nerve pathways within the brain. The connection between input and output is altered: either facilitated or inhibited. Perhaps, as in Chapter 17, we should envisage the brain as initially comparatively undifferentiated and over-provided with pathways between sensory input and motor output. Learning selects between these pathways. It ensures that some become more or less permanently differentiated from others. It ensures that impulses travel preferentially (or the opposite) through these pathways. Thus, in a sense, learning could be seen as an extension into the adult of the lability which we have seen the brain to possess during development.

In previous chapters we have noted that action potentials are all-or-nothing events. The initial segment fires or does not fire. Once the impulse is initiated it propagates without decrement. There is no calling it back, no increasing or decreasing its amplitude or velocity. This is not the case with synapses. We have seen that postsynaptic potentials are graded events. We have seen that the positions where synapses occur on the neuronal soma have a crucial bearing on their effect on the postsynaptic cell. We have seen that the size of the synapse, the amount of transmitter released when an action potential arrives, the type of transmitter, the type and number of receptors in the subsynaptic membrane, all influence the magnitude and duration and type of postsynaptic event. It is not surprising, therefore, that neurobiologists regard the synapse as the most likely locus for the changes underlying and responsible for memory.

And this is where we have, for the moment, to take leave of mammalian systems. They are too complicated. If memory is ultimately an affair of synaptic resistances, which of the mammal's 10^{14} synapses should we look at? There is much evidence to show that neuronal activity leads to biochemical changes indicative of increased protein biosynthesis. There is increased activity of DNA-dependent RNA polymerase and the appearance of increased amounts of mRNA in the perikaryal cytoplasm. Following on from this, increased incorporation of radiolabelled amino acids into protein can be detected. It can also be shown that the density of spines on dendritic trees is significantly increased, just as, in the opposite case, inactivity leads to loss of dendritic spines. These consequences have all been well established—but do they have anything to do with the memory trace? Might they not be just consequences of increased overall cerebral activity? To be sure we have to find systems where learning is occurring in identifiable neurons. Systems in which we can compare the same neuron, the same synapse, when learning is occurring and when it is not. We have thus to turn, initially, to the far simpler systems of the invertebrates.

18.4 INVERTEBRATE SYSTEMS

A number of invertebrate nervous systems are proving themselves invaluable in neurobiological research. Perhaps the simplest nervous system of all is that of the small nematode worm *Caenorhabditis elegans* which, as we noted in Chapter 1, consists of just 302 cells. Its structure has, so to speak, been 'run into the ground' by reconstruction from serial electron micrographs. All its neurons, their shapes, sizes and connections have been mapped. Like many other invertebrates the neurons and their synaptic contacts are identical in isogenic animals. The genetics of the worm are also well researched and many mutants affecting the development and structure of the nervous system have been isolated. To date, however, it has not been used for learning studies.

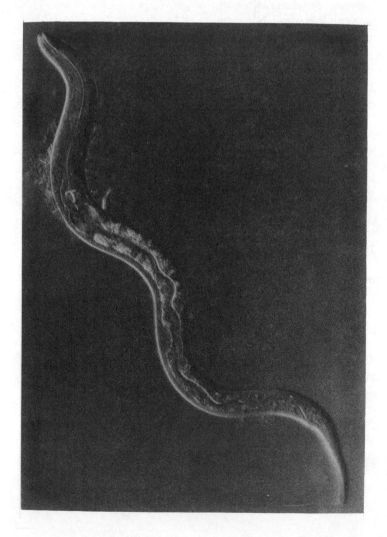

Figure 18.6   *Caenorhabditis elegans*. The worm is about 200 μm in length. It consists of 959 somatic cells of which 302 constitute the nervous system. Many of the nerve cells are large and as the body is translucent can be seen in the living animal. Although there are only 302 neurons they have been grouped into 118 classes on the basis of their shape and connectivity. In spite of this rich variety of different types there does not seem to be a clear distinction between sensory, motor and internuncial neurons: most neurons are polyfunctional. (From White, 1985, *Trends in Neurosciences*, **8**, 277–283; with permission.)

Turning from one of the simplest of invertebrates to some of the most highly evolved we find that the insects provide many useful preparations for the neurobiologist. *Apis mellifica*, the honey bee, *Schistocerca gregaria*, the locust, *Periplaneta americana*, the cockroach, *Phormia regina*, the blowfly, and, finally, *Drosophila melanogaster*, the fruitfly, all have their devotees. *Drosophila*, in particular, because of its extremely well-known genetics, has received much attention.

The experimental approach to learning in *Drosophila* is distinctively different from that used in other organisms. Because of its small genome and the highly developed state of *Drosophila* genetics it is possible to search for single mutations which affect learning and then to search for the gene product involved.

The associative learning test most used with *Drosophila* is to pair an olfactory or electrical stimulus with a gustatory stimulus. The gustatory stimulus (the UCS) is usually sucrose which 'untrained' *Drosophila* will approach and ingest. The olfactory stimulus (the CS) may be one of a number of olfactants to which the insect is sensitive. The aversive electrical stimulus (also a CS) is a grid delivering about 90 V, AC. It is not difficult to condition the fly so that it will approach a source of odorant previously paired with sucrose and avoid an odorant source previously paired with an electric shock.

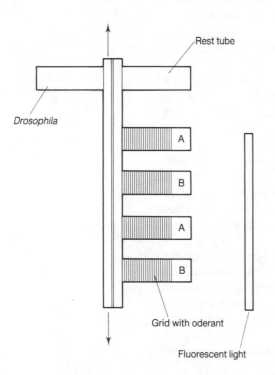

Rest tube

Drosophila

A

B

A

B

Grid with oderant

Fluorescent light

Figure 18.7 Apparatus for conditioning *Drosophila*. The fruit flies are housed in a tube which can be slid back and forth across the openings to a number of other tubes. In the 'rest' position the 'home' tube is opposite a 'rest' tube which is perforated to allow adequate air. The 'test' tubes, A,B,A,B, contain grids coated with oderant. The grids are also connected to a supply to give 90 V, AC, shock. The flies are induced to crawl into the tubes by making use of their photo-taxis towards light. Conditioning may then be carried out by using either an attractive stimulus (sucrose) or an aversive stimulus (electric shock). Memory may then be tested in the second set of tubes (A,B). (After Dudai *et al.*, 1976, *Proceedings of the National Academy of Sciences (USA)*, **73**, 1684–1688.)

This test has been used to isolate mutants deficient in the learning and/or memory mechanisms required for this task. A number of such mutants have been found. Each causes a specific deficit.

Dunce (dnc), the first such mutation to be isolated, shows appreciable learning when tested 30 seconds after training, but after that the memory quickly decays. This mutation can be traced to the X chromosome and appears to affect a **cAMP phospho-diesterase (PDE 2)**. In addition to their memory defect *dnc* flies also show reductions in both **habituation** and **sensitisation**. This perhaps suggests that in *Drosophila*, at least, associative and non-associative memory share a similar mechanism. We shall return to this when we consider *Aplysia* in the next section.

Dopadecarboxylase (Ddc) mutants in contrast to *dnc* mutants fail to learn the associations in the first place. The DOPA decarb-oxylase enzyme (or l-aromatic amino acid decarboxylase) is, as we saw in Chapter 15, required for the synthesis of both **dopamine** and **serotonin**. Flies deficient in these neuro-transmitters thus appear incapable of learning the odour–shock and odour–sucrose pairings. It is moreover possible to breed flies with partial lesions of the gene and to show that they have a **reduced** ability to learn the two associations. There seems, in other words, to be a **dosage** effect. More interesting still it can be shown that such partial (or mild) mutants **do not forget** what they have learned. **The *Ddc* mutation thus affects learning but not recall**. It appears, therefore, that dopamine and/or serotonin are necessary for learning the odour–sucrose, odour–shock paradigm in *Drosophila* but not for retaining or expression/retrieval of that memory.

A number of other mutants have been isolated which affect this and other learning paradigms in *Drosophila*. As in the case of the two mutants described above it is becoming possible to connect the genetic lesion to the biochemical defect and this to very specific deficiencies in either learning or memory. The neural elements of *Drosophila* nervous systems are, however, very small. In order to investigate the molecular biology of learning and memory at the cellular and subcellular level we have to turn to systems whose neurons are orders of magnitude larger. These systems are provided by the last of the invertebrate phyla we shall consider in this Chapter—the **Mollusca**.

A number of molluscan nervous systems have been studied by neurobiologists. They include those of *Limax maximus*, the garden slug; *Pleurobranchaea calfornica*, a marine opisthobranch; *Lymnaea stagnalis*, the pond snail; and, most important of all *Hermissenda crassicornis*, a marine nudibranch; and *Aplysia californica*, the sea hare, a tectibranch.

Although much interesting work has been done on *Hermissenda* we shall concentrate our attention on the best known and most instructive of these organisms: *Aplysia californica*.

18.5 *APLYSIA* AND THE MOLECULAR BIOLOGY OF MEMORY

Figure 18.8 shows a dorsal view of *Aplysia*. It is a large marine mollusc measuring several hundred centimetres from head to tail. The figure shows the position of the **siphon** and **gill**, which play so large a role in the behaviour we are about to examine.

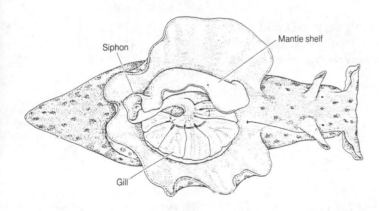

Figure 18.8 *Aplysia californica*. (Reprinted with permission from Kandel, 1979, *Scientific American*, **241**, 60–70; Copyright © 1979 by Scientific American Inc. All rights reserved.)

When a weak mechanical stimulus is applied to the siphon both siphon and gill tend to withdraw beneath the mantle shelf. This is a protective reflex. Habituation, sensitisation and also classical conditioning can be demonstrated.

Habituation. If a sequence of 10–15 weak mechanical stimuli are applied to the siphon the gill withdrawal is much reduced. The response has habituated. Recovery to the original withdrawal magnitude takes about an hour. If, however, the habituating sessions are repeated four or five times then the 'memory' persists for several weeks. During this period the withdrawal is significantly less than normal. All of these characteristics show that *Aplysia* habituation is identical to habituation in vertebrate systems.

Sensitisation. If a noxious stimulus is applied to the animal's head or tail immediately before the siphon is touched then the withdrawal is much enhanced. This sensitisation again lasts about an hour. Long-term sensitisation can be induced in the same way as long term habituation: by repeating the training sessions a number of times.

Classical conditioning. Several conditioning paradigms have proved effective. A weak tactile stimulus to the siphon (such as would normally induce only a tiny gill retraction) can serve as the CS whilst a strong tactile stimulus to the gill itself (normally causing a major retraction) serves as the UCS. After a number of classical CS–UCS pairings the unpaired CS can be shown to elicit an enhanced gill withdrawal. This CR shows all the features of the Pavlovian type of CR. Another means of eliciting a classical CR from the *Aplysia* siphon–gill system is to pair a weak stimulus (CS) to the siphon with a strong stimulus (UCS) to the tail. Once again a number of pairings of CS and UCS leads to a strong withdrawal when the CS is applied alone.

Now all this, the reader may think, is all very well and good— but what's new? What's new is that the neural connections underlying these behavioural responses are very well understood.

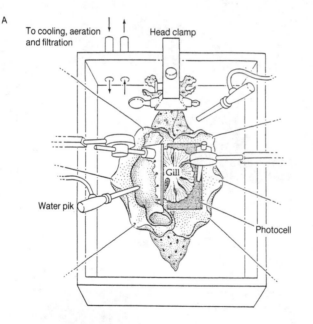

A

To cooling, aeration and filtration

Head clamp

Water pik

Gill

Photocell

Figure 18.9 Experimental arrangement for the study of the gill-withdrawal reflex in *Aplysia*. (A) *Aplysia* is held in a small aquarium in such a way that a water jet can be directed at the siphon (water pik) and the response of the gill detected by the amount of light falling on to a photocell beneath it (dense stipples). (B) Habituation: during some 80 water-jet stimuli to the siphon the gill response gradually habituates. The numbers indicate the number of the trial. After 122 min of rest the response has completely recovered. (C) Sensitisation: habituation is again induced by 18 trials (at 1-min intervals). A strong and prolonged tactile stimulus is then delivered to the neck— time of application indicated by upwardly pointing arrow. The habituated response is immediately restored. This is sensitisation (From Purves and Lichtman, 1985, *Principles of Neural Development*, Sunderland, Mass.: Sinauer; after Kandel, 1976, *Cellular Basis of Behaviour: An Introduction to Behavioural Neurobiology*, New York: Freeman; with permission.)

B   Habituation and recovery

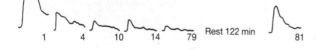

1   4   10   14   79   Rest 122 min   81

C   Sensitization after habituation

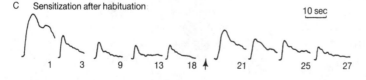

10 sec

1   3   9   13   18 ↑   21   25   27

Aplysia's nervous system is very simple compared with that of
the vertebrates. Like that of *Caenorhabditis* it consists of identifiable
cells and connections. Unlike *Caenorhabditis* or, for that matter,
Drosophila, **these cells are very large**. The largest perikarya are
up to 0.5 mm in diameter. Figure 18.10 shows a diagram of the
abdominal ganglion, in which some of the identifiable cells are
labelled.

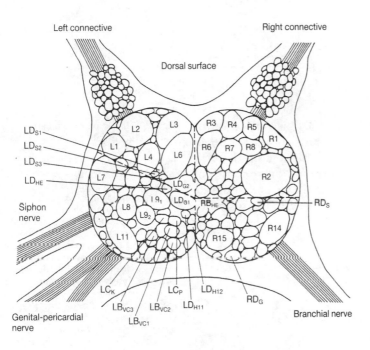

Figure 18.10 Abdominal ganglion of
Aplysia. The abdominal ganglion consists
of about 1500 cells. Identifiable cells are
labelled in the figure. Cells in the left
hemiganglion are prefixed by 'L' and
those in the right hemiganglion by 'R'.
(Reprinted with permission from Kandel,
1979, *Scientific American*, **241**, 60–70.
Copyright © 1979 by Scientific American
Inc. All rights reserved.)

Some of the cells labelled in Figure 18.10 are involved in the
gill withdrawal reflexes we discussed above. It can be shown that
the skin of the siphon contains just 24 sensory neurons and that
these make direct connections to six motor neurons which control
the muscles of the gill. The cell bodies of four of the latter neurons
(L7, LD_{G1}, LD_{G2}, RD_G) can be seen in Figure 18.10. In addition
to this exceedingly simple circuit the sensory cells also synapse
with a small number of interneurons interposed between them
and the motor neurons. The circuit is shown in Figure 18.11.

First let us consider **habituation**. It will be recalled that this
is a reduced gill withdrawal in response to repeated stimuli to
the siphon. This response can be mimicked by stimulating the
sensory neurons from the siphon and recording from the motor
neurons to the gill. In the *Aplysia* system this can be made precise
by stimulating one known sensory fibre and recording from the
perikaryon of a known motor neuron.

Siphon

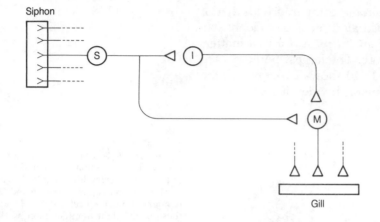

Gill

When the experiment shown in Figure 18.12 is carried out it is clear that although the first stimulus results in a large EPSP in the motor neuron's perikaryon, subsequent stimuli elicit smaller and smaller EPSPs. It can, furthermore, be shown that this is not due to any decrease in sensitivity of the subsynaptic membrane. The habituation is due to a **decrease in the quantity**

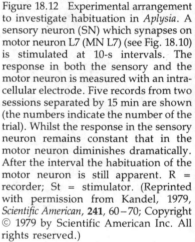

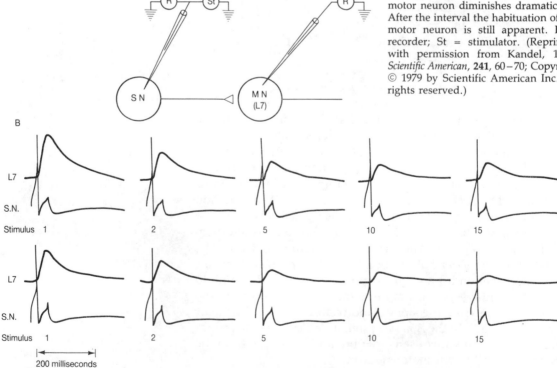

of neurotransmitter released on arrival of an action potential at the presynaptic terminal. There is evidence that this is due to a persistent inactivation of the Ca^{2+} current into the presynaptic terminal. This, as we noted in Chapter 14, would reduce the release of transmitter from synaptic vesicles. Because the effect occurs without the intervention of any second synapse the phenomenon is termed **homosynaptic** depression.

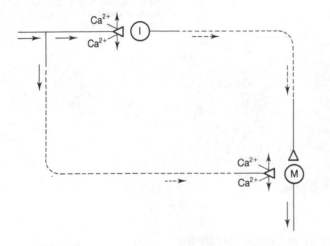

Figure 18.13 Homosynaptic depression causes habituation. A sequence of impulses in the sensory neuron leads to a partial closure of Ca^{2+} gates in the presynaptic terminal. This, in turn, diminishes the amount of transmitter released on to the motor neuron (M). Hence the decreased magnitude of the EPSP in M

Next let us turn to **sensitisation**. Here, it will be remembered, the gill retraction is markedly increased on a second stimulation. The molecular mechanisms underlying this behaviour are, as we shall see, more fully understood than are those underlying habituation. It is, moreover, a more intricate process. Instead of just two neurons—sensory and motor—being involved at least three neurons are implicated.

First let us consider **short-term** sensitisation. Once again the phenomenon can be investigated by stimulating a sensory neuron and recording the response of the subsynaptic motor neuron. In this case the EPSP instead of being smaller when the motor nerve is stimulated a second time is very much larger. Once again, however, it can be shown that this is not due to any increased sensitivity of the subsynaptic membrane but to a **greatly increased release of neurotransmitter**.

How has this come about? The answer is shown in Figure 18.14. The figure shows that when a sensitising stimulus is delivered to the head (or tail) of *Aplysia* 'facilitatory' interneurons are activated. These synapse on the **presynaptic** terminals of the sensory neurons. It is believed that these presynaptic synapses release **serotonin** on to the presynaptic endings of the sensory neurons.

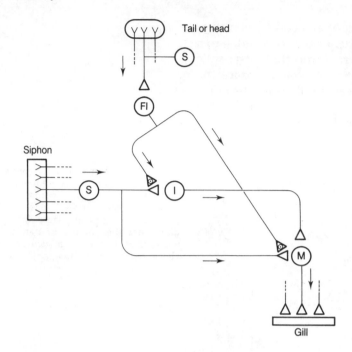

Figure 18.14 'Wiring diagram' for sensitisation in *Aplysia*. Superimposed on the neuronal circuit of Fig. 18.11 is a system of facilitatory interneurons (FI). These neurons are activated by sensory fibres from the tail or head. They make synaptic contact with the presynaptic terminals of the sensory neurons from the siphon. These synapses are believed to be serotoninergic (represented by the cored vesicle). (After Kandel, 1985, in *Principles of Neural Science*, eds E. R. Kandel and J. H. Schwartz, New York: Elsevier, pp. 817–833.)

How does serotonin increase the release of transmitter by the sensory neuron? If we look back to Section 10.2.3 we see that serotonin affects certain potassium channels in the membrane (I_{KS} or S-channels). In *Aplysia* it is believed that this is achieved by serotonin activating membrane-bound adenylate cyclase. The cAMP thus produced initiates a biochemical cascade which via an increased activity of protein kinase C (PKC) leads to phosphorylation of the S-channel protein (or a closely associated protein). The upshot of all this is that the S-channel is blocked and the **outflow of K^+ is reduced**. In Chapter 13 we noted that the outflow of potassium ions was responsible for the 'downward' or recovery phase of the action potential. If the S-channel is blocked the duration of this recovery phase is increased. Finally, turning back to Chapter 14, we recall that the inward flux of Ca^{2+} ions is strongly voltage-dependent. Ca^{2+} channels only open when the membrane is depolarised. Hence if the recovery phase behind an action potential is elongated an **increased amount of Ca^{2+}** can enter. Hence, remembering that vesicle exocytosis is dependent on intraterminal Ca^{2+}, transmitter release is increased. This sequence of events is schematised in Figures 18.15 and 18.16.

Because more than one synapse is involved in sensitisation the neural process is called **heterosynaptic** facilitation. It depends on an activation of the presynaptic serotoninergic synapse

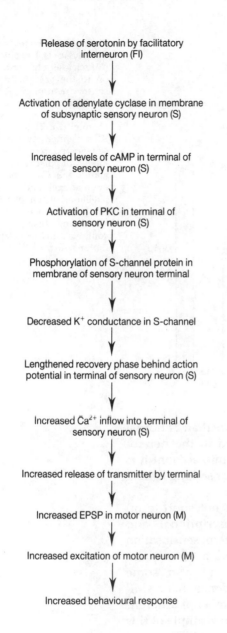

Release of serotonin by facilitatory
interneuron (FI)

Activation of adenylate cyclase in membrane
of subsynaptic sensory neuron (S)

Increased levels of cAMP in terminal of
sensory neuron (S)

Activation of PKC in terminal of
sensory neuron (S)

Phosphorylation of S-channel protein in
membrane of sensory neuron terminal

Decreased K^+ conductance in S-channel

Lengthened recovery phase behind action
potential in terminal of sensory neuron (S)

Increased Ca^{2+} inflow into terminal of
sensory neuron (S)

Increased release of transmitter by terminal

Increased EPSP in motor neuron (M)

Increased excitation of motor neuron (M)

Increased behavioural response

Figure 18.15 Sequence of biochemical events underlying sensitisation in *Aplysia*. For further explanation see text. (After Byrne, 1985, *Trends in Neurosciences*, **8**, 478–482.)

immediately before the arrival of an action potential along the sensory fibre.

Next let us turn to **long-term** sensitisation. It can be shown that the same nerve pathways are involved and that a similar neurological explanation in terms of heterosynaptic facilitation holds. The biochemistry, however, is different. It is possible to show that whereas a single application of serotonin to the presynaptic terminal induces sensitisation of the reflex for a period not exceeding an hour or so, four or more repeated applications

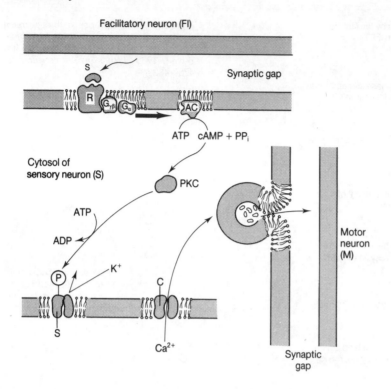

Figure 18.16 Heterosynaptic facilitation in *Aplysia*. The facilitatory interneuron (FI) releases a facilitatory transmitter (S) on to the presynaptic terminal of the sensory neuron (S). A collision-coupling mechanism generates cAMP which activates PKC to phosphorylate the I_{KS} channel (S). This reduces the efflux of K^+ ions after any action potential in the sensory neuron. The consequent prolonged depolarisation of the membrane allows the Ca^{2+} channels (C) to stay open longer and hence increases the likelihood of synaptic vesicles moving to the active zones in the presynaptic membrane, fusing and releasing their contents into the synaptic gap above the motor neuron

of serotonin lead to a sensitisation lasting for more than 24 hours. If the 'half lives' of the biochemicals involved in the heterosynaptic mechanism outlined above are taken into account it is difficult to see how they could be responsible for so long lasting an effect.

It has also been found that long-term (but not short-term) sensitisation can be blocked by both **transcriptional** and **translational** inhibitors. This suggests that long-term sensitisation involves not only the activation of PKC and a consequent phosphorylation of presynaptic S-channels but also some involvement of the genome. There is good evidence that cAMP can stimulate the transcription of genes in a number of different types of eukaryotic cell. We have already met an example of this in Section 16.4, where we noted the way in which cAMP induced the transcription of the mRNA for SNAT in pinealocytes. Other second messengers than cAMP (e.g. Ca^{2+}, IP_3, cGMP) may, of course, also be involved.

What mRNA transcript does the cAMP induce? The short answer is that we do not at present know. It can be shown, however, that the number, size and vesicle complement of sensory neurons involved in long-term sensitisation are all significantly increased. Perhaps the transcript (or transcripts) programmes the synthesis of appropriate enzymes and structural elements. These induced biochemicals would have to be packaged in such a way that they reach and adhere to the appropriate synaptic terminals. For it has to be remembered that neurons in general have many different synaptic terminals. But this, as we saw in Section 14.2 is no new problem in cell biology. How packages budding off the Golgi apparatus find their appropriate location in the cell remains very largely unknown. Recent work on cholinergic vesicles in the electric fish, *Torpedo*, suggests, however, that these, at least, contain synapse-specific glyco-proteins.

The implications of this work on *Aplysia* sensitisation for the relationship between STM amd LTM will not have escaped the reader.

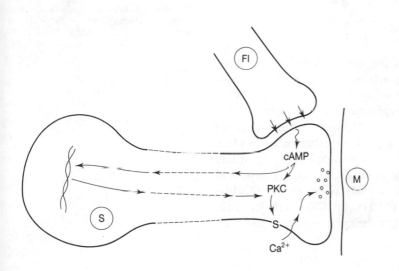

Figure 18.17 Putative mechanisms underlying long-term sensitisation. The same triadic system of facilitatory interneuron (FI), sensory neuron (S) and motor neuron (M) is shown as in previous figures. The same biochemistry obtains as in Fig. 18.16. It is suggested, however, that increased release of facilitatory transmitter on to the sensory terminal generates sufficient second-messenger to affect the genome. The figure shows the second-messenger (cAMP or another) being carried in the retrograde axoplasmic flow to the perikaryon. Here it switches on the protein synthetic machinery so that a factor (or factors) enhancing synaptic activity are manufactured and carried in the anterograde flow to the terminal. For further explanation see text

Finally let us consider **associative learning**. A number of experiments have been carried out in an attempt to discover the molecular basis of associative memory in *Aplysia*. In general it appears that associative memory may make use of the same basic molecular mechanisms as sensitisation. This, it will be remembered, would be consistent with the findings in the *Drosophila dnc* mutants.

One of the more recent experiments used a depolarising stimulus as the CS and and an application of serotonin as the UCS. After a very few pairings it was possible to show that there was a significantly increased level of cAMP in the sensory cells. Neither the CS alone nor the UCS alone nor random applications of CS and UCS led to this outcome.

The model shown in Figure 18.18 builds on the molecular biology worked out for long-term sensitisation (Figure 18.17). It

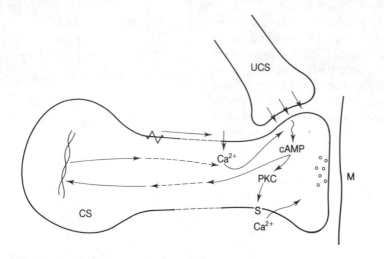

Figure 18.18   Associative learning. The biochemical mechanism is essentially similar to that of Fig. 18.17. The unconditioned stimulus (UCS) causes the release of serotonin. The conditioned stimulus (CS) is a depolarisation. After a few pairings of UCS and CS it is found that there is a significant increase of cAMP in the sensory cells. It is proposed that this is due to the Ca^{2+} influx consequent upon depolarisation potentiating the membrane-bound collision-coupling system. The excess cAMP may then switch on the perikaryal protein-synthetic machinery as proposed in Fig. 18.17. The outcome is that the conditioned stimulus has a greater chance of firing the subsynaptic motor cell than previously. Classical conditioning has occurred. (After Byrne, 1985, *Trends in Neurosciences*, **8**, 478–482.)

suggests that the CS arriving at the terminal will open Ca^{2+} gates in the usual way and that this activates the adenylate cyclase system in the membrane. Arrival of the UCS shortly after enhances this activation. The synergistic interaction between the two events ensures a significantly increased concentration of cAMP. This will lead, in the first instance, to increased release of transmitter, as described above. If the pairings are made sufficiently frequently we can suppose that the long-term effects of cAMP on the genome may begin to make themselves felt, thus ensuring that the CS will normally fire the CR—that, in other words, a new 'low-resistance' path through *Aplysia*'s nervous system is established.

18.6 THE MEMORY TRACE IN MAMMALS

Let us in conclusion return from the simple systems of invertebrates to our 'proper study': mammals and mankind. Does the elucidation of invertebrate memory systems help us to understand what is happening in mammals? We started this chapter by alluding to Occam's razor. Let us use it again here. Let us suppose that the molecular mechanisms underlying memory are much the same throughout the animal kingdom. Let us suppose that the spectacular development of memory in the mammals and especially amongst the primates is due to the vastly increased size and complexity of the nervous system. This great intricacy of structure (we can suppose) allows interaction between neural circuits each of which relies, at bottom, on much the same molecular biology we have seen at work in *Aplysia*. The upshot is the vastly increased range and subtlety of the memory process in the higher animals. In the case of *Homo sapiens*, of course, the situation is complicated yet further by the development of symbolic representation and communication—language.

In previous sections of this chapter we have noted the distinction between short-term and long-term memory and have also given some consideration to where in the mammalian brain the process of consolidation—whereby STM is transformed into LTM—occurs. We noted, in particular, that there is good reason to believe that the hippocampus is deeply implicated in this process. It is thus especially interesting to find that two of the neurophysiological processes which have been thought to underlie consolidation were first detected in the hippocampus, though they have subsequently been shown to occur elsewhere as well. These processes are called **post-tetanic potentiation (PTP)** and **long-term potentiation (LTP)**.

Post-tetanic potentiation has been a candidate for the physical basis of memory for a number of years. It can be shown that after a volley of impulses has been delivered to certain synapses the excitability of the subsynaptic membrane is significantly increased. In other words subsequent impulses in the presynaptic cell induce larger EPSPs in the subsynaptic cell and thus have a greater chance of depolarising its initial segment to threshold and initiating an action potential. PTP generally persists for a few hours and then the subsynaptic membrane returns to normal.

Long-term potentiation differs from PTP in the length of time for which it persists. Instead of a few hours it can be shown to remain for days, weeks and even months. To induce LTP the

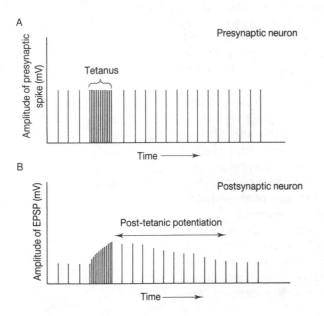

Figure 18.19 Post-tetanic potentiation. (A) Impulses in presynaptic neuron. (B) Amplitude of EPSP in postsynaptic neuron. After the rapid tattoo of tetanic stimulation the magnitude of the EPSP is increased and remains increased for a considerable period of time

stimulation must be of a greater intensity than that required for PTP. It has been found, furthermore, that volleys of impulses impinging on the subsynaptic cell from several brain regions give optimal results.

It is clear that these electrophysiological phenomena are consistent with a memory mechanism. It has been found, more-over, that Ca^{2+} fluxes are once again deeply implicated. If a calcium chelator, EGTA, is injected into subsynaptic cells in the hippocampus it can be shown that LTP is inhibited. Note, however, that it is the **subsynaptic cell** which is affected, not (as in the case of *Aplysia*) the presynaptic ending. This distinction is confirmed by the finding that blocking glutamate receptors on these subsynaptic membranes also blocks LTP. Some form of 'back-reaction' from subsynaptic to presynaptic membrane cannot, however, be ruled out. It is not impossible that the biochemical events induced in the subsynaptic cell by the rain of transmitters from a tetanised presynaptic terminal may lead to some trophic material being released into the synaptic cleft which affects the presynaptic membrane. For, as we shall shortly see, there is also evidence that LTP is associated with an enhanced release of EAAs from presynaptic terminals. Let us, however, look first at the nature of the subsynaptic response to tetanising stimulation.

It will be recalled from Chapter 9 that there are at least three pharmacologically distinct types of glutamate receptor: K, Q and NMDA receptors. It will also be recalled that the NMDA receptor controls a Ca^{2+} channel which can only be opened by glutamate when the membrane has been depolarised by some 30 mV. At present there are no specific antagonists for the K and Q receptors (which induce typical EPSPs); a number of antagonists are, however, known for the NMDA receptor system. Several of the latter, for instance D-2-amino-5-phosphonovalerate (D-AP5) and phenecyclidine (PCP), have been used in an analysis of the molecular basis of LTP in the hippocampus.

It can be shown that both D-AP5 and PCP prevent the induction of LTP in the CA1 and dentate gyrus (DG) regions of the hippocampus. It can be shown, in short, that whilst NMDA antagonists block the response to high-frequency (tetanising) stimulation, the response to low-frequency, non-tetanising, stimuli (presumably mediated by K and Q receptors) is unaffected. These findings have suggested an NMDA-receptor-mediated mechanism for LTP and hence short-term memory.

The suggested mechanism is based on the well-established observation that Mg^{2+} ions block the NMDA receptor at resting potential (Chapter 9). It is suggested, therefore, that low-frequency stimulation, releasing glutamate from presynaptic terminals, whilst activating the non-NMDA receptors and inducing EPSPs in the underlying cell, does not cause sufficient subsynaptic depolarisation to remove the Mg^{2+} blockade on the NMDA receptors. This blockade is, however, removed by the significantly greater subsynaptic depolarisation induced by high-frequency (tetanising) stimulation of the afferent fibres. In this case the presynaptic terminals will release large quantities of glutamate which via the K and Q receptors will cause a large depolarisation of the subsynaptic membrane.

The opening of the NMDA receptor calcium channel is thus dependent on tetanic stimulation. The consequent influx of calcium ions could have a number of consequences. It might affect the excitability of the subsynaptic membrane by acting on **calcium-dependent ion channels** in the membrane, or it could activate a **protein kinase** which might in turn affect membrane excitability by phosphorylating a membrane protein or, lastly, it could act as a 'second-messenger' to trigger some deeper cytosolic or genomic biochemistry.

Lynch and Baudry have proposed a specific theory. They provide evidence which suggests that the influxes of calcium ions at hippocampal synapses activate a membrane-bound enzyme—calpain. This enzyme, they further propose, breaks up the fodrin subsynaptic cytoskeleton (see Chapter 6), thus **unmasking** fresh glutamate receptors. The subsynaptic membrane is thus sensitised (potentiated) for further synaptic activity in response to EAAs. This theory, however, is by no means universally accepted. Indeed it has been impossible to demonstrate an increased binding of labelled glutamate to subsynaptic receptors during LTP as the theory predicts.

An alternative molecular mechanism makes a connection with the observation that NMDA receptors may be involved in the stabilisation of synchronously active synapses (Section 17.8). In Chapter 17 it was suggested that synapses which fired together stayed together, and this was also suggested by the 'wiring diagram' responsible for the eye-blink reflex (Figure 18.4). Synapses which are not synchronised are eliminated or 'down-modulated' by some (as yet unknown) antagonist. In Chapter 17 it was further suggested that NMDA-controlled channels were instrumental in inhibiting the synthesis of this antagonist. In the case of LTP it is similarly suggested that NMDA receptors in tetanised synapses induce (perhaps by a cytosolic second-messenger mechanism) a factor which increases the release of transmitter from the presynaptic terminal. It could be that this is the 'trophic factor' mentioned above which is required to account for the enhanced release of EAAs from tetanised terminals. It could be, in other words, that we have here a case of NMDA-induced 'temporal summation' to put beside the NMDA-induced 'spatial summation' of Chapter 17.

Whether the 'NMDA trophic factor' theory, the calpain theory of Lynch and Baudry, a protein kinase theory, or some totally different interpretation can be sustained, only time will tell. Whatever the underlying biochemical mechanism it does seem that long-term potentiation and its obverse, long-term depression (LTD) (which has also been observed in the brain, especially the cerebellum), provide a means by which certain nerve pathways can become differentiated from the myriads of others which exist in the mammalian brain. It follows that the molecular neurobiology of these pathways could well be the molecular neurobiology of memory. Whether it involves processes restricted to the dendrite or dendritic spine or whether second messengers derepress nuclear DNA and generate new protein, or, more than likely, both, remains a question for future research.

We noted at the end of Section 18.3 above that there is, indeed, much evidence which indicates that in neurons which are physiologically active the protein biosynthetic machinery is switched on and that the synthesis of fresh mRNA and the manufacture of fresh protein can be detected. There is also much evidence for the growth and maintenance of existing synapses and the development of new synapses, especially spine synapses. We discussed some of this evidence in Chapter 17 when considering the various experiments which can be carried out on the vertebrate visual system. The great virtue of studies on LTP and LTD, however, is that they seem to filter out from the mass of ongoing activity just that activity which is arguably related to memory and the consolidation of memory.

The strategy of using ideas generated in the simpler and more easily manipulated nervous systems of invertebrates to set up questions to investigate the immensely more complex nervous systems of vertebrates has in the past proved very fruitful. It is only necessary to remind ourselves of the significance of the squid giant axon in fundamental neurophysiology to assure ourselves of this. *Drosphila* and *Aplysia* suggest what we should be looking for in the brains of mammals and other vertebrates. Their molecular neurobiology suggests the type of molecular biology which may be responsible for mammalian LTP and LTD. The latter, in turn, may allow us to see how the 'negative sculpturing' which we found at work in the embryology of the brain (Chapter 17) may still be at work in the mature mammalian brain, ensuring that a continually updated 'model' of the significant features of the environment crystallises out of a myriad differently weighted synaptic interactions.

Chapter 19
Five pathologies

'Can'st thou not minister to a mind diseased?' Macbeth adjures his physician and, hearing that nothing can be done, retorts: 'Throw physic to the dogs,—I'll none of it.'

This is certainly a major reason for studying molecular neurobiology. Some 10% of the UK population will at some time in their lives be hospitalised for 'mental illness'. For most the period in hospital is short. For some, however, it is lengthy and perhaps permanent. Can an understanding of the molecular biology of the brain help us toward a treatment or, better, a cure?

First of all let us subdivide the term 'mental illness' into two: **neurological** ('organic') and **psychological** (or 'functional') . This subdivision is by no means clear-cut. It is often convenient, however, to distinguish conditions which have a clear anatomical substratum (e.g. multiple sclerosis, Parkinsonism) from those where that substratum is more subtle (e.g. depression, schizophrenia). The latter subdivision (the psychological) is customarily subdivided once again into the **neuroses** and the **psychoses**. Again the basis of this subdivision is far from clear-cut. It is generally held that in the neuroses (such as depression) the sufferer shares the same 'world' as the rest of us but sees it through whatever is the opposite of rose-tinted spectacles. In psychotic conditions (e.g. schizophrenia) the patient seems to live in a different world altogether. He seems to be overcome with delusions and hallucinations. On this classification Lady Macbeth would nowadays be said to be suffering from a (fairly mild) psychotic condition—a species of schizophrenia—induced by 'having known what she should not'.

To those who accept a 'dual-aspect identity' interpretation of the mind/brain relationship there are no sharp discontinuities between neurological and psychotic illnesses. Instead there is a continuum of conditions which extend from phenylketonuria (PKU), say, to paranoid schizophrenia. All have their psychological and their neurological 'aspects', just as (to use a classical metaphor) a curved mathematical surface has a convex face ('aspect') and a concave face ('aspect'). Remember: a 'mathematical' surface has no thickness.

This is not, of course, to say that the entire spectrum of brain/mind disease can be best tackled in the same way. It would be as absurd to try the 'talking cure' (psychoanalysis) with an individual suffering from Huntingdon's disease as to treat one of Freud's Viennese ladies by genetic engineering. The dual-aspect identity interpretation would have it, however, that the talking cure has an effect on the brain's physiology, albeit a subtle and at present untraceable effect, just as altering the neuronal genome would have a massive effect on the brain's functioning—and hence its 'owner's' subjectivity.

In this chapter we shall look at some of the brain/mind pathologies which have an identifiable molecular aetiology. In a recent paper Martin has identified 22 neuropathologies of this type. We shall, however, only consider five: we shall start with one of the pathologies of the developing brain, **phenylketonuria (PKU)**, move on to some of the conditions which affect the mature brain, **Huntingdon's disease (HD) (= Huntingdon's chorea)** and **depression**, and end by considering two of the degenerative conditions which affect the elderly: **Parkinson's disease (PD)**, and **Alzheimer's disease (AD)**. There are, of course, a multitude of other ills which can affect the brain: birth mishaps, infections by various agents, dietary deficiencies, cardiovascular accidents, etc. The reader should consult one of the standard textbooks in neurology.

19.1 PHENYLKETONURIA (PKU)

A large number of congenital defects in amino acid metabolism are now known to affect the brain. The most important of these are shown in Table 19.1. These metabolic defects are expressed in many of the body's organs but the major symptoms are neurological: mental retardation, convulsions, ataxia. The infant brain is particularly sensitive to any abnormal biochemistry. We noted the significance of sensitive periods in Chapter 17 when we discussed the brain's development. In children this period lasts for the first few years of life and different brain regions enter and leave their sensitive periods independently of each other. Because the defects are widespread the biochemical abnormality can normally be detected in the urine and/or the blood. An early diagnosis generally means that a satisfactory treatment is possible.

The most well known of these congenital defects is that responsible for **phenylketonuria (PKU)**. The defect is in the enzyme system catalysing the transformation of **phenylalanine**

Table 19.1 Amino acid metabolism and mental defect

Disease	Amino acid	Enzyme defect	Symptom
Arginosuccinic aciduria	Arginine	Arginosuccinase	Severe mental retardation, abnormal EEG
Cystathionuria	Methionine	Cystathionase	Mental retardation
Histidinaemia	Histidine	Histidase	Mental retardation
Homocystinuria	Methionine	Cystathione synthetase	Lens dislocations, osteoporosis, mental retardation
Hyperammonaemia	Ornithine	Ornithine transcarbamylase, Argininsuccinase	Nausea, vomiting, mental retardation
Maple syrup urine disease (MSUD)	Leucine Isoleucine Valine	Oxidative decarboxylases	Seizures, death in infancy
Phenylketonuria	Phenylalanine	Phenylalanine hydroxylase co-factors	Severe mental defect
Tyrosinanaemia	Tyrosine	Tyrosine transaminase	Mental retardation

Many of these lesions also affect other bodily systems; the central nervous system (perhaps because it is the most delicately poised) is commonly the system which is most severely upset

to **tyrosine**. We saw in Chapter 15 (Figure 15.17) that this transformation requires **phenylalanine hydroxylase** and **tetrahydrobiopterin (BH$_4$)** as a co-factor.

Figure 19.1 shows that the failure to transform phenylalanine to tyrosine leads to the build up of **phenylpyruvic acid**. This can readily be detected in the urine. PKU is inherited in a Mendelian fashion. It is carried in the heterozygous form in 1–2% of the white population of the UK. Adult heterozygotes show some penetrance of the defect. It can be shown that after ingesting a quantity of phenylalanine the quantity of the amino acid detect-

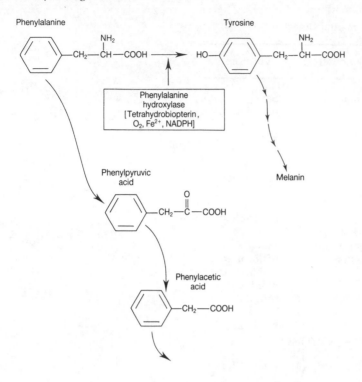

Figure 19.1 Metabolic defect in PKU. The enzyme system responsible for catalysing the step from phenylalanine to tyrosine is defective in phenylketon-uriacs. In consequence the little-used pathway to phenylpyruvic acid is opened up and the latter can soon be detected in the urine. As tyrosine is a precursor for melanin it is found that phenylketon-uriacs are usually albino

able in their blood is significantly greater than in normal individuals. PKU, for reasons we shall see below, is hardly present at all in black populations.

The transformation of phe to tyr is, of course, particularly important in catecholamineric neurons (see Chapter 15). The metabolic defect, however, is believed to have a general affect throughout the brain. As tyrosine is a starting point in the synthesis of the pigment **melanin** it is clear that pigmentation will be affected. Phenylketonuriacs consequently tend to be flaxen-haired and blue-eyed. This relationship between the PKU lesion and pigmentation explains its vanishingly small representation amongst black populations.

It must not be supposed, however, that the neurological consequences of PKU are due to deficiencies in catecholaminergic or indoleaminergic transmitter systems. Such deficiencies, of course, occur but the neurological defect—profound mental retardation—is due to the accumulation of phenylpyruvate in the brain. This seems to have a number of metabolic effects, which include interference with **mitochondrial oxidation, DOPA decarboxylase** and **5-HT decarboxylase**. At the anatomical level it can be shown that **myelination** is defective in the brains of phenylketonurics.

Fortunately treatment of the condition is routine, provided an early diagnosis (before 6 months of age) has been made.

Restriction of dietary phenylalanine has proved effective. Some phenylalanine must, of course, be allowed as it is an essential amino acid. The restricted diet can be discontinued when the child reaches an age of 4–10 years. The age range for discontinuation is due to the fact that there seem to be a number of varieties of PKU. But once the brain's development has passed beyond the 'sensitive period' elevated levels of phenylalanine are no longer harmful.

19.2 HUNTINGDON'S DISEASE (= CHOREA) (HD)

Huntingdon's disease (= Huntingdon's chorea) is one of a group of disorders of the basal ganglia which lead to jerky, rapid involuntary movements. The word chorea is, indeed, derived from a Greek root meaning 'dance' and an earlier name for the condition was 'St Vitus' dance'. It has been found that in many cases agents such as L-dopa aggravate the symptoms whilst drugs which block dopaminergic synapses, for instance haloperidol, or inhibit dopamine synthesis, for example reserpine, are able to reduce the symptoms. It seems, therefore, that the symptoms of HD are the consequence of an excess of dopamine. We shall see in Section 19.4 that Parkinsonism is, in contrast, due to lack of dopamine. The choreas are thus often regarded as **inverse Parkinsonisms**.

Huntingdon's disease is one of the most tragic of this group of disorders. It is tragic because it is **inherited**. It is doubly tragic as its clinical onset is usually during the fourth or fifth decade of life. The other choreas are usually associated with the degenerations of old age in the seventh and eighth decades. Finally it is triply tragic as it usually only shows itself when a family has been started. The sufferer may thus have unwittingly passed on this inexorable and incurable disease to his/her own sons and daughters.

Huntingdon's disease normally starts in a very small way as a facial twitch but this gradually spreads to all parts of the body. Speech and walking gradually become more difficult and then impossible. Ultimately loss of memory, hallucinations, delusions, disorientations, disorders of mood and emotion make the sufferer's life intolerable. Death normally intervenes about 15 years after the onset of the first symptoms.

In recent years some progress has been made in determining the genetic basis of the disease. It affects 5–10 people in every 100 000 and is inherited as an autosomal dominant. But because of its late onset it has proved very difficult to locate the gene. Moreover as the primary biochemical defect is as yet unknown it has not been possible to 'fish' for the gene with synthetic oligonucleotide probes.

However, another technique has become available. This depends on the finding that human DNA is highly polymorphic. Indeed it has been calculated that the human haploid genome contains one variant (polymorphism) for every 100 base pairs. Many of these variant sequences will fall at the cleavage sites of one or other of the 200+ different restriction endonucleases. In consequence these polymorphisms will reveal themselves as differences in the lengths of the resultant restriction fragments. This is shown in Figure 19.2.

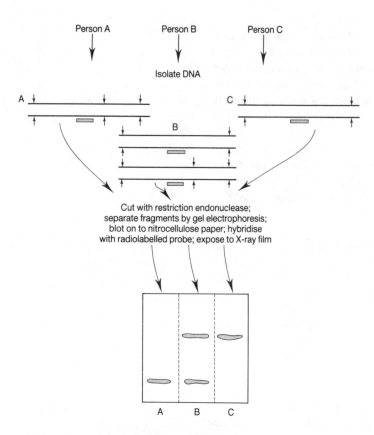

Cut with restriction endonuclease; separate fragments by gel electrophoresis; blot on to nitrocellulose paper; hybridise with radiolabelled probe; expose to X-ray film

Figure 19.2 Detection of DNA polymorphisms in the human genome. In this example it is supposed that DNA is isolated from three individuals. Person C possesses a mutant DNA lacking a restriction site; person A is normal; person B is heterozygous: one chromosome possesses the restriction site, the other does not. Restriction sites are represented by arrows. The DNA is exposed to the restriction enzyme, which cuts it at the arrowed sites. The different sized fragments are separated by gel electrophoresis. A radiolabelled probe is made from a clone of the critical region (shown by stippled rectangle) and hybridised with the blot on the nitrocellulose paper. The position of the gene under investigation can thus be narrowed down to a manageable fragment of the genome. For further explanation see text. (After Shows, Sagaguchi and Naylor, 1983, in *Advances in Human Genetics*, **12**, New York: Plenum Press, Chapter 5.)

The different restriction fragment lengths shown in Figure 19.2 are called **restriction fragment length polymorphisms (RFLPs)**. They are inherited in a Mendelian fashion. If an RFLP can be shown to be inherited in the same way as the gene under investigation—in this case the putative gene for HD—then the location of the latter can be determined. This was achieved for HD by Gusella and co-workers in 1983. The HD gene was mapped to the short arm of chromosome 4.

This does not mean to say that the gene itself has been found—only that it is linked to a particular RFLP. The situation is, moreover, complicated by the finding that the RFLP exists in a number of different varieties—'haplotypes'. Nevertheless the application of recombinant DNA techniques is opening up possibilities of detecting the HD gene itself with all that that entails for understanding, treatment and, ultimately, cure.

19.3 DEPRESSION

The cases considered so far in this chapter have been fairly clearcut instances of so-called 'upward' causation. A defect in metabolism is magnified up through the intricate pathways of the brain to affect the whole. But, of course, as we noted in the introduction to this chapter this is not always the case. In normal life mood does not change **because** of random variations in the brain's chemical base but usually because of changes in the circumstances of our everyday life. In other words in normal life causation often starts at the 'top' and works 'downwards'. It is important to recognise that this is the case. Too exclusive a concentration on upward causation, from molecule to man, leads to the absurdity of extreme 'reductionism': that we are 'nothing but' molecules.

One of the most interesting cases of the complex interaction between upward and downward causation is provided by the linkage between stress, anxiety and depression (= affective disorder). This topic has engendered a vast literature spanning the subject areas of psychiatry, neuroanatomy and neuropharmacology. Before embarking on this subject, however, we need to make some important distinctions. First we need to separate **endogenous** from **exogenous** or **reactive** depression. Both may involve the same neurochemical mechanisms but clearly the endogenous type is less dependent upon environmental triggering. Second, within each category of the foregoing classification, it is important to distinguish between '**monopolar**' and '**bipolar**' affective disorder. The first condition is commonly known simply as major depression and the second as manic-depression.

Endogenous depression. Endogenous depressions seem to afflict the sufferer without any obvious cause in his or her external circumstances. Frequently (by no means always) they are of the '**bipolar**' or '**manic-depressive**' type. The mood oscillates between extreme elation and extreme depression. The depression is often so deep that suicide is attempted.

There is evidence that bipolar depression has a genetic basis. One study involved the **Old Order Amish** society of Pennsylvania. This very tightly-knit society has strict rules of inbreeding so that the gene pool is effectively closed. Most members of the society are equable and well balanced. But every so often manic-depressives appear—often ending in suicide. Because the society is so closely knit the family trees can be examined in detail. It can be shown that the trait is inherited as if it were determined by an autosomal dominant gene. The penetrance, however, is only 63%. In other words an individual inheriting the gene only has a 63% chance of expressing it, i.e. of suffering bipolar depression.

We noted in Section 19.2 how recombinant DNA techniques had allowed the gene coding for Huntingdon's disease to be traced to chromosome 4. A similar technique has been used to search for the locus of the gene responsible for endogenous depression in the Old Order Amish people. The RFLP markers indicated that the gene was located on chromosome 11. However, similar techniques applied to other populations (three Icelandic and three North American families) did not home in on the same locus. It is likely, therefore, that more than one gene is responsible. Yet another study suggests that a third gene for the condition is located on the X chromosome. This would be consistent with the finding (noted below) that twice as many women as men suffer monopolar depression.

The implication that three (or perhaps more) genes are involved in affective disorder need not surprise us. We have still no idea at all how the defective gene or genes exert their catastrophic effects. We shall see below that the biochemical causation of depressions is thought to lie in imbalances of a 'cocktail' of neurotransmitters. It is likely that the defective genes are responsible for one or another of the many enzymes and co-enzymes in the synthesis and degradation of these neuro-transmitters. In this regard it is suggestive to find that the segment of chromosome 11 marked in the Old Order Amish study is close to the gene for **tyrosine hydroxylase (TH)**. We shall see below that the catecholamines are deeply implicated in the pharma-cology of depression. TH, it will be recalled from Chapter 15, is a rate-limiting enzyme in the synthesis of these transmitters.

Exogenous depression. Exogenous depression again may be either monopolar (i.e. 'major depression') or bipolar (i.e. 'manic-depression'). It should not be thought, however, that the symptoms and symptom-patterns are at all clear-cut. They have, in fact, been long known to constitute 'an extraordinarily heterogeneous syndrome'. It is interesting to note, however, that major studies in the United States have shown that whereas male and female Americans suffer bipolar depression in about equal numbers, twice as many females as males suffer monopolar depression.

Exogenous depressions are customarily associated with major events in the patient's socio-cultural environment: bereavement, divorce, redundancy, post-natal, post-menopausal, etc. All these events are more or less 'stressful'. Obviously what is stressful to one individual may not be stressful to another. Stress, however (to use the physicist's definition), produces 'strain'. This strain may also take many forms. But if the stress is long continued the strain very frequently takes the form of anxiety and/or depression.

Animal experimentation can to some extent mimic the human experience. If an animal is subjected to noxious but escapable stimuli it reacts vigorously and makes its escape. If it is subjected to the same stimuli in a situation from which there is no escape it ultimately becomes lethargic and 'despairing'. We shall return to these animal experiments later when we have looked briefly at the underlying neurochemistry.

Neurochemistry of depression. There is little doubt that a neurotransmitter imbalance is associated with both types of endogenous and exogenous depression. Noradrenaline, dopamine, serotonin and acetylcholine are all probably implicated in one way or another. The evidence for this belief comes mainly from neuropharmacology.

Agents which deplete monoamines such as reserpine (see Chapter 15) tend to induce depressive illness whilst agents which

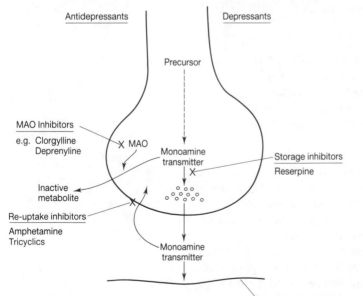

Figure 19.3 Neuropsychopharmacology of the monoaminergic synapse. Reference back to Chapter 15 shows that monoaminergic synapses can be influenced at three major points. The quantity of monoamine transmitter at the synapse can be increased by inhibiting the breakdown enzyme, MAO, or by inhibiting the re-uptake system. Conversely the concentration of the transmitter may be reduced by interfering with the mechanism leading to the monamine becoming sequestered within synaptic vesicles. If this step is inhibited the resulting free monamine in the terminal is exposed to MAO

have the opposite effect, most importantly the MAO inhibitors (MAOIs) such as clorgyline and deprenyline, are antidepressants. The important tricyclic antidepressants (e.g. imipramine and amitryptiline) act by blocking re-uptake of monoamines from the synaptic cleft.

This evidence suggests that depression occurs when the subsynaptic membranes of monoaminergic synapses are exposed to insufficient concentrations of their accustomed neurotransmitter. Remember that many monoaminergic synapses are made 'en passant' and thus release their transmitter to influence comparatively large volumes of grey matter (see Figure 15.19).

Acetylcholine, on the other hand, tends to act in an opposite sense to the central monoamines. Most antidepressants seem to have an anticholinergic action; vice versa reserpine potentiates central cholinergic activity. This could further enhance the depression.

The suggestion is, therefore, that depression may result from an imbalance between central monoaminergic and cholinergic systems. It may also be supposed that the cycling of manic-depressive illness is due to first one and then the other system gaining the upper hand.

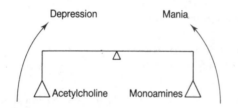

Figure 19.4 Neurotransmitter balance and depression. In manic-depressive illness first one neurochemical system then the other gains an ascendency

However, the situation is not quite as simple as this analysis suggests. The major difficulty is that whereas the drugs exert their effects within seconds or minutes the psychological depression may takes several weeks to lift. Perhaps this is not surprising for, as we have seen, the neuropharmacology is very far from being simple and straightforward.

It has been proposed, however, that the difference in time scales between the pharmacological action and the psychological consequence can be accounted for if the notion of denervation supersensitivity is invoked. It will be recalled that we introduced this idea in Section 15.5 when we discussed the withdrawal symptoms addicts experience when an exogenous opiate is removed. The same argument applies here, only the other way about. Just as decreased impulse traffic leads to a compensatory increase in synaptic sensitivity, so an overworked pathway is likely to adapt by **decreasing** the number of receptors in its synaptic membranes. It is found that most antidepressants '**down-regulate**' monoamine receptors after a few weeks of treatment. If these monoamine receptors are comparable to the α_2 receptors in the **presynaptic membranes** of adrenergic neurons then their 'down-regulation' would increase the quantity of monoamine in the synaptic cleft. For it will be remembered from Section 15.4 that these presynaptic receptors respond to high synaptic concentrations of norepinephrine by inhibiting the presynaptic terminal from releasing any more. The time period for this type of effect coincides with the lifting of the depression.

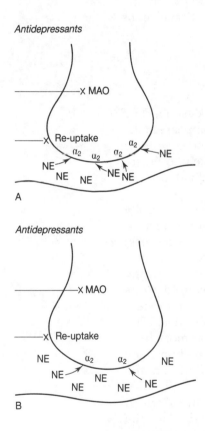

Figure 19.5 Antidepressants down-regulate presynaptic monoamine receptors. This schematic diagram shows (A) that in the presence of anti-depressants the concentration of norepinephrine (NE) in the synaptic gap increases and tends to saturate the α_2 presynaptic receptors. It will be recalled that these have an inhibitory effect on the presynaptic terminal. It is suggested (B) that over a period of time the number and/or sensitivity of the α_2 receptors decreases, thus reducing the inhibition on the presynaptic terminal. For further explanation in text

Stress and depression. We noted at the end of the section on 'exogenous depression' above that animal experimentation suggests that it is **inescapable** stress which leads to the symptoms of reactive depression. This would seem to be a good model for exogenous depression in humans. If stress is long continued and unavoidable, depression is often the outcome.

In animal experiments it appears that during the initial stress the monoaminergic synapses are overworked. The brain contains more than its usual quantity of monoamines. This readies the animal to react quickly and vigorously to its difficult situation. If the stress is continued, however, the monoaminergic synapses are depleted. Their output, so to speak, exceeds their synthetic capacity. They fall into comparative quiescence. But (it is speculated) this period of quietude has the inverse effect to that described above. If the α_2 adrenoreceptors respond to unusually large quantities of noradrenaline in the synaptic gap by a 'down regulation' then might they not respond to unusually small quantities by an 'up regulation'? If this is the case then when monoamines are once more released into the synaptic gap they will have more than their usual inhibitory feedback on the presynaptic terminal. Hence the onset and continuance of depression.

19.4 PARKINSON'S DISEASE (PD)

The symptoms of 'the shaking palsy' were first described by James Parkinson in 1817. The disease most usually appears in the sixth decade of life though it may occur earlier. If the symptoms have not appeared by the age of 70 they are unlikely to do so. It is relatively common, affecting some 200 individuals per 100 000.

The symptoms (like those of Huntingdon's disease) normally start in a small way. Often the initial sign is a tremor in a hand. But they progress to give uncontrollable shaking of (sometimes) all the limbs. The tremor is due to the alternate contraction of opposing muscle groups. In addition to tremor, patients normally suffer from rigidity about a joint (sometimes referred to as 'cogwheeling' where a joint under an applied force seems to jerk from one position to another) and, most difficult of all, an inability to initiate a voluntary movement (akinesia). Furthermore once a movement has been started it often shows 'festination'—the walk, for instance, becomes more and more a shuffling run, the steps becoming shorter and shorter.

Clearly all these symptoms and the many others which textbooks of neurology describe indicate a defect in the neurological control of movement. It has been known since the end of the last century that the control centres affected are deep in the brain stem and basal ganglia. The principal sites involved are the **substantia nigra** and the pathway from this nucleus to the **corpus striatum**.

It is now known that the nigro-striatal pathway is severely affected in Parkinsonism, up to 70% of nigral cells disappearing in severe cases. It is known, further, that this pathway is **dopaminergic**. Could the distressing symptoms be treated by supplying extra dopamine? Unfortunately it turns out that

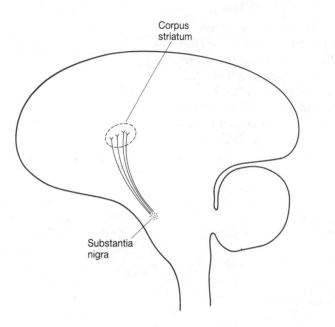

Corpus
striatum

Substantia
nigra

Figure 19.6 Nigro-striatal pathway. Schematic diagram to show the position of the substantia nigra in the midbrain and the course of the dopaminergic fibres to the corpus striatum in the telencephalon

dopamine does not pass the blood–brain barrier. On the other hand it is found that **L-dopa (laevodopa)** (a precursor, see Figure 15.17) does. Hence, in the late 1960s, a treatment became available. L-Dopa can be given orally. The effects on the symptoms are dramatic. In some cases it is only when the drug is removed that the patient appears anything other than normal.

However, the treatment *is* only of the symptoms. The underlying cause—the death of the nigral cells—remains untouched. Moreover as the disease progresses larger and larger doses of L-Dopa are required to control the symptoms. Furthermore unpleasant side effects commonly manifest themselves: nausea, anorexia, odd writhing movements, tachycardia.

What, then, causes the death of the nigral cells? Here one of the most remarkable instances of serendipity has provided a clue. The breakthrough happened in one of the most unlikely places— the Californian 'drug culture'. Addicts taking an illegally manufactured synthetic heroin developed severe neuropathological symptoms which strikingly resembled those shown in advanced states of Parkinson's disease. When samples of the synthetic heroin were analysed they were shown to contain a contaminant—**1-methyl-4-phenyl-1,2,3,6-tetrahydopyridine (MPTP)**. When tested on experimental animals (squirrel monkeys and mice) it was shown that MPTP induces symptoms which closely mimic the symptoms of human PD. Furthermore although there are some differences of detail (no Lewy bodies) the neuropathology of MPTP intoxication is remarkably similar to true PD—the selective elimination of nigral cells.

It was quickly shown that it is not MPTP itself which does the damage but its oxidation product **MPP⁺**. In the brain MPTP is oxidised by MAO B first to MPDP⁺ and this rearranges to form the stable metabolite MPP⁺. This oxidation appears to take place in the supporting astrocytes and the resultant MPP⁺ is carried into the nigral cells by their own dopamine uptake system. Alternatively, and in addition, the MPP⁺ may be bound by the pigment which has given the nigral cells their name. It is known that MPP⁺ is strongly bound by neuromelanin which is present in these cells.

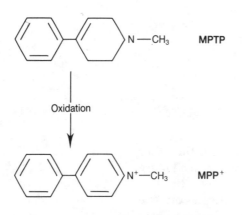

Figure 19.7 Oxidation of MPTP to MPP⁺

Is all this just a lucky accident (lucky for some, unlucky for others) or does it point to the cause of Parkinsonism? The jury is still out. But one very interesting observation has been made. This is the marked similarity of MPP⁺ to the herbicide **paraquat** (Figure 19.8).

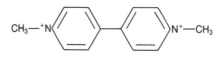

Figure 19.8   Paraquat

Could at least some Parkinsonism have an environmental cause? There is some evidence that this might indeed be the case. A survey in the province of Quebec showed a remarkably high correlation (0.967) between the incidence of the disease and the use of herbicides and pesticides. Paraquat is, of course, not the only pyridine compound in the environment—either as a pesticide or as a byproduct of the chemical industry. It has thus been further suggested that PD is a disease of industrialisation. Although cases of 'the shaking palsy' have been described as far back as Galen in the second century AD it has only become well known since the onset of the industrial revolution. The case against the environment is, however, not yet proven. Historical evidence is always open to criticism. There is also evidence for genetic and developmental defects which predispose towards PD.

Research over the next few years is likely to disentangle the environmental and genetic causes and, hopefully, point towards a means of curing sufferers and protecting those at risk. The MPTP work has, for example, suggested that antioxidants such as vitamin E might act as protectants. A very different approach also seems promising for the more distant future. This involves the replacement of degenerating nigral cells by transplantation of fresh dopaminergic cells into the brain. This has already been tried with some success in experimental animals, and there have also been some attempts with humans. In the case of experimental animals embryonic tissue has been used to transplant into brains made Parkinsonian by MPTP. The grafts have 'taken' and in some cases the dopamine metabolites have recovered to within 5% of pre-MPTP levels. In the case of humans tissue has been taken from the patient's own adrenal medulla, a good source of dopaminergic cells, and surgically implanted into the brain. More recently disaggregated cells from the brains of aborted human fetuses have been introduced into the brains of Parkinsonian patients. It is too early to be sure how effective these treatments will turn out to be. It is likely to be many years before they become routine. Clearly they raise important ethical questions. The human shipwreck of the Parkinsonian condition suggests, however, that carefully controlled work should continue.

19.5 ALZHEIMER'S DISEASE (AD)

The first description of AD was given by Alois Alzheimer in 1907. His words are worth quoting:

> A woman of 51 years old, showed jealousy towards her husband as the first noticeable sign of the disease. Soon a rapidly increasing loss of memory could be noticed. She could not find her way around in her own apartment. She carried objects back and forth and hid them. At times she would think that someone wanted to kill her and would begin shrieking loudly.
> In the Institution her entire behaviour bore the stamp of utter perplexity. She was totally disorientated to time and place. Occasionally she stated she could not understand and did not know her way around. At times she greeted the doctor like a visitor, and excused herself for not having finished her work; at other times she shrieked loudly that he wanted to cut her, or she repulsed him with indignation,

saying that she feared something against her chastity. Periodically she was totally delirious, dragged her bedding around, called her husband and her daughter, and seemed to have auditory hallucinations. Frequently, she shrieked with a dreadful voice for many hours...

Her ability to remember was severely disturbed. If one pointed to objects, she named most of them correctly, but immediately afterwards she would forget everything. When reading she went from one line to another, reading the letters or reading with a senseless emphasis... When talking she used perplexing phrases and some periphrastic expressions (milk-pourer instead of cup). Sometimes one noticed her getting stuck. Some questions she obviously did not understand. She seemed no longer to understand the use of some objects...

The generalised dementia progressed. After 4½ years of the disease death occurred. At the end the patient was completely stuporous; she lay in her bed with ther legs drawn up under her, and in spite of all precautions she acquired decubitus ulcers.

Alzheimer's disease is without doubt one of the most terrible afflictions of late-middle age to old age. It has often (on the analogy of heart failure) been termed 'brain failure'. Others have referred to it as amentia—death of the mind. At present there is nothing that can be done. The disease must run its course. It is debatable whether the patient or his/her carers suffer most: for both it is a near intolerable condition.

In the West the demographic trends point to an increasingly elderly population. In 1950 there were about 214 million people older than 60 world-wide; in 2025 there will be 1000 million. Alzheimer's disease shows a penetrance of about 5% in those over 65. In the mid-1980s in the US alone some $25 billion were spent per year on the institutional care of demented patients. These statistics show the immensity of the problem. But there is hope. Advances at the molecular level are beginning to clarify the aetiology. If the causation can be understood relief, protection and even cure may become possible.

First of all it should be said that diagnosis is a problem. The condition rarely presents itself in quite so clear-cut a way as Alzheimer described above. There are often confounding factors. Frequently there is some Parkinsonism. Often there is (quite understandably) exogenous depression. In most cases the only certain diagnosis is post-mortem. Here the classical signs are **neurofibrillary tangles (NFTs)** in cortical pyramidal cells and elsewhere; areas of degenerating neurites known as **plaques**; single electron-dense granules within neuronal perikarya termed **granulovacuolar degeneration (GVD)**; rod-shaped eosinophilic inclusions known as **Hirano bodies**. In addition the gross appearance of the brain shows considerable atrophy and an enlargement and coarsening of the sulci.

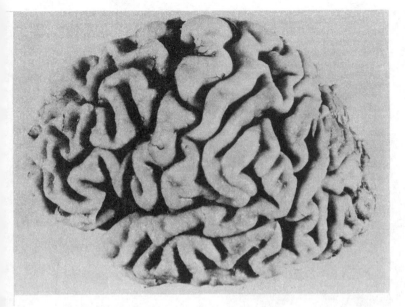

Figure 19.9 Lateral view of the cerebrum of a patient with Alzheimer's disease. Note the greatly enlarged sulci. (From Terry in Davis and Robertson, 1985, *Textbook of Neuropathology* , Baltimore: Williams & Wilkins; with permission.)

The condition appears to be restricted to humans and perhaps the higher primates. This makes it difficult to study. There are no good animal models. There are, however, a number of analogies, and a number of different causes have been suggested.

Is it, like HD, an **inherited** condition? Or, like PD, can we suggest an **environmental cause**? Alternatively could it be due to an **infective agent**? Or again, like PD, is it due to the degeneration of a particular population of neurons, in this case the **cholinergic** neurons in Meynert's and other brain stem nuclei? Or, finally, could there be some breakdown of the blood – brain barrier and some **autoimmune** reaction occurring? It will probably turn out that the cause is multifactorial. It is likely that more than one of the above mechanisms is at work and, quite probably, some additonal ones we have not thought of. Indeed it is probable that there is more than one variety of the disease itself.

Recently, however, significant progress has been made at the molecular level. It was indicated above that one of the consistent histological signs of AD is an accumulation of patches of degenerating axon terminals and dendritic branches (neurites)— the so-called plaques. These occur in large numbers in the cerebral cortex, in the hippocampus and elsewhere. They also occur in smaller numbers in the brains of all aged humans. At the centre of these plaques there is usually a core of **amyloid**.

Another, and related, histological feature of AD is, as we have already noted, the presence of neurofibrillary tangles (NFTs) in the cell bodies and processes of many neurons. Electron microscopical examination of these NFTs shows them to consist largely

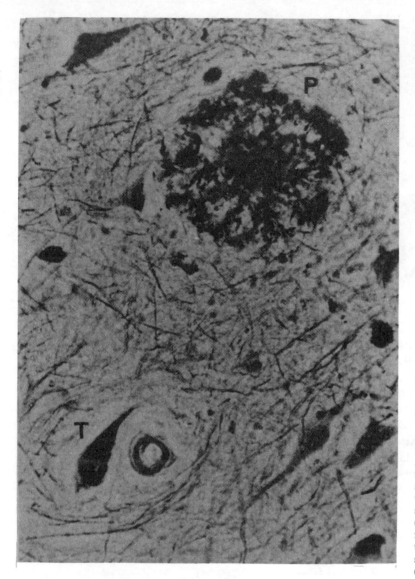

Figure 19.10 Alzheimer plaque. The large dark circular object (P) at the top right-hand corner is an Alzheimer plaque. It consists of degenerating nerve processes and often has a central core of amyloid. The black triangular objects (T) are nerve cell bodies filled with neurofibrillary tangles (NFTs). Some unaffected neurons can also be seen. The preparation is from the hippocampus of an Alzheimer patient and has been stained with a silver stain. (From Wischik and Crowther, 1986, *British Medical Bulletin*, **42**, 51–56; with permission.)

Figure 19.11   Paired helical filaments. (A) EM of a thin section of a nerve cell body at ×10 000. Numerous neurofibrils can be seen weaving through the cytoplasm. The black objects are lipofuchsin granules and the white spaces are vacuoles. The vacuoles often contain a small densely staining body (only the remnants of this can be seen in the figure) and this 'granulovacuolar degeneration' is also diagnostic of Alzheimer's disease. (B) The neurofibrils can be extracted from Alzheimer neurons and viewed in isolation. This negative contrast EM shows that they consist of two strands twisted around each other forming the so-called 'paired helical filaments' (PHFs). Scale bar 100 nm. (C) Computer modelling of the PHFs of (B) show that the best fit is achieved if two strap-like strands are twisted around each other. (D) Each 'strap' of the PHF is believed to consist of three spherical subunits. When these are twisted around each other they yield the image shown in (C). ((A) Courtesy Dr D.J. Selkoe; (B) from Wischik and Crowther, 1986, *British Medical Bulletin*, **42**, 51–56; with permission; (C) and (D) reproduced from Wischik *et al.*, 1985, *The Journal of Cell Biology*, **100**, 1905–1912, by copyright permission of the Rockefeller University Press.) →

of pairs of 10 nm filaments twisted around each other with a periodicity of 80 nm. These helices of old age are called **paired helical filaments (PHFs)**.

Not only are NFTs found within neurons but they are also much in evidence in the plaques. It has been suggested that the amyloid protein at the centre of plaques is identical (though different in three-dimensional conformation) to the protein of NFTs. However, careful immunological studies suggest that this is not the case and that the original identifications were due to contamination of NFTs with amyloid.

A

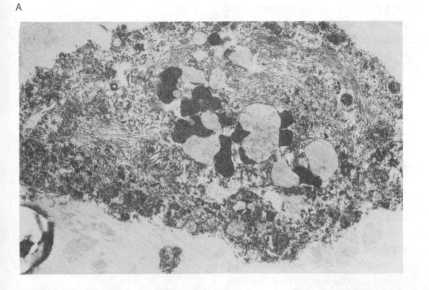

B

C

D

The amyloid protein—called the **A4 protein**—has been isolated and sequenced. It consists of 42–43 amino acid residues and is closely similar (if not identical) to an amyloid protein obtained from the cerebral blood vessels of AD and Down's syndrome patients. The A4 protein appears to be present in the β-pleated sheet form (see Chapter 2) in plaque centres.

Using the recombinant DNA techniques described in Chapter 5 an oligonucleotide probe complementary to a seven-residue sequence of the A4 protein was prepared. This was used to screen a cDNA 'library' constructed from the total mRNA from the cerebral cortex of a 5-month aborted human fetus. The probe picked out a large cDNA stretch of some 3353 base pairs. This cDNA, without its leader and tail sequences, codes for a 695-residue protein with a molecular weight of about 79 kDa.

The 42/43 amino acid A4 protein (the cDNA sequence for which was recognised by the oligonucleotide probe) is found incorporated in the 695 residue protein towards the C-terminal end (residues 597–638 inclusive). Hydrophobic analysis of the the 695 residue protein shows that it probably contains a membrane-spanning segment from residue 625 to 648. The C-terminal is in the cytoplasmic domain, the lengthy N-terminal sequence in the extracellular domain. The A4 protein, on this analysis, is thus half in and half out of the membrane—half in and half out of the extracellular domain.

Computer searches of databases in which the amino acid sequences of proteins are stored has not revealed any similar sequences. The A4 precursor protein thus seems to be a **new** membrane-spanning protein. Its extracellular domain contains two potential *N*-glycosylation sites and other features which suggest that it may be a receptor protein.

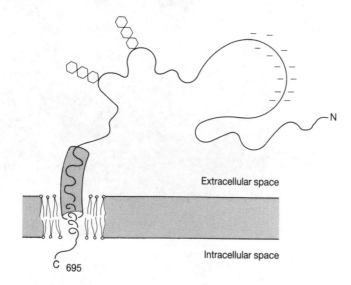

Figure 19.12   Location of the A4 protein and the A4 precursor protein in a neuronal membrane. The A4 (amyloid) protein is shown (enclosed in a cylinder) half in and half out of the membrane. The major part of the 695-residue amyloid-precursor protein is located in the extracellular space. As shown it possess two *N*-glycosylation sites and a negatively charged domain (45% asp and glu). For further explanation see text. (After Kang *et al.*, 1987, *Nature*, **325**, 733–736.)

The first tentative conclusion from this detailed molecular biology is that in AD the A4 precursor protein is disrupted, perhaps because its surrounding membrane disintegrates, or because the protein itself is attacked, and the A4 fragment is released to stack up in the β-sheet conformation of amyloid.

Further research has shown that the A4 precursor protein comes in at least three different varieties. This is due to the presence of two additional exons in its gene: the so-called Alzheimer disease amyloid polypeptide (AD-AP) gene. Variable splicing of the primary transcript gives three different mRNAs, which vary from tissue to tissue. Of particular interest is the finding that in one case a sequence of 56 residues interpolated at residue 289 of the A4 precursor protein is strongly homologous to the active sites of certain well-known protease inhibitors—the protease nexins. It is known that these inhibitors (by blocking protease activity) promote outgrowth of neurites from neurons. It is thus speculated that the break-up of the A4 precursor protein during the formation of a plaque deposits this domain in the plaque core. This would then account for the common observation that such cores are frequently invaded by neurites from the surrounding tissue.

The next important finding from the molecular biology laboratories is that the AD-AP gene is located on chromosome 21. Chromosome 21, it will be recalled, is the chromosome triplicated in Down's syndrome (trisomy 21). Individuals suffering from Down's syndrome thus have three copies of the AD-AP gene. It has long been known that practically all individuals afflicted with Down's syndrome seem to show the symptoms of AD if they live beyond the age of about 40. The AD-AP gene is not, however, located on the section of chromosome 21 which is responsible for Down's syndrome.

The idea that AD has a hereditary dimension thus seems to have some basis in fact. But it is likely that there is an environmental factor at work also. It may be that the AD-AP gene product reacts with some other factor or factors within the brain to initiate plaque formation.

One of the factors which has often been implicated is **aluminium**. Electron probe microanalysis and nuclear magnetic resonance (NMR) have shown aluminosilicate deposits in the centres of Alzheimer plaques. Natives of Guam and some of the other islands of the western Pacific who show a type of early-onset dementia resembling AD and/or PD can be shown to live in areas where aluminium concentrations in the soil are unusually high and calcium and magnesium levels unusually low. But whether aluminium deposits in AD plaques is a cause or a consequence of plaque formation remains very much an open question.

In conclusion we can perhaps begin to draw the evidence together into a preliminary hypothesis. This would suggest that the primary lesion is the disruption of the amyloid precursor protein either by increased dosage, or by some environmental stress (perhaps aluminium, perhaps the hard knocks which boxers endure and which induces the somewhat similar condition of **dementia pugilistica**, perhaps just the wear and tear of a long life). Clearly if there is more precursor-protein present then the quantity of amyloid released when it is disrupted will be greater. Hence the genetic dimension. The break up of the precursor-protein leads (we may suppose) to the disintegration of the neuronal membrane in which it is embedded (or, conceivably, the sequence is the other way about). This results in the formation of a plaque.

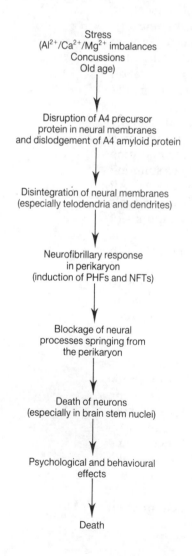

Stress
($Al^{2+}/Ca^{2+}/Mg^{2+}$ imbalances
Concussions
Old age)

Disruption of A4 precursor
protein in neural membranes
and dislodgement of A4 amyloid protein

Disintegration of neural membranes
(especially telodendria and dendrites)

Neurofibrillary response
in perikaryon
(induction of PHFs and NFTs)

Blockage of neural
processes springing from
the perikaryon

Death of neurons
(especially in brain stem nuclei)

Psychological and behavioural
effects

Death

Figure 19.13 A theory of Alzheimer's disease. The sequence of events shown in the figure starts with some form of stress. This does not side-line genetics. As explained in the text the quantity of A4 precursor protein present in neural membranes may well be under genetic control. A dosage effect may lead to more A4 precursor being present in some individuals than others and hence render them more susceptible to the initial plaque-forming event in the cascade

The formation of a plaque (a region of necrotic neurites) has very significant consequences. The most important of these may be the induction of the neurofibrillary change which we observe as the PHFs of NFTs. We examined the filamentous and micro-tubular components of axons and dendrites in Chapter 14. We noted how central they were in the life of the neuron. If axoplasmic (and dendroplasmic) transport is blocked the perikaryon would be unable to obtain its trophic factors (by retrograde transport) or send out the necessary materials to axon and dendrite terminals by anterograde transport. The cell would soon die.

The loss of the cell bodies of the cholinergic neurons in Meynert's and other brain stem nuclei is one of the recognised signs of AD. It is known that the fibre projections from cholinergic nuclei are directed to wide areas of the cortex and especially the hippocampus. The latter, we have noted, is one of the major regions of plaque development. It is also the case that choline acetyl transferase (CAT), the major marker of cholinergic terminals, is dramatically lost from the hippocampi of AD patients. At the psychological plane we recall that there is good reason to believe that the hippocampus is deeply involved in short term memory (Chapter 18). Short-term memory is dramatically destroyed in AD. It also, of course, proverbially tends to weaken in all elderly brains.

The above analysis shows how unified neurobiology is becoming. In order to achieve an understanding of the human catastrophe of Alzheimer's disease we need to bring together data from a large percentage of all the various sub-disciplines into which the subject has fragmented. Underpinning all these sub-disciplines is our growing insight at the molecular level. This therefore forms a suitable place to finish this book.

We started this chapter with Shakespeare. Let us complete it by quoting his famous lines describing man's seventh age:

> Last scene of all,
> That ends this strange eventful history,
> Is second childishness, and mere oblivion,
> Sans teeth, sans eyes, sans taste, sans everything.

Our hope is that molecular neurobiology may make this seventh age (and indeed the ills of the other six) less burdensome.

Appendix 1
Units

1. SI PREFIXES AND MULTIPLICATION FACTORS

Multiplication factor		Prefix	Symbol
1 000 000 000 000	$= 10^{12}$	tera	T
1 000 000 000	$= 10^{9}$	giga	G
1 000 000	$= 10^{6}$	mega	M
1 000	$= 10^{3}$	kilo	k
100	$= 10^{2}$	hecto	h
10	$= 10^{1}$	deca	da
0.1	$= 10^{-1}$	deci	d
0.01	$= 10^{-2}$	centi	c
0.001	$= 10^{-3}$	milli	m
0.000 001	$= 10^{-6}$	micro	μ
0.000 000 001	$= 10^{-9}$	nano	n
0.000 000 000 001	$= 10^{-12}$	pico	p
0.000 000 000 000 001	$= 10^{-15}$	femto	f
0.000 000 000 000 000 001	$= 10^{-18}$	atto	a

2. SI UNITS

A (ampere): SI unit of current—the constant current which, if maintained in each of two infinitely long straight parallel wires of negligible cross sectional area placed in a vacuum, 1 metre apart, would produce between the wires a force of 2×10^{-7} newtons per metre length.

Bq (Becquerel): SI unit of radioactivity—one nuclear transformation per second. 1 Bq $= 2.7 \times 10^{-11}$ Ci (q.v.).

C (coulomb): SI unit of electrical charge—the quantity of electricity transported per second by a current of 1 ampere.

Da (dalton): unit of atomic mass—defined as 1/12 the mass of $^{12}_{6}C$.

F (farad): the SI unit of capacitance—the capacitance of a capacitor between whose plates a potential of 1 V appears when a charge of 1 C is held.

F (faraday): 9.649×10^4 C mol^{-1}.

J (joule): SI unit of energy (= 0.24 cal).

M (mole): SI unit of substance—defined as the same number of entities as there are in 0.012 kg of carbon isotope $^{12}_{6}C$ (see N_A, Avogadro's number).

m (metre): SI standard of length.

N_A (Avogadro's number): the number of entities in a mole = 6.022×10^{23}.

R (gas constant): 8.314 J K^{-1} mol^{-1} (1.987 cal K^{-1} mol^{-1}).

S (siemens): SI unit of conductance (= a reciprocal ohm (i.e. 1/ohm)). Defined as the electrical conductance between two points of a conductor when a constant potential difference of 1 V applied between these points produces a current of 1 A in the conductor.

s (second): SI standard of time.

V (volt): unit of potential difference between two points—the volt is defined as the potential difference between two points on a conductor when a constant current of 1 A leads to a power dissipation of 1 W between those points.

3. OTHER UNITS

Å (Angstrom): 10^{-10} m.

a (annum): year.

bp (base pair): nucleotide base pair (measure of the length of a nucleic acid or polynucleotide).

cal (calorie): the quantity of heat required to raise 1 g of water from 14.5 °C to 15.5 °C.

Ci (curie): unit of radioactivity—1 Ci = 3.7×10^{10} nuclear transformations per second.

S (svedberg): sedimentation coefficient in a centrifugal field of force.

Appendix 2
Data

BIOPHYSICS OF NEURONS

Datum	Squid (giant axon)	Frog (node)	Frog (myelin)	Cat (spinal motor neuron)
R_i	30 Ω cm	110 cm		70 Ω cm
R_m	1 $\times$ 103 Ω cm^2	10–20 Ω cm^2	0.1 MΩ cm^2	2500 Ω cm^2
τ	1 ms			5 ms
C_m	1 μF cm^{-2}	3–7 μF cm^{-2}	0.004 μF cm^{-2}	2 μF cm^{-2}

where C_m is the capacitance of unit area of membrane, R_i is the resistance of unit volume of cytoplasm, R_m is the resistance of unit area of membrane, and τ is the membrane time constant.

Rall, W. (1977) in *Handbook of Physiology*, Section 1: The Nervous System, Vol. 1, Cellular Biology of Neurons, Part 1, ed. by J.M.Brookhart, V.B.Mountcastle, E.R.Kandel, and S.R.Geiger, Bethseda: American Physiological Society, pp. 39–97.

GENOMES

E.coli: 5 $\times$ 10^6 bp; 3–4 $\times$ 10^3 genes.
Drosophila: 1.65 $\times$ 10^8 bp; 1–2 $\times$ 10^5 genes.
Homo sapiens: 3 $\times$ 10^9 bp; 2–20 $\times$ 10^5 genes.

MOLECULAR WEIGHTS

Molecule	Molecular weight (Da)
Amino acid (average)	100
Nucleotide pair (average)	600
Rhodopsin	40 000

Molecule	Molecular weight (Da)
Haemoglobin	68 000
Amyloid precursor	79 000
Glycine receptor (GlyR)	93 000
Muscarinic acetylcholine receptor (mAChR)	51 400
Nicotinic acetylcholine receptor (nAChR)	268 000
Potassium channel (*Drosophila*)	70 200
Sodium channel (glycosylated)	260 000
$Na^+ + K^+$ pump (α-subunit)	100 000

DENSITIES OF CHANNELS AND RECEPTORS

	$(\mu m^2$ membrane$)^{-1}$
$Na^+ + K^+$ pump (rabbit vagus)[a]	750
$Na^+ + K^+$ pump (inner segment of rod cell)[b]	3 400
Ca^{2+} pump (rabbit SR)[c]	8 700
nAChR (motor endplate)[c]	10 000
Na^+ channels (squid giant axon)[c]	300
Na^+ channels (frog node of Ranvier)[c]	3 000
Na^+ channels (rat node of Ranvier)[c]	2 100
Na^+ channels (rabbit unmyelinated vagus nerve)[c]	110
Na^+ channels (frog twitch muscle)[c]	650
K^+ channels (squid axon)[a]	70

Data: [a] K.H.Pfenninger (1978) *Annual Review of Neuroscience*, **1**, 455–471; [b] W.Almers and C.Stirling (1984) *Journal of Membrane Biology*, **77**, 169–186; [c] B.Hille (1984) *Ionic channels in Excitable Membranes*, Sinauer. For further discussion see D.C.Chang *et al.*, eds (1983), *Structure and Function of Excitable Cells*, New York: Plenum. It should be noted that as these data have been assembled from different sources which have used different counting techniques the results are not strictly comparable.

NEURONS

Sizes

Smallest perikarya: d = c. 5 μm (cerebellar granule cells).[a]
Largest perikarya: d = c. 100 μm (cerebral Betz cells). Mauthner
  cells and some reticular formation cells are also extremely large.
  In the invertebrates cells in the visceral ganglia of *Aplysia* may
  be up to 1000 μm in diameter.[a]
A large dorsal root ganglion cell may be 120 μm in diameter with
  an axon 12 μm in diameter and up to 1 m in length. The
  perikaryon of such a cell may have a volume of 864 000 μm^3
  and a surface area of 43 200 μm^2 (assuming sphericity). Its
  axon, however, can be calculated to have a volume of 108 M
  μm^3 and a total surface area of 36 M μm^2.[a]
Extent of dendritic arborisations [b]: pyramidal cells (mouse
  cortex), c. 3200 μm; stellate cells (mouse cortex), c. 5000 μm.
Pyramidal dendrites develop about two spines per micrometre.[b]

Data: [a] W.Rall (1977), *Ibid.*; [b] V. Braitenberg (1978), 'Cortical
architectonics: general and areal' in *Architectonics of the Cerebral
Cortex*, ed. by M.A.B.Brazier and H.Petsche, New York: Raven
Press.

Numbers

Numbers of neurons per cubic millimetre of cerebral cortex

	Visual cortex	Motor cortex
Mouse	100 000	60 000
Rat	47 000	25 000
Rabbit	42 000	26 000
Monkey (macaque)	115 000	18 000
Human	50 000	

Neuronal densities decrease as brain size increases; the Indian
elephant, for instance, only musters about 7000 neurons per cubic
millimetre of cortex.

Numbers of synapses per cubic millimetre of cerebral cortex

	Visual cortex	Motor cortex
Mouse	6.6×10^8	8.5×10^8
Monkey (macaque)	6.2×10^8	9.6×10^8

Synapses per neuron

	Visual cortex	Motor cortex
Mouse	7000	13 000
Monkey	5600	60 000

Well over 100 000 synaptic contacts are made on typical cerebellar Purkinje cells. Axon densities in the mouse have been computed at 1 to 2×10^6 mm axon per cubic millimetre of cerebral cortex.

Data from B.G.Cragg (1967), 'The density of synapses and neurones in the motor and visual areas of the cerebral cortex', *Journal of Anatomy*, **101**, 639–654; S.M.Blinkov and I.I.Glezer (1968), *The Human Brain in Figures and Tables*, New York: Plenum Press; V.Braitenberg (1978), *Ibid*.

Acronyms and abbreviations

A: adenine

α-BuTX: α-bungarotoxin

α-TX: α-toxin—a neurotoxin which attaches to the α-subunit of nAChR

Ac: acetyl

ACh: acetylcholine

AChE: acetylcholinesterase

AChR: acetylcholine receptor

ACTH: adrenocorticotrophic hormone

AD: Alzheimer's disease

AD-AP: Alzheimer's disease amyloid polypeptide

ADP: adenosine diphosphate

AHP: afterhyperpolarisation

AMP: adenosine monophosphate

AMPT: α-methyl-p-tyrosine

ATP: adenosine triphosphate

AVEC: Allen enhanced video contrast (microscopy)

β-AR: β-adrenergic receptor

BBB: blood–brain barrier

BH$_4$: tetrahydrobiopterin

BP: before present

bp: base pair (i.e. nucleotide base pair)

C: cytosine

CAM: cell adhesion molecule

cAMP: cyclic adenosine monophosphate

CAT: choline acetyltransferase

CCK: cholecystokinin

cDNA: complementary DNA

cGMP: cyclic guanosine monophosphate

CGRP: calcitonin-gene related peptide

CLIP: corticotropin-like intermediate lobe protein

COMT: catechol-o-methyl transferase

Con-A: concanavalin A

CR: conditioned response

CS: conditioned stimulus

Da: dalton—a unit of molecular mass defined as 1/12 the mass of $^{12}_{6}C$

D-AP5: D-2-amino-5-phosphonovalerate

DA: dopamine

DAG: diacylglycerol

ddNTP: dideoxynucleotide

DNA: deoxyribonucleic acid

DOPA: 3,4-dihydroxyphenylalanine

EAA: excitatory amino acid

EcoR1: much used restriction endonuclease derived from *E.coli*

ECS: electro-convulsive shock

EM: electron microscope

EPP: end-plate potential

EPSP: excitatory postsynaptic potential

ER: endoplasmic reticulum

G: guanine

GABA: γ-aminobutyric acid

GABA-T: GABA aminotransferase

GAD: glutamic acid decarboxylase

Gal: galactose

GDP: guanosine diphosphate

Glc: glucose

GlyR: glycine receptor

GMP: guanosine monophosphate

GTP: guanosine triphosphate

GVD: granulovacuolar degeneration

Hb: haemoglobin

HD: Huntingdon's disease

HIAA: hydroxyindoleacetic acid

hnRNA: heteronuclear RNA

I_{Ca}**:** calcium current

I_{KCa}**:** calcium-dependent potassium current

I_{K}**:** delayed potassium current

I_{KA}**:** early potassium current

I_{KM}**:** muscarinic potassium current

I_{KS}**:** serotonin-dependent potassium current

IP$_3$: inositol triphosphate

IF: intermediate filament or initiation factor (context will decide)

Ig: immunoglobulin

IPSP: inhibitory postsynaptic potential

IS: insertion sequence

ISI: interstimulus interval

L-AP4: L-2-amino-4-phosphonobutyrate

LSD: lysergic acid diethylamide

LTD: long-term depression

LTM: long-term memory

LTP: long-term potentiation

Ma: million years
mAChR: muscarinic acetylcholine receptor
MAO: monoamine oxidase
MAOI: monoamine oxidase inhibitor
MAP: microtubule accessory protein
Mb: myoglobin
MPP$^+$: 1-methyl-4-phenylpyridinium ion
MPTP: 1-methyl-4-biphenyl-1,2,3,6-tetrahydropyridine
M_r: molecular weight, relative molecular mass—the ratio of the
    mass of a molecule to 1/12 the mass of $^{12}_6$C
mRNA: messenger RNA
MS: multiple sclerosis
MSH: melanophore stimulating hormone
MT: microtubule
najaTX: neurotoxin derived from the cobra *Naja naja siamensis*
nAChR: nicotinic acetylcholine receptor
NAG: *n*-acetylglucosamine
N-CAM: neural cell adhesion molecule
Ng-CAM: neuron–glia cell adhesion molecule
NE: norepinephrine
NMDA: *n*-methyl-*d*-aspartate
NFT: neurofibrillary tangle
NGF: nerve growth factor
OHDA: hydroxydopamine
P_i: inorganic phosphate
PAGE: polyacrylamide gel electrophoresis
PCP: phencyclidine
PD: Parkinson's disease
PDE: phosphodiesterase
PGF: polypeptide growth factor
PHF: paired helical filament
POMC: pro-opiomelanocortin
PI: phosphatidyl inositol
PKC: protein kinase C
PKU: phenylketonuria
PP_i: inorganic pyrophosphate
PTP: post-tetanic potentiation
RA: retrograde amnesia
RER: rough endoplasmic reticulum
RF: receptive field
RFLP: restriction fragment length polymorphism
RNA: ribonucleic acid
rNTP: ribonucleotide triphosphate
rRNA: ribosomal RNA
SDAT: senile dementia of the Alzheimer type
SEM: scanning electron microscope
SI: Système Internationale d'Unités

SK: substance K
SP: substance P
SR: sarcoplasmic reticulum
STM: short term memory
T: thymine or transducin (context will decide)
T_m: the temperature at which the two strands in a double-stranded nucleic acid are 50% dissociated
TEA: tetraethylammonium chloride
TEM: transmission electron microscope
TH: tyrosine hydroxylase
Tn: transposon
tRNA: transfer RNA
TTX: tetrodotoxin
U: uracil
UCR: unconditioned reflex
UCS: unconditioned stimulus
VAS: vesicle attachment site
VIP: vasoactive intestinal peptide
V_m: resting potential across a membrane

Glossary

Aetiology: the cause of a disease.

Afferent: fibres conducting *toward* some region.

Afterhyperpolarisation: period during which an excitable cell's membrane is hyperpolarised in an action potential.

Agonist: drug which mimics a hormone or neurotransmitter, binding to the receptor and causing the normal response.

Allele: one of two or more alternative forms of a gene.

Amphipathic: applied to molecules (especially proteins) in which one part of the molecule is water-soluble and the other water-insoluble.

Anosmia: loss of olfactory sense.

Antagonist: drug which binds to the receptor of a hormone or neurotransmitter and does *not* induce the normal response.

Anterograde: movement from the perikaryon towards the terminal.

Antibody: a protein produced by the immune system in response to a foreign substance (usually a protein). It is synthesised in such a way that it reacts with the foreign substance (antigen, q.v.) which led to its synthesis and no other.

Antigen: any substance (usually a protein) capable of eliciting an immune response, i.e. the synthesis of a specific antibody (q.v.).

Anxiolytic agent: a drug such as valium (diazepam) which reduces anxiety.

Aphasia: loss of power to communicate in speech or writing.

Ataxia: lack of muscular co-ordination

Autonomic nervous system: that part of the peripheral nervous system which controls the 'automatic' activity of the body's systems, e.g. heart beat, blood pressure, movement of the alimentary tract, respiratory movements. It is divided into two sub-systems: the **sympathetic** and the **parasympathetic** systems. The sympathetic system is generally regarded as involved in response to emergencies ('fight and flight') and operates with noradrenaline; the parasympathetic system is involved in more quiescent, vegetative, functions and uses acetylcholine as a transmitter.

Avogadro's number (*N*): the number of particles in a mole or gram ion of substance, i.e. 6.023×10^{23}.

Axolemma: boundary membrane of an axon.

Axoneme: central core of a flagellum or cilium consisting of an outer ring of nine microtubular doublets and a central pair of microtubules.

Baroreceptor: pressure receptor.

Biotinylation: attachment of biotin to a molecule.

Bouton: expansion at the termination of an axon specialised for transmitter release.

Capsid: the proteinaceous coat of a virus.

Caudal: towards the posterior.

cDNA (complementary DNA): a stretch of DNA which faithfully copies a particular stretch of RNA.

Chiasmata (sing. chiasma): a zone of contact along a chromosome pair (visible at meiotic diplotene) which represents where a cross-over is occurring.

Chorea: involuntary jerking movements of the skeletal muscles.

Chromatid: one of the daughters of a replicated chromosome still joined to its sister chromatid at the centromere.

Clone: colony of cells formed by successive division of a single parent cell.

Coated pit: depression in the plasma membrane lined on the cytoplasmic surface with bristle-like clathrin or synapsin molecules. After endocytosis these pits form coated vesicles.

Conservative substitution: the substitution during evolutionary development of a protein of one amino acid by another which resembles the original in its physico-chemical characteristics.

Contralateral: relating to the opposite side of the body.

Cross-over: exchange of information between non-sister chromatids during meiotic division.

Cytoplasm: see **Cytosol**.

Cytosol: colloidal material contained within the plasma membane and outside the nuclear membrane.

Dementia: an acquired global impairment of intellect, memory, and personality but without impairment of consciousness.

Depolarisation: transmembrane voltage less than normal resting potential (V_m).

Diencephalon (= thalamencephalon): posterior part of forebrain.

Dominant: an allele (q.v.) which is expressed whether it is present in the homozygous or the heterozygous form (compare recessive, q.v.).

Down-modulation: see 'modulation'.

Efferent: fibres conducting *away from* some region.

End plate: area of vertebrate striped muscle lying beneath a motor nerve terminal.

Endocytosis: uptake of material from the extracellular space by membrane invagination and budding off as an intracytoplasmic vesicle.

Endogenous: caused from within the organism.

Eukaryocyte: cell characterised by possessing a separate membrane-bound nucleus and cytoplasmic organelles such as mitochondria.

Exocytosis: fusion of vesicle membrane with plasma membrane so that contents of vesicle are voided to the extracellular space.

Exogenous: caused from outside the organism.

Exon: sequence of nucleotides in an initial mRNA transcript which is preserved in the mRNA translated at the ribosome.

Expression vector: a means of inserting a gene into a cell so that on receipt of an appropriate signal the cell will manufacture large amounts of the protein for which the gene codes.

Fasciculation: aggregation of a number of nerve fibres in parallel to form a bundle.

Festination: an involuntary quickening of steps when walking.

Gene, structural: nucleotide sequence coding for a specific polypeptide or protein.

Genome: the total complement of genetic material in a cell or individual.

Glycosylation: addition of monosaccharide units to a polypeptide chain—usually begins in the lumen of the endoplasmic reticulum and completed in the Golgi body.

Goldman equation: an equation which relates the electrical potential across a membrane to the distribution and permeability constants of the ions which that membane separates.

Heterozygous: having two different alleles (q.v.) for the same trait.

Homopolymer: polymer built of only one type of subunit.

Homopolymer tailing: a procedure by which a string of identical nucleotides is added (by terminal transferase) to the end of one strand of a DNA molecule. This tail (e.g. A-A-A-A-A-) will readily stick to a complementary tail (e.g. T-T-T-T-T-) affixed to another single strand of DNA.

Homozygous: having identical alleles (q.v.) for a given trait.

Hyperpolarisation: transmembrane voltage greater than resting potential (V_m).

Hydropathy: disliking water—applied to those segments of a polypeptide chain which are hydrophobic and for this reason often found buried in the lipid core of biomembranes.

In vitro: a biological process studied outside the organism (i.e. 'in glass').

In vivo: a biological process studied within the living organism.

Intron (= intervening sequence): a sequence of nucleotides in the primary mRNA transcript which are excised and are no longer present when the mRNA is translated into polypeptide.

Ionotropic: the action of a neurotransmitter which directly opens ion channels in a subsynaptic membrane.

Ipsilateral: same side of the body.

Klenow fragment (enzyme): fragment of *E.coli* DNA polymerase 1 which lacks the 5'-3' exonuclease activity of the entire enzyme. Alternative to reverse transcriptase in the preparation of cDNA.

Krebs cycle: series of biochemical reactions whereby acetyl coenzyme A is fully oxidised to carbon dioxide and water with the release of energy. The energy is used to synthesise ATP from ADP and P_i. Also known as the tricarboxylic acid cycle and the citric acid cycle.

Leader sequence: nucleotide sequence at the 5' end of a mRNA primary transcript which is important in the regulation of transcription. Usually removed before translation occurs.

Leaflet: one monolayer of a biomembrane's lipoprotein bilayer.

Meiosis: two successive nuclear divisions but only one duplication of the chromosomes thus leading to the production of four haploid gametes (also called 'reduction division').

Mesencephalon: midbrain.

Metabotropic: the action of a neurotransmitter which works through a membrane-bound collision-coupling system and usually involves second messengers such as cAMP, cGMP, PI, etc.

Metencephalon: anterior division of hindbrain.

Mitosis: eukaryotic cell division whereby the chromosomes of the parent cell replicate and segregate to form two daughter nuclei.

Modulation: alteration of a membrane channel's conductance. 'Up-modulation': increased conductance; 'down-modulation': decreased conductance.

Müller cells: large neuroglial cells found in vertebrate retina.

Multimeric protein: a protein which consists of two or more subunits.

Multivesicular body: vacuolated body formed by the inward budding of the membrane of an uncoated vesicle.

Myotube: a developing muscle fibre formed by the fusion of myoblasts.

Native: normal *in vivo* conformation of a biological macromolecule.

Nernst equation: an equation which relates the electrical potential across a membrane to the distribution across that membrane of a single ionic species.

Neurilemma: the plasma membrane of a neuron.

Neurite: a nerve cell process—axon or dendrite.

Neuroleptic: a drug which has an antipsychotic action.

Neuropil: densely intertwined network of axons, dendrites and synapses.

Nucleoplasm: colloidal fluid contained within the nuclear membrane.

Oocyte: egg cell.

Palindromic sequence: DNA sequence which reads identically forwards and backwards (i.e. $5' \to 3'$ or $3' \to 5'$).

Paranoid: exhibiting unnecessary suspicion, fear of persecution, etc.

Parasympathetic nervous system: see **Autonomic nervous system.**

Phosphodiester: any molecule which contains the group

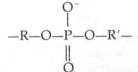

where R and R' are carbon containing groups.

Phosphodiesterase: an enzyme which attacks the phosphate linkage joining the two R groups of a phosphodiester (q.v.).

Pia mater: the innermost of the three membranes (meninges) covering the brain and spinal cord.

Pial: see **pia mater**.

Plasma membrane: the boundary membrane of a cell.

Plexiform layer: the vertebrate retina has two plexiform layers. The outer plexiform layer consists of the layer of synapses between the photoreceptor cells and the bipolars, the inner plexiform layer consists of the layer of synapses bewtween the bipolars and the ganglion cells.

Prokaryocyte: a cell which lacks a membrane-bound nucleus and other membrane-bound organelles, such as mitochondria.

Protein family: proteins with primary sequences differing by less than 50%.

Protein superfamily: proteins whose primary sequences can be shown by statistical analysis to be significantly alike.

Protein kinase: an enzyme which catalyses the transfer of a phosphate group from ATP to a protein to form a phosphoprotein.

Pseudogene: gene having sequence homology with an active gene but which contains mutations which prevent its expression.

Recessive: although the allele (q.v.) is present in the genome it is only expressed when it is in the homozygous condition. Its influence is masked by the dominant allele in a heterozygote.

Recombinant DNA: hybrid DNA formed by fusing DNA fragments obtained from different sources.

Refractory period: the time following an action potential during which the neuronal membrane cannot carry another.

Resting potential: electrical potential across a nerve or other cell membrane when an action potential is *not* being conducted. Depending on cell type it may range from -50 mV to -75 mV (interior negative).

Restriction map: diagrammatic map showing how the DNA fragments produced by restriction endonclease digestion could best be ordered. The map shows the relation of the sites cleaved by restriction endonucleases with respect to each other.

Retrograde: movement from a terminal toward perikaryon.

Retrovirus: a virus which uses RNA as its genetic material but which possesses a reverse transcriptase enabling it to synthesise a DNA copy of the whole or part of its RNA within a cell.

Rostral: towards the anterior.

Sarcolemma: the plasma membrane of a muscle fibre or cell.

Schizophrenia (= dementia praecox): a group of conditions in which the individual feels 'split off' from the rest of humanity, unable to relate to his fellows, sometimes apathetic, sometimes suffering from overwhelming hallucinations and delusions.

Soma: sometimes just the perikaryon, sometimes perikaryon plus dendrites.

Spacer DNA: lengths of DNA between genes (especially rRNA genes) which are not transcribed into mRNA (cf. intron (q.v.)).

Spike: Action potential minus the 'afterhyperpolarisation' (q.v.).

Stop codon: mRNA triplets which signal end of message— UAG, UAA, UGA.

Structural gene: see **gene**.

Svedberg: unit for the sedimentation coefficient of macro-molecules—in general the greater the particle mass the greater the sedimentation coefficient, but the relationship is not linear.

Sympathetic nervous system: see **autonomic nervous system**.

Telencephalon: anterior part of forebrain.

Transducer: a device for transforming energy in one form into another.

Transduction: (genetics) the transfer of genes between bacteria.

Transfection: insertion of DNA into a cell without the use of a vector (q.v.) and leading to the integration of that DNA into the host genome.

Transposon: stretch of DNA (gene) which can move around within the genome rather than, like most genes, remaining fixed.

Tricarboxylic acid cycle: see **Krebs cycle**.

Trophic: nutritional support of a cell or organism.

Tropic: an influence which guides the growth or movement of a cell or organism.

Up-modulation: see **modulation**.

Vector: a device used to introduce recombinant DNA into a host cell; examples of vectors are phage, plasmids, cosmids.

Wild-type: normal, i.e. non-mutant form; in other words the usual type found in nature.

Bibliography

Molecular neurobiology is a huge and very rapidly developing subject. The following lists are intended both as references for the chapters and to provide an entrée to the literature. Starred (*) publications are sources of in-text illustrations. Wherever possible review articles and texts available in most college and university libraries have been cited. Students interested in following a topic to greater depth can use the references listed at the end of these publications to check the primary sources.

Most scientific libraries now possess extensive bibliographic resources to help the student cope with the avalanche of scientific information. These resources range from electronic databases (*Medline, Excerpta Medica, Life Sciences*) to abstracting services (*Index to Scientific Reviews,Biological Abstracts, Index Medicus*) to the useful aids published by the Institute for Scientific Information: *Current Contents—Life Sciences* and the *Science Citation Index (SCI)*. The latter two publications make it possible to keep abreast of what is being published from week to week and to follow the development of a topic once a reference has been located.

CHAPTER 1: INTRODUCTORY ORIENTATION

1. History

Brazier, M.A.B. (1959) 'The historical development of neurophysiology', in *Handbook of Physiology*, Washington: American Physiological Society, vol.1, pp. 1–58.

Clarke, E. and C.D.O'Malley (1968) *The Human Brain and Spinal Cord*, Berkeley: University of California Press.

McIlwain, H. (1958) 'Thudichum and the medical chemistry of the 1850s and 1860s', *Proceedings of the Royal Society of Medicine*, **51**, 127–132.

Reichardt, L.F. (1984) 'The emergence of molecular neurobiology', *Trends in Biochemical Sciences*, **9**, 173–176.

Smith, C.U.M. (1976), *The Problem of Life: an Essay in the Origins of Biological Thought*, London: Macmillan.

Tower, D.B. (1958) 'Origins and development of neurochemistry' *Neurology*, **8**, Suppl. 1: 3–31.

2. Molecular Neurobiology

Bradford, H.F. (1986) *Chemical Neurobiology*, New York: Freeman.

Kay, J., ed. (1986) *Molecular Neurobiology: Biochemical Society Symposia, 52*, London: Biochemical Society.

Siegel, G.J. *et al.*, eds (1981) *Basic Neurochemistry*, Boston: Little Brown and Co.

Soreq, H. (1984) *Molecular Biology Approach to the Neurosciences*, Chichester: John Wiley.

Watson, J.D. and R.McKay, eds (1983) 'Molecular Neurobiology' in *Cold Spring Harbor Symposia on Quantitative Biology*, **XLVIII**, Cold Spring Harbor, NY: Cold Spring Harbor Laboratory.

Various (1982) 'Trends in molecular neuroscience', *Trends in Neurosciences*, **9**, 295–322.

3. Outline of Nervous Systems

(a) Invertebrate nervous systems

Bullock, T.H. and G.A.Horridge (1965) *Structure and Function in the Nervous Systems of Invertebrates* (2 vols), San Francisco: Freeman.

Usherwood, P.N.R. and D.R.Newth, (1975) *Simple Nervous Systems*, London: Edward Arnold.

Wiersma, C.A.G., ed. (1967) *Invertebrate Nervous Systems*, Chicago: University of Chicago Press.

(b) Vertebrate nervous systems

*Kalat, J.W. (1981) *Biological Psychology*, Belmont: Wadsworth Publishing Co.

Kandel, E.R. and J.H.Schwarz (1985), *Principles of Neural Science*, New York: Elsevier Publishing Co.

*Nauta, W.J.H. and M.Feirtag (1986), *Fundamentals of Neuroanatomy*, New York: Freeman.

*Paten, B.M. and B.M.Carlson (1974) *Foundations of Embryology*, New York: McGraw Hill.

Shepherd, G.M. (1983) *Neurobiology*, Oxford: Oxford University Press.

Thompson, R.F. (1985) *The Brain: an Introduction to Neuroscience*, New York: Freeman.

*Warwick, R. and P.L. Williams, eds (1973) *Gray's Anatomy*, Edinburgh: Churchill Livingstone.

4. Cells of the Nervous System

Ramón y Cajal, S. (1911) *Histologie de Système Nerveux de l'Homme et des Vertèbres*, Paris: Maloine.

Schmitt, F.O., F.G.Worden, G.Adelman and S.G.Dennis, eds (1981) *The Organisation of the Cerebral Cortex*, Cambridge, Mass.: MIT Press.

Shepherd, G.M. (1979), *The Synaptic Organisation of the Brain* 2nd edition, Oxford: Oxford University Press.

Szentágothai, J. (1978) 'The neuron network of the cerebral cortex: a functional interpretation', *Proceedings of the Royal Society of London B*, **201**, 219–248.

Watson, W.E. (1976), *The Cell Biology of Brain*, London: Chapman & Hall.

5. Organisation of neurons in the brain

Braitenberg, V. (1977), *On the Texture of Brains*, Heidelberg: Springer-Verlag.

Freeman, W.J. (1975), *Mass Action in the Nervous System*, New York: Academic Press.

Lorente de No, R. (1938) 'The cerebral cortex: architecture, intracortical connections and motor projections', in *Physiology of the Nervous system*, ed. J.Fulton, Oxford: Oxford University Press.

*Nauta, W.J.H. and M.Feirtag (1979), 'The organisation of the brain', *Scientific American*, **241**(3), 78–105.

*Pappas, G.D. and S.G.Waxman (1972) 'Synaptic structure—morphological correlates of chemical and electrotonic transmission', in *Structure and Function of Synapses*, ed. G.D.Pappas and D.P.Purpura, Amsterdam: North Holland.

*Poritsky, R. (1969) 'Two and three dimensional ultrastructure of boutons and glial cells on the motoneuronal surface of cat spinal cord', *Journal of Comparative Neurology*, **135**, 423–452.

*Szentágothai, J. (1979), 'Local neuron circuits of the neocortex', in *The Neurosciences: Fourth Study Program*, eds. F.O.Schmitt and F.G.Worden, Cambridge, Mass. MIT Press, pp. 399–415.

6. Laboratory techniques

Miller, C., ed. (1986), *Ion Channel Reconstitution*, New York: Plenum Press.

Pritchard, R.H. and I.B.Holland (1985) *Basic Cloning Techniques*, Oxford: Blackwell.

Rodriguez, R.L. and R.C.Tait (1983), *Recombinant DNA Techniques: An Introduction*, Reading, Mass.: Addison-Wesley.

Sakmann, B. and E. Neher eds, 1983, eds., *Single Channel Recording*, New York: Plenum Press.

Turner, A.J. and H.S.Bachelard (1987), *Neurochemistry: A Practical Approach*, Oxford: IRL Press.

CHAPTER 2: THE CONFORMATION OF INFORMATIONAL MACROMOLECULES

1. General

Alberts, B., D.Bray, J.Lewis, M.Raff, K.Roberts and J.D.Watson (1984) *The Molecular Biology of the Cell*, New York: Garland Publishing Inc.

Avers, C.J., 1986, *Molecular Cell Biology*, Reading, Mass.: Addison-Wesley.

*Becker, W.M. (1986), *The World of the Cell*, Menlo Park, California: Benjamin/Cummings Publishing Co., Inc.

*Darnell, J., H.Lodish and D.Baltimore (1986) *Molecular Cell Biology*, New York: Scientific American Books Inc.

*Rees, A.R. and M.J.E.Sternberg (1984), *From Cells to Atoms*, Oxford: Blackwell Scientific Publications.

2. Proteins

Blake, C.C.F. and L.N.Johnson (1984), 'Protein structure', *Trends in Biochemical Sciences*, **9**, 147–151.

Cohen, C. and D.A.D.Parry (1986), 'Interlocking α-helices, related to the coiled-coil structure, are a common stablising motif in proteins of all types', *Trends in Biochemical Sciences*, **11**, 245–248.

*Dickerson, R.E. and I.Geis (1969), *The Structure and Action of Proteins*, Menlo Park, California: Benjamin/Cummings Publishing Co., Inc.

Doolittle, R. (1985) 'Proteins', *Scientific American*, **253**(4), 88–96.

Massouliè, J. and S.Bon (1982) 'The molecular forms of cholinesterase and acetylcholinesterase in vertebrates', *Annual Review of Neuroscience*, **5**, 57–106.

Rossman. M. G. and P.Argos (1981) 'Protein folding', *Annual Review of Biochemistry*, **50**, 497–532.

Richardson, J.S. (1981), The anatomy and taxonomy of protein structure, *Advances in Protein Chemistry*, New York: Academic Press, pp. 168–339.

*Taylor, P *et al.* 1986, 'A molecular perspective on the polymorphisms of acetylcholinesterase', *Trends in Pharmacological Science*, **7**, 321–323.

3. Nucleic acids

Avery, O.T, C.M.McLeod and M.McCarty (1944) 'Studies on the chemical nature of the substance inducing transformation of pneumococcal types', *Journal of Experimental Medicine*, **79**, 137–158.

Felsenfeld, G. (1983) 'DNA', *Scientific American*, **253**(4), 58–66.

Rich, A. and S.H.Kim (1978) 'The three-dimensional structure of transfer RNA', *Scientific American*, **238**(1), 53–62.

Watson, J.D. and F.H.C.Crick (1953), 'Molecular structure of nucleic acids. A structure for deoxyribose nucleic acid', *Nature*, **171**, 737–738.

Watson, J.D. and F.H.C.Crick (1953), 'Genetic implications of the structure of deoxyribonucleic acid', *Nature*, **171**, 964–967.

CHAPTER 3: INFORMATION PROCESSING IN CELLS

1. General

Watson, J.D., N.H. Hopkins, J.W. Roberts, J.A. Steitz and A.M. Weiner (1987) *Molecular Biology of the Gene* (fourth edition), vol. 1, Menlo Park, California: Benjamin/Cummings Publishing Co. Inc.

Otherwise as for Chapter 2.

2. The genetic code

Crick, F.H.C. (1966) 'The genetic code', *Scientific American*, 215(4), 55–62.

Dickerson, R.E. (1983) 'The DNA helix and how it is read', *Scientific American*, 249(6), 87–102.

Ycas, M. (1969), *The Biological Code*, New York: Wiley.

3. 'DNA makes RNA and RNA makes protein'

Abei, M. and C.Weissmann (1987) 'Precision and orderliness in splicing', *Trends in Genetics*, 3, 102–107.

Abelson, J. (1979) 'RNA processing and the intervening sequence problem', *Annual Review of Biochemistry*, 48, 1035–69.

Brown, D.D. (1981) 'Gene expression in eukaryotes', *Science*, 211, 667–674.

Darnell, J.E. (1982) 'Variety in the level of gene control in eukaryotic cells', *Nature*, 297, 365–371.

Darnell, J.E. (1983) The processing of RNA, *Scientific American*, 249(4), 72–82.

Lake, J.A. (1981) 'The ribosome', *Scientific American*, 245(2), 56–67.

Moldave, K. (1985), 'Eukaryotic protein synthesis', *Annual Review of Biochemistry*, 54, 1109–1150.

Ogden, R.C. *et al.*, (1981), 'The mechanism of tRNA splicing', *Trends in Biochemical Sciences*, 6, 154–158.

4. Control of the expression of genetic information

Beckwith, J.J., J.Davies and J.Gallant, eds (1983), *Gene Functions in Prokaryotes*, Cold Spring Harbor, NY: Cold Spring Harbor Laboratory.

Beerman, W. and U.Clever (1964), 'Chromosomal puffs', *Scientific American*, 210(4), 50–58.

Brown, D.D. (1981), 'Gene expression in eukaryotes', *Science*, 211, 667–674.

Hudson, L. *et al.* (1987) 'Aberrant splicing of proteolipid protein mRNA in the dysmyelinating jimpy mutant mouse', *Proceedings of the National Academy Sciences (USA)*, 84, 1454–1458.

*Karpati, G. (1984), 'Three tachykinins in the human brain', *Trends in Neurosciences*, 7, 57–59.

Lynch, D.R. and S.H.Snyder (1986), 'Neuropeptides: multiple molecular forms, metabolic pathways and receptors', *Annual Review of Biochemistry*, 55, 773–799.

*Nawa, H., K.Kotani and S.Nakashani (1984) 'Tissue-specific generation of two preprotachykinin mRNAs from one gene by alternative RNA splicing', *Nature*, 312 729–734.

Ptashne, M. (1984) 'Repressors', *Trends in Biochemical Sciences*, 9, 142–145.

Stark, G.R. (1984), 'Gene amplification', *Annual Review of Biochemistry*, 53, 447–491.

Sutcliffe, J.G. *et al.* (1984), 'Control of neuronal gene expression', *Science*, 225, 1308–1315.

CHAPTER 4: MOLECULAR EVOLUTION

1. General

Nei, M. and R.K.Koehn, eds (1983) *Evolution of Genes and Proteins*, Sunderland, Mass.: Sinauer.

Watson, J.D., N.H. Hopkins, J.W. Roberts, J.A. Steitz and A.M. Weiner (1988) *Molecular Biology of the Gene* (fourth edition), vol. 2, Menlo Park, California: Benjamin/Cummings Publishing Co., Inc.

Wilson, A.C., S.S.Carlson and T.J.White (1977) 'Biochemical evolution', *Annual Review of Biochemistry*, 46, 573–639.

2. Mutation

Jeffreys, A.J. and S.Harris (1982) 'Processes of gene duplication', *Nature*, 296, 9–10.

3. Transposons

McClintock, B. (1984) 'The significance of responses of the genome to challenge', *Science*, 226, 792.

Cold Spring Harbor Symposium XLV (1980) *Movable Genetic Elements*, Cold Spring Harbor, NY: Cold Spring Harbor Laboratory.

Starlinger, P. (1984) 'Transposable elements', *Trends in Biochemical Sciences*, 9, 125–127.

4. Protein Evolution

*Avers, C.J. (1986) *Molecular Cell Biology*, Reading, Mass.: Addison-Wesley.

Dayhoff, M.O. (1978) *Atlas of Protein Sequence and Structure*, vol. 5, suppl. 3, Washington: National Biomedical Research Foundation.

Deschenes, R.J. *et al.* (1984) 'Cloning and sequence analysis of a cDNA encoding rat preprocholecystokinin', *Proceedings of the National Academy of Science USA*, 81, 726–730.

*Doolittle, R.F. (1985) 'The genealogy of some recently evolved vertebrate proteins', *Trends in Biochemical Sciences*, 10, 233–237.

Doolittle, W.F. (1985) 'Protein evolution', in *The Proteins* eds Neurath and Hills, 3rd edition, vol. 4, New York: Academic Press, pp. 1–118.

*Douglass, J., O.Civelli and E.Herbert (1984) 'Polyprotein gene expression', *Annual Review of Biochemistry*, 53, 665–715.

Hanke, W. and H. Breer (1986) 'Channel properties of an insect neuronal acetylcholine receptor protein reconstituted in planar lipid bilayers', *Nature*, 321, 171–174.

Herbert, E. *et al.* (1983) 'Generation of diversity of evolution of opioid peptides', *Cold Spring Harbor Symposium on Quantitative Biology*, **XLVIII**, 375–384.

Lunt, G.G. (1986) 'Is the insect neuronal nAChR the ancestral ACh receptor protein?, *Trends in Neurosciences*, **9**, 341–342.

*Lynch, D.R. and S.H.Snyder (1986) 'Neuropeptides: multiple molecular forms, metabolic pathways and receptors', *Advances in Biochemistry*, **55**, 773–799.

CHAPTER 5: MANIPULATING BIOMOLECULES

Abelson, J. and E. Butz, eds (1980) 'Recombinant DNA', *Science*, **209**, 1317–1338.

Emery, A.E., (1984) *An Introduction to Recombinant DNA*, Chichester: John Wiley.

Glover, D.M. (1980) *Gene Cloning: The Mechanics of DNA Manipulation*, London: Chapman & Hall.

Maniatis, T., E.F.Fritsch and J.Sambrook (1982) *Molecular Cloning*, Cold Spring Harbor, NY: Cold Spring Harbor Laboratory.

Old, R.W. and S.B.Primrose (1985) *Principles of Gene Manipulation*, Oxford: Blackwell.

Pritchard, R.H. and I.B.Holland, eds (1985) *Basic Cloning Techniques*, Oxford: Blackwell.

Ptashne, M. (1986) *A Genetic Switch: Gene Control and Phage* λ, Cambridge, Mass. and Palo Alto: Cell Press and Blackwell Scientific Publications.

Smith, M. (1982) 'Site-directed mutagenesis', *Trends in Biochemical Sciences*, **7**, 440–442.

Uhl, G.R., ed. (1987) *In situ Hybridisation in Brain*, New York: Plenum Press.

Watson, J.D., J.Tooze and D.T.Kurtz (1983), *Recombinant DNA: A Short Course*, New York: Freeman.

*Watson, J.D., N.H.Hopkins, J.W.Roberts, J.A.Steitz and A.M.Weiner (1987) *Molecular Biology of the Gene* (fourth edition), vol 1, Menlo Park, California: Academic Press.

White, M.M. (1985) 'Designer channels: site-directed mutagenesis as a probe for structural features of channels and receptors', *Trends in Neurosciences*, **8**, 364–368.

Williamson, R., ed. (1979, 1981, 1982) *Genetic Engineering*, vols. 1, 2, 3, New York: Academic Press.

Williamson, R., ed. (1985) 'Techniques of genetic engineering' (videotape set) Oxford: IRL Press.

Yellen, G. (1984) 'Channels from genes: the oocyte as an expression system', *Trends in Neurosciences*, **7**, 457–458.

CHAPTER 6: BIOMEMBRANES

1. General

Alberts, B., D. Bray, J. Lewis, M. Raff, K. Roberts and J.D. Watson (1984) *The Molecular Biology of the Cell*, New York: Garland Publishing Co.

Bradford, H.F. (1985) *Chemical Neurobiology*, New York: Freeman.

Bretscher, M.S. (1985) 'The molecules of the cell membrane', *Scientific American*, **253**(4), 100–109.

Cotman, C.W. and W.B.Levy (1975) Membranes in nerve impulse conduction, in *MTP International Review of Science, Biochemistry Series 1*, vol. 2, pp. 187–205.

*Darnell, J., H.Lodish and D.Baltimore (1986) *Molecular Cell Biology*, New York: Scientific American Books.

Fernández-Morán, F. (1968) 'Membrane structure in nerve cells', in *The Neurosciences, a Survey for Synthesis*, New York: Rockefeller Press.

Karp, G (1979) *Cell Biology*, New York: McGraw Hill.

Robertson, R.N. (1983) *The Lively Membranes*, Cambridge: Cambridge University Press.

Siegel, G.J., R.W.Albers, B.W.Agranoff and R.Katzman (1981) *Basic Neurochemistry*, Boston: Little Brown, Co.

Singer, S.J. and G.L.Nicolson (1972) 'The fluid-mosaic model of the structure of cell membranes', *Science*, **175**, 720–731.

2. Membrane fluidity

Quinn, A.J. and D.Chapman (1980) 'The dynamics of membrane structure', *CRC Critical Reviews of Biochemistry*, **8**, 1–117.

3. Membrane asymmetry

Rothman, J. and J. Lenard (1977) 'Membrane asymmetry', *Science*, **195**, 743–753.

4. Membrane proteins

Almers, W. and C.Stirling (1984) 'Distribution of transport proteins over animal cell membranes', *Journal of Membrane Biology*, **77**, 169–186.

Anderson, D.J. (1984) 'New clues to protein localisation in neurons', *Trends in Neurosciences*, **7**, 355–357.

Carruthers, A. and D.L.Melchior (1986) 'How bilayer lipids affect membrane protein activity'. *Trends in Biochemical Sciences*, **11**, 331–335.

*Jay, D. and L. Cantley (1986) 'Structural aspects of red cell anion exchange protein', *Annual Review of Biochemistry*, **55**, 511–538.

Unwin, N. and R.Henderson (1984) 'The structure of proteins in biological membranes', *Scientific American*, **250**(2), 78–94.

5. Mobility of membrane proteins

Jacobson, K, A.Ishihara and R.Inman (1987) 'Lateral diffusion of proteins in membranes', *Annual Review of Physiology*, **49**, 163–175.

Vaż, W., F.Goodsaid-Zaldvondo and K.Jacobson (1984) 'Lateral diffusion of lipids and proteins in bilayer membranes', *FEBS Letters*, **174**, 199–207.

6. Synthesis of biomembranes

Besharse, J.C. (1986) 'Photosensitive membrane turnover: differentiated membrane domains and cell-cell interaction', in *The Retina: A Model for Cell Biology Studies*, eds. R.Adler and D.Farber, Orlando: Academic Press.

7. Myelin and myelination

*Laursen, R.A., M.Samiullah and M.B.Lees (1984) 'The structure of bovine brain myelin proteolipid and its organisation in myelin', *Proceedings of the National Academy of Science (USA)*, **81**, 2912–2916.

Morell, P., ed. (1984) *Myelin*, New York: Plenum Press.

Morell, P. and W.T.Norton (1980) 'Myelin', *Scientific American*, **242**(5), 88–118.

Newman, S., K.Kitamura and A.T.Campagnoni (1987) 'Identification of cDNA coding for a fifth form of myelin basic protein in mouse', *Procedings of the National Academy of Science USA*, **84**, 886–890.

Takahashi, N. *et al.* (1985) 'Cloning and characterisation of the myelin basic protein gene from mouse: one gene can encode both 14 kd and 18.5 kd MBPs by alternate use of exons', *Cell*, **42**, 138–148.

8. The sub-membranous cytoskeleton

Bennett, V. (1985) 'The membrane skeleton of human erythrocytes and its implication for more complex cells', *Annual Review of Biochemistry*, **54**, 273–304.

Chasis, J.A. *et al.* (1987) 'Red cell biochemical anatomy and membrane proteins', *Annual Review of Physiology*, **49**, 237–248.

Fulton, A.B. (1984) *The Cytoskeleton*, London: Chapman & Hall.

9. Junctions between cells

Abbott, N.J. (1985) 'Are glial cells excitable after all?', *Trends in Neurosciences*, **8**, 141–142.

Anon. (1986) 'Structure–function relationships in vertebrate retina—an introduction', *Trends in Neurosciences* **9**, 214.

Fraser, S.E. (1985) 'Gap junctions and cell interactions during development', *Trends in Neurosciences*, **8**, 3–4.

Gold, G.H. (1981) 'Photoreceptor coupling: its mechanism and consequences' *Current Topics in Membranes and Transport*, **15**, 59–89.

*Gold, G.H and J.E.Dowling (1979) 'Photoreceptor coupling in the retina of the Toad', *Bufo marinus*, 1, Anatomy', *Journal of Neurophysiology*, **42**, 292–310.

Hertzberg, E.L., T.S.Lawrence and N.B.Gilula (1981) 'Gap junctional communication', *Annual Review of Physiology*, **43**, 579–491.

Kumar, N.M. and N.B.Gilula (1986) 'Cloning and characterisation of human and rat liver cDNAs coding for gap-junction protein', *Journal of Cell Biology*, **103**, 767–776.

Marc, R.E. (1986) 'The development of retinal networks' in *The retina: A Model for Cell Biology Studies*, eds R.Adler and D.Farber, Orlando: Academic Press.

Neyton, J. and A.Trautmann (1985) 'Single currents of an intercellular junction', *Nature*, **317**, 331–335.

Unwin, N. (1986) 'Is there a common design for cell membrane channels?', *Nature*, **323**, 12–13.

CHAPTER 7: G-COUPLED RECEPTORS

1. General

Dunlap, K., G.G.Holz and S.G.Rane (1987) 'G proteins as regulators of ion channel function', *Trends in Neurosciences*, **10**, 241–244.

Gilman, A.G. (1986) 'Receptor-regulated G proteins', *Trends in Neurosciences*, **9**, 460–463.

Gilman, A.G. (1987) 'G-proteins: transducers of receptor-generated signals', *Annual Review of Biochemistry*, **56**, 615–649.

Neer, E.J. and D.E.Clapham (1988) 'Roles of G-protein subunits in transmembrane signalling', *Nature*, **333**, 129–134.

Snyder, S.H. (1985) 'The molecular basis of communication between cells', *Scientific American*, **253**(4), 114–121.

Strange, P.G. (1988) 'The structure and mechanism of neurotransmitter receptors', *Biochemical Journal*, **249**, 309–318.

2: Messengers and receptors

Foster. A.C. and G.E.Fagg (1988) 'Acidic amino acid receptor nomenclature: time for a change', *Trends in Neurosciences*, **11**, 17–18.

Kruk. Z.L. and C.J.Pycock (1983) *Neurotransmitters and Drugs*, London: Croom Helm.

Triggle, D.J. (1978) 'Receptor theory', in *Receptors in Pharmacology*, eds J.R.Smythies and R.J.Bradley, New York: Marcel Dekker.

3. The beta-adrenergic receptor

Dixon, R.A.F. *et al.* (1986) 'Cloning of the gene and cDNA for mammalian β-adrenergic receptor and homology with rhodopsin', *Nature*, **321**, 75–79.

4. The muscarinic acetylcholine receptor

Bonner, T.I. *et al.* (1987) 'Identification of a family of muscarinic acetylcholine receptor genes', *Science*, **237**, 527–532.

Kerlavage, A.R., C.M.Fraser and J.Venter (1987) 'Muscarinic cholinergic receptor structure: molecular biological support for subtypes', *Trends in Pharmacological Science*, **8** 426–431.

Kubo, T. (1986) 'Cloning, sequencing and expression of complementary DNA encoding the muscarinic acetylcholine receptor', *Nature*, **323**, 411–416.

*Kubo, T. *et al.* (1986) 'Primary structure of porcine cardiac muscarinic acetylcholine receptor deduced from cDNA sequence', *FEBS Letters*, **209**, 367–372.

Noma, A. (1986) 'GTP-binding proteins couple cardiac muscarinic receptors to potassium channels', *Trends in Neurosciences*, **9**, 142–143.

5. The substance-K receptor

*Masu, Y. *et al.* (1987) 'cDNA cloning of bovine substance-K receptor through oocyte expression system', *Nature*, **329**, 836–838.

6. Rhodopsin

Baehr, W. and M.L.Applebury (1986) 'Exploring visual transduction with recombinant DNA techniques', *Trends in Neurosciences*, **9**, 198–203.

Hargreave, P.A. (1986) 'Molecular dynamics of the rod cell' in *The Retina: a Model for Cell Biology Studies*, eds R.Adler and D.Farber, part 1, pp. 207–237.

*Lefkowitz, R.J. *et al.* (1986) 'β-adrenergic receptors: shedding light on an old subject', *Trends in Pharmacological Sciences*, **7**, 444–448.

Stryer, L. (1987) 'The molecules of visual excitation', *Scientific American*, **257**(1), 32–40.

7. Cone opsins

*Nathans, J., D.Thomas and D.Hogness (1986) 'Molecular genetics of human color vision: the genes encoding blue, green and red pigments', *Science*, **232**, 193–202.

Nathans, J. (1987) 'Molecular biology of visual pigments', *Annual Review of Neuroscience*, **10**, 163–194.

CHAPTER 8: PUMPS

1. General

Cantley, L. (1986) 'Ion transport systems sequenced', *Trends in Neurosciences*, **9**, 1–3.

Christensen, H.N. (1975) *Biological Transport*, Reading, Mass.: Benjamin.

Tanford, C. (1983) 'The mechanism of free energy coupling in active transport', *Annual Review of Biochemistry*, **52**, 399–409.

2. Energetics

Lehninger, A.L. (1982) *Principles of Biochemistry*, New York: Worth.

Spanner, D.C. (1964) *Introduction to Thermodynamics*, New York: Academic Press.

3. The sodium/potassium pump

Bronner, F. and A.Kleinzeller, eds (1983) 'Structure, mechanism and function of the Na/K pump', *Current Topics in Membranes and Transport*, **19**, 1–1043.

Kawakami, K. *et al.* (1985) 'Primary structure of the α-subunit of *Torpedo californica* (Na$^+$+K$^+$) ATPase deduced from cDNA sequence', *Nature*, **316**, 733–736.

*Shull, G.E., A.Schwartz and J.B.Lingrel (1985) 'Amino-acid sequence of the catalytic subunit of the (Na$^+$+K$^+$) ATPase deduced from complementary DNA', *Nature*, **316**, 691–695.

Taniguchi, K. *et al.* (1984) 'Conformational change of sodium- and potassium-dependent adensoine triphosphatase', *Journal of Biological Chemistry*, **259**, 15228–15233.

4. The calcium pump

*MacLennan, D.H. *et al.* (1985) 'Amino-acid sequence of Ca^{2+}+Mg^{2+}- dependent ATPase from rabbit muscle sarcoplasmic reticulum, deduced from its complementary DNA sequence', *Nature*, **316**, 696–700.

5. Other pumps and transport mechanisms

West, I.C. (1983) *The Biochemistry of Membrane Transport*, London: Chapman & Hall.

Wilson, D.B. (1978) 'Cellular transport mechanisms', *Annual Review of Biochemistry*, **47**, 933–965.

CHAPTER 9: LIGAND-GATED CHANNELS

1. General

Miller, C. ed. (1986) *Ion Channel Reconstitution*, New York: Plenum Press.

Persigian, V.A., ed. (1984) 'Biophysical discussions: ionic channels and membranes', *Biophysical Journal*, **45**, 1–359.

Sakmann, B. and E. Neher, eds (1983) *Single-Channel Recording*, New York: Plenum Press.

Sakmann, B. and E. Neher (1984) 'Patch clamp for studying ionic channels in excitable membranes', *Annual Review of Physiology*, **46**, 455–472.

Sakmann, B., J. Bormann and O.P. Hamill (1983) 'Ion transport by single receptor channels', *Cold Spring Harbor Symposium on Quantitative Biology*, **XLVIII**, 247–257.

Stevens, C.F. (1987) 'Channel families in the brain', *Nature*, **328**, 198–199.

2. The nicotinic acetylcholine receptor

Anon. (1985) 'Understanding acetylcholine receptor structure', *Trends in Neurosciences*, **8**, 355.

*Barrantes, F.J. (1983) 'Recent developments in the structure and function of the acetylcholine receptor', *International Review of Neurobiology*, **24**, 259–341.

*Brisson, A. and P.N.T. Unwin (1985) 'Quarternary structure of the acetylcholine receptor', *Nature*, **315**, 474–477.

Clark, P.B.S. (1987) 'Recent progress in identifying nicotinic receptors in the mammalian brain', *Trends in Pharmacological Sciences*, **8**, 32–35.

Colquhoun, D., D.C. Ogden and A. Mathie (1987) 'Nicotinic acetylcholine receptors of nerve and muscle: functional aspects', *Trends in Pharmacological Sciences*, **8**, 465–472.

*Hirokawa, N. (1983) 'Membrane specialisation and cytoskeletal structures in the synapse and axon revealed by the quick-freeze, deep-etch method', in D.C. Chang *et al.* eds, *Structure and Function of Excitable Cells*, New York: Plenum Press, pp. 113–141.

*Merlie, J.P. *et al.* (1983) 'The regulation of acetylcholine receptor expression in mammalian muscle' in *Cold Spring Harbor Symposia on Quantitative Biology*, **XLVIII**, 135–146.

Mishima, M. *et al.* (1985) 'Location of functional regions of acetylcholine receptor α-subunit by site-directed mutagenesis', *Nature*, **313**, 364–369.

Mishima, M. *et al.* (1986) 'Molecular distinction between foetal and adult forms of muscle acetylcholine receptor', *Nature*, **321**, 406–411.

Neher, E. and Sakmann, (1976) 'Single-channel currents

recorded from membrane of denervated frog muscle fibres', *Nature*, **260**, 779 – 802.

*Noda. M. *et al.* (1983) 'Structural homology of *Torpedo californica* acetylcholine receptor subunits', *Nature*, **302**, 528 – 532.

*Numa, S., *et al.* (1983) 'Molecular structure of the nicotinic acetylcholine receptor', in *Cold Spring Harbor Symposia on Quantitative Biology*, **XLVIII**, 57 – 69.

Stevens, C.F. (1985) 'AChRs: five-fold symmetry and the ε-subunit', *Trends in Neurosciences*, **8**, 335 – 336.

*Stroud, R.M. (1981) 'Structure of an ACh receptor, a hypothesis for a dynamic mechanism of its action' in *Proceedings of Second SUNYA Conversation in the Discipline of Biomolecular Stereodynamics*, ed. R.H.Sarma, vol. 2, New York: Adenine Press.

*Zingsheimer, H.P. *et al.* (1982) 'Direct structural localisation of two toxin-recognition sites on an ACh receptor protein', *Nature*, **299**, 81 – 84.

3. The GABA$_A$ receptor

Barnard, E.A., M.G.Darlison and P.Seeburg (1987) 'Molecular biology of the GABA$_A$ receptor: the receptor/channel superfamily', *Trends in Neurosciences*, **10**, 502 – 509.

*Schofield, P.R. *et al.* (1987) 'Sequence and functional expression of the GABA$_A$ receptor shows a ligand-gated receptor superfamily', *Nature*, **328**, 221 – 227.

Stevenson, F.A. (1988) 'Understanding the GABA$_A$ receptor: a chemically gated ion channel', *Biochemical Journal*, **249**, 21 – 32.

4. The glycine receptor

Betz, H. (1987) 'Biology and structure of the mammalian glycine receptor', *Trends in Neurosciences*, **10**, 113 – 117.

*Greeningloh, G. *et al.* (1987) 'The strychnine-binding subunit of the glycine receptor shows homology with the nicotinic acetylcholine receptor', *Nature*, **328**, 215 – 220.

*Triller, A. *et al.* (1985) 'Distribution of glycine receptors at central synapses: an immunogold study', *Journal of Cell Biology*, **101**, 683 – 688.

5. Receptors for excitatory amino acids

Barnes, D.M. (1988) 'NMDA receptors trigger excitement', *Science*, **239**, 254 – 256.

Cotman, C.W. and L.L.Iverson (1987) 'Excitatory amino acids in the brain: focus on NMDA receptors', *Trends in Neurosciences*, **10**, 263 – 265.

Cull-Candy, S.G. and M.M.Usowicz (1987) 'Multiple-conductance channels activated by excitatory amino acids in cerebellar neurons', *Nature*, **325**, 525 – 528.

Jahr, C.E. and C.F.Stevens (1987) 'Glutamate activates multiple single channel conductances in hippocampal neurons', *Nature*, **325**, 522 – 525.

Johnson, J.W. and P.Ascher (1987) 'Glycine potentiates the NMDA response in cultured mouse brain neurons', *Nature*, **325**, 529 – 531.

MacDermott, A.B. and N.Dale (1987) 'Receptors, ion channels and synaptic potentials underlying the integrative actions of excitatory amino acids', *Trends in Neurosciences*, **10**, 280 – 284.

CHAPTER 10 VOLTAGE-GATED CHANNELS

1. General

Hodgkin, A.L. and A.F.Huxley (1952) 'Currents carried by sodium and potassium ions through the membrane of the giant axon of *Loligo*', *Journal of Physiology (London)*, **116**, 449 – 472.

Pfenninger, K.H. (1978) 'Organisation of neuronal membranes', *Annual Review of Neuroscience*, **1**, 445 – 471.

Poo, M.-M. (1985) 'Mobility and localisation of proteins in excitable membranes', *Annual Review of Neuroscience*, **8**, 369 – 406.

Stevens, C.F. (1984) 'Biophysical studies of ion channels', *Science*, **225**, 1346 – 1350

Various (1984) 'Biophysical discussions: ionic channels and membranes', *Biophysical Journal*, **45**, 1 – 337.

2. The sodium channel

Agnew, W.S. *et al.* (1986) 'The structure and function of the voltage sensitive Na channel', *Annals of the New York Academy of Science*, **479**, 238 – 256.

Barchi, R.L. (1987) 'Sodium channel diversity: subtle variations on a complex theme', *Trends in Neurosciences*, **10**, 221 – 222.

Catterall, W.A. (1985) 'The electroplax sodium channel revealed', *Trends in Neurosciences*, **8**, 1 – 3.

Caterall, W.A. (1986) 'Molecular properties of voltage-sensitive sodium channels', *Annual Review of Biochemistry*, **55**, 953 – 985.

*Noda, M. *et al.* (1984) 'Primary structure of *Electrophorus electricus* sodium channel deduced from cDNA sequence', *Nature*, **312**, 121 – 127.

Numa, S. and M. Noda (1986) 'Molecular structure of sodium channels', *Annals of the New York Academy of Science*, **479**, 338 – 355.

*Sigworth, F.J. and E.Neher (1980) 'Single Na$^+$-channel currents observed in cultured rat muscle cells', *Nature*, **287**, 447 – 449.

3. Potassium channels

Jan, L.Y. *et al.* (1985) 'Application of *Drosophila* molecular genetics in the study of neural function—studies of the *Shaker* locus for a potassium channel', *Trends in Neurosciences*, **8**, 234 – 238.

Salakoff, L. (1983) 'Genetic and voltage-clamp analysis of a *Drosophila* potassium channel', *Cold Spring Harbor Symposia on Quantitative Biology*, **XLVIII**, 221 – 231.

*Schwarz, T.L. *et al.* (1988) 'Multiple potassium-channel components are produced by alternative splicing at the *Shaker* locus in *Drosophila*', *Nature*, **331**, 137 – 142.

Tempel, B.L. *et al.* (1987) 'Sequence of a probable potassium channel component encoded at *Shaker* locus in *Drosophila*', *Science*, **237**, 770 – 775.

4. Calcium channels

Alsobrook, J.P. and C.F.Stevens (1988) 'Cloning the calcium channel', *Trends in Neuroscience*, **11**, 1 – 2.

*Tanabe, T. *et al.* (1987) 'Primary structure of the receptors for the Ca^{2+} channel blockers from skeletal muscle', *Nature*, **328**, 313–318.

5. Conclusion

Stevens, C.F. (1987) 'Channel families in the brain', *Nature*, **328**, 198–199.

CHAPTER 11: RESTING POTENTIALS AND CABLE CONDUCTION

1. General

Aidley, D.J. (1978) *The Physiology of Excitable Cells*, Cambridge: Cambridge University Press.

Kandel, E.R. and J.H. Schwarz (1985) *Principles of Neural Science*, New York: Elsevier.

*Katz, B. (1966) *Nerve, Muscle and Synapse*, New York: McGraw Hill.

Matthews, G.G. (1986) *Cellular Physiology of Nerve and Muscle*, Palo Alto: Blackwell Scientific Publications.

Murray, R.W. (1983) *Test Your Understanding of Neurophysiology'*, Cambridge: Cambridge University Press.

2. Measurement of the resting potential

Hodgkin, A.L., A.F.Huxley and B.Katz (1952) 'Measurement of current voltage relations in the membrane of the giant axon of *Loligo*', *Journal of Physiology*, **116**, 424–448.

3. The origin of the resting potential

Goldman, D.E. (1943) 'Potential, impedance and rectification in membranes', *Journal of General Physiology*, **27**, 37–60.

Hille, B. (1977) 'Ionic basis of resting and action potentials' in *Handbook of Neurophysiology*, vol.1, section 1, Bethesda, Maryland: American Physiological Society, pp. 99–136.

Hodgkin, A.L. and P.Horowicz (1959) 'The influence of potassium and chloride ions on the membrane potential of single muscle fibres', *Journal of Physiology*, **148**, 127–160.

Kandel, E.R. (1985) *Principles of Neural Science*, eds. E.R. Kandel and J.H. Schwarz, New York: Elsevier, pp. 13–24.

Newman, E.A. (1985) 'Regulation of potassium levels by glial cells in the retina', *Trends in Neurosciences*, **8**, 154–159

4. Electrotonic potentials and cable conduction

Dodge, F.A. (1979) 'The nonuniform excitability of central neurons as exemplified by a model spinal neuron', in *The Neurosciences: Fourth Study Program*, eds F.O.Scmitt and F.G.Worden, New York: Rockefeller Press, 423–437.

Jack, J. (1979) 'An introduction to linear cable theory' in *The Neurosciences: Fourth Study Program*, eds F.O.Schmitt and F.G.Worden, New York: Rockefeller University Press, 439–455.

Rall, W. (1962) 'Theory of the physiological properties of dendrites', *Annals of the New York Academy of Science*, **96**, 1071–1092.

Rall, W. (1977) 'Core conductor theory and cable properties of neurons' in *Handbook of Neurophysiology*, vol.1, section 1, Bethesda, Maryland: American Physiological Society, pp. 39–97.

*Shepherd, G.M. (1979) *The Synaptic Organisation of the Brain*, Oxford: Oxford University Press.

CHAPTER 12 SENSORY TRANSDUCTION

1. General

Barlow, H.B. and J.D.Mollon, eds (1982) *The Senses*, Cambridge: Cambridge University Press.

Becker, W.M. (1986) *The World of the Cell*, Menlo Park, California: Benjamin/Cummings Publishing Co. Inc.

Frisch, L., ed. (1965) 'Sensory Receptors', *Cold Spring Harbor Symposia in Quantitative Biology*, **XXX**, New York: Cold Spring Harbor Laboratory.

2. Chemoreception

Adler, J. (1983) 'Bacterial chemotaxis and molecular neurobiology' *Cold Spring Harbor Symposia in Quantitative Biology*, **XLVIII**, 803–804.

Koshland, D.E.Jr. (1981) 'Biochemistry and adaptation in a simple bacterial system', *Annual Review of Biochemistry*, **50**, 765–782.

Lancet, D. (1986) 'Vertebrate olfactory reception', *Annual Review of Neuroscience*, **9**, 329-355.

McNab, R.N. (1984) 'The bacterial flagellar motor', *Trends in Biochemical Sciences*, **9**, 185–186.

Nakamura, T. and G.H.Gold (1987) 'A cyclic nucleotide-gated conductance in olfactory receptor cilia', *Nature*, **325**, 442–446.

*Simon, M.I. *et al.* (1985) 'Sensory transduction in bacteria', *Current Topics in Membranes and Transport*, **23**, 3–15.

Teeter, J. and G.H.Gold (1988) ' A taste of things to come', *Nature*, **331**, 298–299.

3. Photoreceptors

Adler, R. and D.Farber (1986) *The Retina: A Model for Cell Biology Studies*, Orlando: Academic Press.

*Baylor, D.A., T.D.Lamb and K.-W. Yau (1979) 'The membrane curent of single rod outer segments', *Journal of Physiology*, **288**, 589–611.

*Besharse, J.C. (1986) 'Photosensitive membrane turnover: differentiated membrane domains and cell–cell interaction', in R.Adler and D.Farber, eds *The Retina: A Model for Cell Biology Studies*, Orlando: Academic Press, pp.297–352.

*Hogan, M.J., J.A.Alverado and J.E.Weddell (1971) *Histology of the Human Eye*, Philadelphia: Saunders.

Lamb, T.D. (1986) 'Transduction in vertebrate photoreceptors: the roles of cyclic GMP and calcium', *Trends in Neurosciences*, **9**, 224–228.

Liebman, P.A., K.R.Parker and E.A.Dratz (1987) 'The molecular mechanism of visual excitation and its relation to the structure and function of the rod outer segment', *Annual Review of Physiology*, **49**, 765–791.

*Penn, R.D. and W.A.Hagins (1969) 'Signal transmission along retinal rods and the origin of the electroretinographic a-wave', *Nature*, **223**, 201–205.

4. Mechanoreceptors

*Flock, A. (1965) 'Transducing mechanisms in lateral line canal organ receptors', in L.Frisch, *Cold Spring Habor Symposia in Quantitative Biology*, **XXX**, pp. 133–145.
*Hudspeth, A.J. (1983a) 'The hair cells of the inner ear', *Scientific American*, **248**(1), 42–52.
Hudspeth, A.J. (1983b) 'Transduction and tuning by vertebrate hair cells', *Trends in Neurosciences*, **6**, 366–369.
Hudspeth, A.J. (1985) 'The cellular basis of hearing: the biophysics of hair cells', *Science*, **230**, 745–752.

CHAPTER 13 THE ACTION POTENTIAL

1. General

Adley, D.J. (1978) *The Physiology of Excitable Cells*, Cambridge: Cambridge University Press.
*Hille, D. (1984) *Ionic Channels of Excitable Membranes*, Sunderland, Mass.: Sinauer.
*Hodgkin, A.L. and A.F.Huxley (1939) 'Action potentials recorded from inside a nerve fibre', *Nature*, **144**, 710–711.
Matthews, G.G. (1986) *Cellular Physiology of Nerve and Muscle*, Palo Alto: Blackwell Scientific Publications.
Ruch, T.C. and H.D.Patton (1974), *Physiology and Biophysics*, Philadelphia: Saunders.
Sakmann, B. and E.Neher, eds (1983) *Single-Channel Recording*, New York: Plenum Press.
Sherrington, C.S. (1951) *Man on his Nature*, Harmondsworth: Penguin Books.

2. Voltage-clamp analyses

Brismar, T. and B.Frankenhaeuser (1981) 'Potential clamp analysis of mammalian myelinated fibres', *Trends in Neurosciences*, **4**, 68–70.
*Hodgkin, A.L. and A.F.Huxley (1952) 'A quantitative description of membrane current and its application to conduction and excitation in nerve', *Journal of Physiology*, **117**, 500–544.
*Hodgkin, A.L., A.F.Huxley and B.Katz (1952) 'Measurement of current-voltage relations in the membrane of the giant axon of *Loligo*', *Journal of Physiology*, **116**, 424–448.

3. Patch-clamp analyses

*Patlak, J. and R.Horn (1982) 'Effect of N-bromoacetamide on single sodium channel currents in excised membrane patches', *Journal of General Physiology*, **79**, 333–351.
Sakmann, B. and E.Neher (1984) 'Patch clamp techniques for studying ionic channels in excitable membranes', *Annual Review of Physiology*, **46**, 455–472.
Sigworth, F.J. and E.Neher (1980) 'Single Na$^+$ channel currents observed in cultured rat muscle cells', *Nature*, **287**, 447–449.

4. Propagation of the action potential

Hodgkin, A.L. (1964), *The Conduction of the Nerve Impulse*, Springfield, Ill.: Thomas.
Poo, M.M. (1985) 'Mobility and localisation of proteins in excitable membranes', *Annual Review of Neuroscience*, **8**, 369–406.
Stevens, C.F. (1979) 'The neuron', *Scientific American*, **241**(3), 49–59.

5. Initiation of the action potential

Combs, J.S., D.R.Curtis and J.C.Eccles (1957) 'The generation of impulses in motoneurones', *Journal of Physiology*, **139**, 232–249.

6. Rate of impulse propagation

Hodgkin, A.L. (1964) *The Conduction of the Nerve Impulse*, Springfield, Ill.: Thomas.
*Livingstone, R.B. *et al.* (1973) 'Specialised paranodal and interparanodal glial–axonal junctions in the peripheral and central nervous system: a freeze-etching study', *Brain Research*, **58**, 1–24.

CHAPTER 14 THE NEURON AS A SECRETORY CELL

1. General

*Alberts, B., D.Bray, J.Lewis, M.Raff, K.Roberts and J.D.Watson (1984) *Molecular Biology of the Cell*, New York: Garland Publishing Inc.
Castel, M., H.Gainer and H.D.Dellmann (1984) 'Neuronal secretory systems', *International Review of Cytology*, **88**, 303–459.
Darnell, J., H.Lodish and D.Baltimore (1986) *Molecular Cell Biology*, New York: Scientific American Books Inc.

2. Neurons and secretions

Dale, H.H. (1935) 'Pharmacology and nerve endings', *Proceedings of the Royal Society of Medicine*, **28**, 319–332.
Donovan, B.T. (1970) *Mammalian Neuroendocrinology*, London: McGraw-Hill.

3. Synthesis in the perikaryon

Farquhar, M.G. (1985) 'Progress in unravelling pathways of Golgi traffic', *Annual Review of Cell Biology*, **1**, 447–488.
Kelly, R.B. (1985) 'Pathways of protein secretion in eukaryotes', *Science*, **230**, 25–32.
Steiner, D.F. *et al.* (1980) 'Processing mechanisms in the biosynthesis of proteins', *Annals of the New York Academy of Science*, **343**, 1–16.
Walter, P.R., R.Gilmore and G.Blobel (1984) 'Protein translocation across the endoplasmic reticulum', *Cell*, **38**, 5–8.
Wickner, W. and H.F.Lodish (1985) 'Multiple mechanisms of

insertion of proteins into and across membranes', *Science*, **230**, 400–407.

4. Transport along the axon

Allen, R.D. (1987) 'The microtubule as an intracellular engine', *Scientific American*, **256**(2), 26–33.

*Hirokawa, N. (1986) 'Quick-freeze, deep-etch visualisation of the axonal cytoskeleton', *Trends in Neurosciences*, **9**, 67–71.

*Lasek, R.J. (1986) 'Polymer sliding in axons' in *The Cytoskeleton: Cell Function and Organisation*, eds C.Lloyd, J.Hyams and R.Warn, *Journal of Cell Science*, Supplement 5, 161–179.

Osborn, M. and K.Weber (1986) 'Intermediate filament proteins: a multigene family distinguishing major cell lineages', *Trends in Biochemical Sciences*, **11**, 469–472.

Schnapp, B.J. and T.S.Reese (1986) 'New developments in understanding rapid axonal transport', *Trends in Neurosciences*, **9**, 155–162.

Vale, R.D., J.M.Scholey and M.P.Scheetz (1986) 'Kinesin: possible biological roles for a new microtubule motor', *Trends in Biochemical Sciences*, **11**, 464–468.

Wang, E. *et al.* (1985) 'Intermediate filaments: part IV, Neurocytoskeleton', *Annals of the New York Academy of Science*, **455**, 462–596.

*Weiss, D.G. (1986) 'Visualisation of the living cytoskeleton by video-enhanced microscopy and digital image processing', in *The Cytoskeleton: Cell Function and Organisation*, eds C.Lloyd, J.Hyams and R.Warn, *Journal of Cell Science*, Supplement 5, 1–15.

5. Exocytosis and endocytosis at the synaptic terminal

*Akert, K. *et al.* (1972) 'Freeze etching and cytochemistry of vesicles and membrane complexes in synapses of the central nervous system', in *Structure and Function of Synapses*, eds G.D.Pappas and G.D.Purpura, New York: Raven Press, pp. 67–86.

Baines, A.J. and V.Bennett (1985) 'Synapsin 1 is a spectrin-binding protein immunologically related to erythrocyte protein 4.1', *Nature*, **315**, 410–413.

*Heuser, J.E. and T.S.Reese (1979) 'Synaptic-vesicle exocytosis captured by quick freezing' in *The Neurosciences: Fourth Study Program*, eds F.O.Schmitt and F.G.Worden, Cambridge, Mass.: MIT Press, pp. 573–600.

Lentz, T.L. (1983) 'Cellular membrane reutilisation and synaptic vesicle recycling', *Trends in Neurosciences*, **6**, 48–53.

Rothman, J.E. and J.Leonard (1984) 'Membrane traffic in animal cells', *Trends in Biochemical Science*, **9**, 176–178.

Stevens, C.F. (1979) 'The neuron', *Scientific American*, **241**(3), 48–59.

CHAPTER 15 NEUROTRANSMITTERS AND NEUROMODULATORS

1. General

*Bradford, H.F. (1986) *Chemical Neurobiology*, New York: Freeman.

Brown, D.A. (1986) 'Synaptic mechanisms', *Trends in Neurosciences*, **9**, 468–470.

*Cooper, J.R., F.E.Bloom and R.H.Roth (1985) *The Biochemical Basis of Neuropharmacology*, New York: Oxford University Press.

Hökfelt, T., O.Johansson and M.Goldstein (1984) 'Chemical anatomy of the brain', *Science*, **225**, 1326–1334.

Kruk, Z.L. and C.L.Pycock (1983) *Neurotransmitters and Drugs*, London: Croom Helm.

McGeer, P.L., J.C.Eccles and E.G.McGeer (1978) *Molecular Neurobiology of the Mammalian Brain*, New York: Plenum Press.

McIlwain, H. and H.S.Bachelard (1985) *Biochemistry and the Central Nervous System*, Edinburgh: Churchill Livingstone.

Various (1983) 'Neurotransmitters and their actions', *Trends in Neurosciences*, **6**, 293–349.

2. Acetylcholine

*Cuello, A.C. and M.V.Sofroniew (1984) 'The anatomy of CNS cholinergic neurons', *Trends in Neurosciences*, **7**, 74–78.

Dunant, Y. and M.Israel (1985) 'The release of acetylcholine', *Scientific American*, **252**(4), 40–48.

3. Amino acids

Fagg, G.E. and A.C.Foster (1983) 'Amino acid neuro-transmitters and their pathways in the mammalian central nervous system', *Neuroscience*, **9**, 701–719.

Tallman, J.F. and D.W.Gallagher (1985) 'The GABA-ergic system: A locus of benzodiazepine action', *Annual Review of Neuroscience*, **8**, 21–44.

Watkins, J.C. (1984) 'Excitatory amino acids and central synaptic transmission', *Trends in Pharmacological Sciences*, **5**, 373–376.

4. Serotonin

Fuller, R.W. (1980) 'Pharmacology of central serotonin neurons', *Annual Review of Pharmacology and Toxicology*, **20**, 111–127.

Richardson, B.P. and G.Engel (1986) 'The pharmacology and function of 5-HT$_3$ receptors', *Trends in Neurosciences*, **9**, 424–428.

5. Catecholamines

Fuller, R.W. (1982) 'Pharmacology of brain epinephrine neurons', *Annual Review of Pharmacology and Toxicology*, **22**, 31–55.

Lindvall, O. and A. Björklund (1983) 'Dopamine and norepinephrine containing neuron systems: Their anatomy in the rat brain', in *Chemical Neuroanatomy*, ed. P.C.Emson, New York: Raven Press, pp. 229–255.

Minneman, K., R.N.Pitmann and P.B.Molinoff (1981), 'β-adrenergic receptor subtypes: properties, distribution and regulation', *Annual Review of Neuroscience*, **4**, 419–461.

*Morrison, J.H., M.G.Molliver and R.Grzanna (1979) 'Noradrenergic innervation of cerebral cortex: widespread effects of local cortical lesions', *Science*, **205**, 313–316.

Roth, R.H. (1984) 'CNS dopamine autoreceptors: distribution, pharmacology and function', *Annals of the New York Academy of Science*, **430**, 27–53.

6. Peptides

Hökfelt,T., O.Johansson, A.Ljungdahl, J.M.Lundberg and M.Schultzberg (1980) 'Peptidergic neurons', *Nature*, **284**, 515–524.

Lundberg, J.M. and T.Hökfelt (1983) 'Coexistence of peptides and classical neurotransmitters', *Trends in Neurosciences*, **6**, 325–332.

*Iverson, L.L. (1979) 'The chemistry of the brain', *Scientific American*, **241**(3), 118–129.

Iverson, L.L. (1984) 'Amino acids and peptides: Fast and slow chemical signals in the nervous system?', *Proceedings of the Royal Society B (London)*, **221**, 245–260.

*Schwarz, J.H. (1985), in *Principles of Neural Science*, eds. E.R.Kandel and J.H.Schwarz, New York: Elsevier, pp. 148–158.

Mansour, A. *et al.* (1988) 'Anatomy of CNS opioid receptors', *Trends in Neurosciences*, **11**, 308–314.

Miller, R.J. (1986) 'Peptides as neurotransmitters: focus on the encephalins', in *Neuropeptides and Behaviour*, vol.1, eds D.De Wied, W.H.Gispen and Tj. B. Van Wimersma Greidamus, Oxford: Pergamon Press.

Palkovits, M. (1984) 'Distribution of neuropeptides in the central nervous system: A review of biochemical mapping studies', *Progress in Neurobiology*, **23**, 151–189.

*Tsunoo, A., S.Konishi and M. Otsuka (1982) 'Substance P as an excitatory transmitter of primary afferent neurons in guinea pig sympathetic ganglia', *Neuroscience*, **7**, 2025–2037.

Vale, W. and M.Brown (1979) 'Neurobiology of peptides', in *The Neurosciences: Fourth Study Program*, eds F.O.Schmitt and F.G.Worden, Cambridge, Mass.: MIT Press, pp. 1027–1041.

CHAPTER 16 THE SUBSYNAPTIC MEMBRANE

1. General

Bradford, H.F. (1986) *Chemical Neurobiology*, New York: Freeman.

*Csillig, A. and F.Hajos (1980) 'Potassium movements in relation to synaptosomal morphology', *Journal of Neurochemistry*, **34**, 493–503.

2. Electrophysiology of the subsynaptic membrane

Eccles, J.C. (1964) 'Ionic mechanisms and post-synaptic inhibition', *Science*, **145**, 1140–1147.

Matthews, G.G. (1986) *Cellular Physiology of Nerve and Muscle*, Palo Alto: Blackwell.

3. Ion channels in the subsynaptic membrane

*McBurney, R.N. (1983) 'New approaches to the study of rapid events underlying neurotransmitter action', *Trends in Neurosciences*, **6**, 297–302.

4. Modulation of ion channels by second messenger systems

Brown, D.A. (1983) 'Slow cholinergic excitation—a mechanism for increasing neuronal excitability', *Trends in Neurosciences*, **6**, 301–306.

Siegelbaum, S.A. and R.W.Tsien (1983) 'Modulation of gated ion channels as a mode of transmitter action', *Trends in Neurosciences*, **6**, 307–313.

5. Other effects of second messengers

*Berridge, M.J. (1985) 'The molecular basis of communication within the cell', *Scientific American*, **253**(4), 124–136.

Miller, R.J. (1986) 'Protein kinase C: a key regulator of neuronal excitability?', *Trends in Neurosciences*, **9**, 538–541.

Morrisey, J.J. (1981) 'The neuronal induction of pineal gland n-acetyl-transferase activity' in *Essays in Neurochemistry and Neuropharmacology*, vol. 5, eds M.B.H.Youdin, W.Lovenberg, D.F.Sharman and J.R.Lagnano, Chichester: John Wiley.

Reiter, R. (1980) 'The pineal gland: a regulator of regulators', *Progress in Psychobiology and Physiological Psychology*, **9**, 323–356.

Worley, P.F. *et al.* (1988) 'Lithium blocks a phosphoinositide-mediated cholinergic response in hippocampal slices', *Science*, **239**, 1428–1429.

6. The subsynaptic density

Froehner, S.C. (1986) 'The role of the postsynaptic cytoskeleton in AChR organisation', *Trends in Neurosciences*, **9**, 37–41.

*Kelly, P.T. and C.W.Cotman (1977) 'Identification of glycoproteins and proteins at synapses in the central nervous system', *Journal of Biological Chemistry*, **252**, 786–793.

*Sealock, R., B.E.Wray and S.C.Froehner (1984) 'Ultrastructural localisation of the M_r 43 000 protein and the acetylcholine receptor in *Torpedo* postsynaptic membranes using monoclonal antibodies', *Journal of Cell Biology*, **98**, 2239–2244.

CHAPTER 17 EPIGENETICS OF THE BRAIN

1. General

*Cowan, W.M. (1979) 'The development of the brain', *Scientific American*, **241**(3), 107–117.

*Jacobson, M. (1978) *Developmental Neurobiology*, New York: Plenum.

Malimski, G. and S. Bryant, eds (1984) *Pattern Formation: A Primer in Developmental Biology*, London: Macmillan.

*Purves, D. and J.W.Lichtman (1985) *Principles of Neural Development*, Sunderland, Mass.: Sinauer.

Ribchester, R.R. (1986) *Molecule, Nerve and Muscle*, Glasgow: Blackie.

Various (1985) 'Developmental neurobiology—special issue', *Trends in Neurosciences*, **8**, 229–300.

Waddington, C.H. (1957) *The Strategy of the Genes*, London: Allen & Unwin.

2. The origins of neurons and glia

*Hatten, M.E and C.A.Mason (1986) 'Neuron-astroglial interactions *in vitro* and *in vivo*', *Trends in Neurosciences*, **9**, 168–174.

3. Morphogenesis of neurons

*Altman, J. (1967) 'Postnatal growth and differentiation of the mammalian brain, with implications for a morphological theory of memory', in G.C.Quarton, T.Melnechuk and F.O.Schmitt, eds, *The Neurosciences*, New York: Rockefeller Press.

Thoen, H., U.Otten and M.Schwab (1979) 'Orthograde and retrograde signals for the regulation of neuronal gene expression: the peripheral sympathetic nervous system as a model', in *The Neurosciences: Fourth Study Program*, eds F.O.Schmitt and F.G.Worden, Cambridge, Mass.: MIT Press, pp. 911–928.

*Racik, P. (1979) 'Genetic and epigenetic determinants of local neuronal circuits in the mammalian central nervous system' in *The Neurosciences, Fourth Study Program*, eds F.O.Schmitt and F.G.Worden, Cambridge, Mass.: MIT Press, pp. 109–127.

Banker, G.A. and W.M.Cowan (1979) 'Further observations on hippocampal neurons in dispersed cell culture', *Journal of Comparative Neurology*, **187**, 469–494.

4. Growth cones

Manson, C. (1985) 'How do growth cones grow?', *Trends in Neurosciences*, **8**, 304–306.

5. Pathfinding

*Angelletti. R.H. and R.A.Bradshaw (1971) 'Nerve growth factor from mouse submaxillary gland: amino acid sequence', *Proceedings of the National Academy of Science (USA)*, **68**, 2417–2420.

*Campenot, R.B. (1982) 'Development of sympathetic neurons in compartmentalised cultures', *Developmental Biology*, **93**, 1–21.

*Davis, G.E., S.Varon, E.Engvall and M.Manthorpe (1985) 'Substrate-binding neurite-promoting factors: relationships to laminin, *Trends in Neurosciences*, **8**, 528–532.

Edgar, D. (1985) 'Nerve growth factors and molecules of the extracellular matrix in neuronal development', *Journal of Cell Science: Supplement 3*, 107–113.

*Gundersen, R.W. and J.N.Barrett (1979) 'Neuronal chemotaxis: chick dorsal root axons turn toward high concentrations of nerve growth factor', *Science*, **206**, 1079–1080.

*Letourneau, P.C. (1975) 'Cell-to-substratum adhesion and guidance in neuronal morphogenesis', *Developmental Biology*, **44**, 77–91.

Levi-Montalcini, R. and P.Calissano (1986) 'Nerve growth factor as a paradigm for other polypeptide growth factors', *Trends in Neurosciences*, **9**, 473–477.

6. Cell adhesion molecules (CAMs)

Cunningham, B.A. (1986) 'Cell adhesion molecules: a new perspective on molecular embryology', *Trends in Biochemical Sciences*, **11**, 423–426.

*Edelman, G.M. (1984) 'Modulation of cell adhesion during induction, histogenesis and perinatal development of the nervous system', *Annual Review of Neuroscience*, **7**, 339–377.

Edelman, G.M. (1986) 'Cell adhesion molecules in neural histogenesis', *Annual Review of Physiology*, **48**, 417–430.

Rutishauser, U. (1986) 'Differential cell adhesion through spatial and temporal variations of NCAM', *Trends in Neurosciences*, **9**, 374–378.

Rutishauser. U. and G.Goridis (1986) 'N-CAM the molecule and its genetics', *Trends in Genetics*, **2**, 72–76.

7. Differential survival

Clarke, P.G.H. (1985) 'Neuronal death in the development of the vertebrate nervous system', *Trends in Neurosciences*, **8**, 345–349.

Cowan, W.M. (1979) 'Selection and control in neurogenesis' in *The Neurosciences, Fourth Study Program*, eds F.O.Schmitt and F.G.Worden, Cambridge, Mass.: MIT Press.

Cowan, W.M. *et al.* (1984) 'Regressive events in neurogenesis' *Science*, **225**, 1258-1265.

8. Morphopoietic fields

Wolpert, L. (1978) 'Pattern formation in biological development', *Scientific American*, **239**(4), 153–164.

9. Functional sculpturing

Barlow, H.B. (1975) 'Visual experience and cortical development', *Nature*, **258**, 199–204.

Blaisdel, G.G. and J.D.Pettigrew (1979) 'Degree of interocular synchrony required for maintenance of binocularity in the kitten's visual cortex', *Journal of Neurophysiology*, **42**, 1692–1710.

*Constantine-Paton, M. (1981) 'Induced ocular-dominance zones in tectal cortex', in *The Organisation of the Cerebral Cortex*, eds F.O.Schmitt, F.G.Worden, G.Adelman and S.G.Dennis, Cambridge, Mass.: MIT Press: pp. 47–67.

Cotman, C.W. and L.L.Iverson (1987) 'Excitatory amino acids in the brain—focus on NMDA receptors', *Trends in Neurosciences*, **10**, 263–265.

*Hubel, D.H., T.N.Wiesel and S. LeVay (1977) 'Plasticity of ocular dominance columns in monkey striate cortex', *Philosophical Transactions of the Royal Society (B)*, **278**, 377–409.

Hubel, D.H. and T.N.Wiesel (1979) 'Brain mechanisms of vision', *Scientific American*, **241**(3), 130–144.

Jacobson, M. (1970) 'Development, specification and diversification of neuronal connections' in *The Neurosciences: Second Study Program*, ed. F.O.Schmitt, New York: Rockefeller Press, pp. 116–129.

CHAPTER 18 MEMORY

1. General

Power, G.H. and E.R.Hilgard (1981) *Theories of Learning*, Engelwood Cliffs, NJ: Prentice Hall.

Eccles, J.C. (1977) *The Understanding of the Brain*, New York: McGraw Hill.

Hilgard, E.R. and D.G.Marquis (1940) *Conditioning and Learning*, New York: Appleton-Century-Crofts.

*Thompson, R.F. (1986) 'The neurobiology of learning and memory', *Science*, **233**, 941–947.

2. Some definitions

Bower, G.H. and E.R.Hilgard (1981) *Theories of Learning*, Englewood Cliffs, NJ: Prentice-Hall.

3. Short and long term memory

Entingh, D. *et al.* (1975) 'Biochemical approaches to the biological basis of memory', in *Handbook of Psychobiology*, ed. M.S.Gazziniga and C.Blakemore, New York: Academic Press, pp. 201–238.

Goelet, P., V.F.Castellucci, S.Schacher and E.R.Kandel (1986) 'The long and the short of long-term memory—a molecular framework', *Nature*, **322**, 419–422.

4. Where is the memory trace located

Lashley, K. (1950) 'In search of the Engram', *Symposium of Society of Experimental Biology*, **4**, 454–482.

Thompson, R.F. *et al.* (1983) 'The engram found? Initial localisation of the memory trace for a basic form of associative learning', *Progress in Psychobiological Physiological Psychology*, **10**, 167–196.

5. Invertebrate systems

Alkon, D.L. (1984) 'Calcium-mediated reduction in ion channels: a biophysical memory trace (Hemissenda)', *Science*, **226**, 1037–1045.

Carew, T.J and C.L.Sahley (1986) 'Invertebrate learning and memory: from behaviour to molecules', *Annual Review of Neuroscience*, **9**, 435–487.

Dudai, Y. (1985) 'Genes, enzymes and learning in *Drosophila*', *Trends in Neurosciences*, **8**, 18–22.

*Dudai, Y. *et al.* (1976) 'Dunce, a mutant of *Drosophila* deficient in learning', *Proceedings of the National Academy of Sciences (USA)*, **73**, 1684–1688.

*White, J.G. (1985) 'Neuronal connectivity in *Caenorhabditis elegans*', *Trends in Neurosciences*, **8**, 277–283.

6. *Aplysia* and the molecular biology of memory

Bailey, C.H. and M.Chen (1983) 'Morphological basis of long-term habituation and sensitisation in *Aplysia*', *Science*, **220**, 91–93.

*Byrne, J.H. (1985) 'Neural and molecular mechanisms underlying information storage in *Aplysia*: implications for learning and memory', *Trends in Neurosciences*, **8**, 478–482.

Dale, N., S,Schacher and E.R.Kandel (1988) 'Long-term facilitation in *Aplysia* involves increase in transmitter release', *Science*, **239**, 282–284.

Frost, W.N., V.F.Castellucci, R.D.Hawkins and E.R.Kandel (1985) 'Monosynaptic connections made by the sensory neurons of the gill- and siphon-withdrawal reflex in *Aplysia* paticipate in the storage of long-term memory for sensitisation', *Proceedings of National Academy of Sciences (USA)*, **82**, 8266–8269.

*Kandel, E.R. (1976) *Cellular Basis of Behaviour: An Introduction to Behavioural Neurobiology*, New York: Freeman.

*Kandel, E.R. (1979) 'Small systems of neurons', *Scientific American*, **241**(3), 60–70.

*Kandel, E.R. (1985) 'Cellular mechanisms of learning and the biological basis of individuality' in *Principles of Neural Science*, eds E.R.Kandel and J.H.Schwartz, New York: Elsevier: pp. 817–833.

Ocorr, K.A., E.T.Walters and J.H.Byrne (1985) 'Associative conditioning analog selectively increases cAMP levels of tail sensory neurons in *Aplysia*', *Proceedings of the National Academy of Sciences (USA)*, **82**, 2538–2552.

7. The memory trace in mammals

Anderson, P. (1983) 'Possible cellular basis for prolonged changes of synaptic efficiency: a simple case of learning', in J.-P. Changeux, J. Glowinski, M.Imbert and F.E.Bloom, eds, *Progress in Brain Research*, **58**, 419–426.

Barnes, D.M. (1988) 'NMDA receptors trigger excitement', *Science*, **239**, 254–256.

Collingridge, G.L. and T.V.P.Bliss (1987) 'NMDA receptors— their role in long-term potentiation', *Trends in Neurosciences*, **10**, 288–293.

Lynch, G. and M.Baudry (1984), 'The biochemistry of memory: a new and specific hypothesis', *Science*, **224**, 1057–1063.

Waterman, M., G.H.Murdoch, R.M.Evans, M.G.Rosenfeld (1985) 'Cyclic AMP regulation of eukaryotic gene transcription by two discrete mechanisms', *Science*, **229**, 267–269.

CHAPTER 19: FIVE PATHOLOGIES

1. General

Breakefield, X.O. and F.Cambi (1987) 'Molecular genetic insights into neurological diseases', *Annual Review of Neurosciences*, **10**, 535–594.

*Davis, R.L. and D.M. Robertson (1985) *Textbook of Neuropathology*, Baltimore: Williams & Wilkins.

Martin, J.B. (1987) 'Molecular genetics: Applications to clinical neurosciences', *Science*, **238**, 765–772.

Kety, S.S. (1979) 'Disorders of the human brain', *Scientific American*, **241**(3), 172–179.

Sacks, O.W. (1973) *Awakenings*, London: Duckworth.

Sarason, I.G. and B.R.Sarason (1984) *Abnormal Psychology*, Englewood Cliffs, NJ: Prentice-Hall, Inc.

Smith, C.U.M. (1988) 'Biology and psychiatry', *Journal of the Royal Society of Medicine*, **81**, 439–440.

Tsuang, M.T. and R.Vandermey (1980) *Genes and the Mind*, Oxford: Oxford University Press.

Walton, J.N. (1985) *Brain's Diseases of the Nervous System*, Oxford: Oxford University Press.

2. Phenylketonuria (PKU)

McIlwain, H. and H.S.Bachelard (1985) *Biochemistry and the Central Nervous System*, Edinburgh: Churchill Livingstone.
Walton, J.N. (1985) *Brain's Diseases of the Nervous System*, Oxford: Oxford University Press.

3. Huntingdon's disease (=chorea) (HD)

Gusella, J.F. (1986) 'DNA polymorphism and human disease', *Annual Review of Biochemistry*, **55**, 831–854.
Gusella, J.F. *et al.* 'A polymorphic DNA marker genetically linked with Huntingdon's disease', *Nature*, **306**, 234–238.
Harper, P.S. (1984) 'Localisation of the gene for Huntingdon's chorea', *Trends in Neurosciences*, **7**, 1–2.
*Shows, T.B., A.Y.Sakaguchi and S.L.Naylor (1983) 'Mapping the human genome, cloned genes, DNA polymorphisms and inherited disease' in *Advances in Human Genetics*, **12**, New York: Plenum Press, Chapter 5.

4. Depression

Egeland, J.A. *et al.* (1987) 'Bipolar affective disorders linked to DNA marker on chromosome 11', *Nature*, **325**, 783–787.
Paykel, E.S. ed. (1982) *Handbook of Affective Disorders*, New York: Guildford Press.
Shows, T.B., A.Y.Sakaguchi and S.L.Naylor (1983) 'Mapping the human genome, cloned genes, DNA polymorphisms and inherited disease' in *Advances in Human Genetics*, **12**, New York: Plenum Press, Chapter 5.
Van Praag, H.M. (1982) 'Neurotransmitters in CNS disease: Depression', *Lancet*, **2**, 1259–1264.

5. Parkinson's disease (PD)

Lewin, R. (1985) 'Parkinson's disease: an environmental cause', *Science*, **229**, 257–258.
Lewin, R. (1988) 'Cloud over Parkinson's therapy', *Science*, **240**, 390-392.

6. Alzheimer's disease (AD)

Carrell, R.W. (1988) 'Alzheimer's disease: enter a protease inhibitor', *Nature*, 478–479.
Delabar, J.-M. (1987) 'β amyloid gene duplication in Alzheimer's disease and karyotypically normal Down syndrome', *Science*, **235**, 1390–1392.
Goldgaber, D. *et al.* (1987) 'Characterisation and chromosomal localisation of a cDNA encoding brain amyloid of Alzheimer's disease', *Science*, **235**, 877–880.
Kang, J. *et al.* (1987) 'The precursor of Alzheimer's disease amyloid A4 protein resembles a cell-surface receptor', *Nature*, **325**, 733–736.
Price, D.L. (1986) 'New Perspectives on Alzheimer's disease', *Annual Review of Neuroscience*, **9**, 489–512.
Roth, M. and L.L. Iverson, eds (1986) 'Alzheimer's disease and related disorders', *British Medical Bulletin*, **42**, 1–115.
St George-Hyslop, P.H. (1987) 'The generic defect causing familial Alzheimer's disease maps on chromosome 21', *Science*, **235**, 885–889.
*Terry, R.D. (1985) 'Alzheimer's disease', in Textbook of Neuropathology, eds R.L. Davis and D.M.Robertson, Baltimore: Williams & Wilkins, pp. 824–841.
*Wischik, C.M. *et al.* (1985) 'Subunit structure of paired helical filaments in Alzheimer's Disease', *Journal of Cell Biology*, **100**, 1905–1912.
*Wischik, C.M. and R.A.Crowther (1986) 'Subunit structure of the Alzheimer tangle', *British Medical Bulletin*, **42**, 51–56.
Wurtman, R.J. (1985) 'Alzheimer's disease', *Scientific American*, **252**(1), 48–56.

Index

F = figure; T = table